Hospice

Complete Care for the Terminally Ill

Hospice

Complete Care for the Terminally Ill

Jack McKay Zimmerman, M.D., F.A.C.S.
Church Hospital, Baltimore

Second Edition

Contributions by

Milton Buschman, M.D.
Gloria R. Cameron, M.H.A.
Paul S. Dawson, M.S.
Marjorie M. Lamb, R.N., B.S.
Yvonne M. Leacock, M.S.
Maureen Mason
Lucy B. McBee
Kathleen A. Roche, R.N., M.A.
Frederick T. Wehr, A.B.

Foreword by
Dame Cicely Saunders

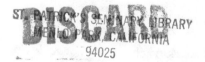

Urban & Schwarzenberg
Baltimore-Munich • 1986

Urban & Schwarzenberg, Inc.
7 E. Redwood Street
Baltimore, Maryland 21202
USA

Urban & Schwarzenberg
Pettenkoferstrasse 18
D-8000 München 2
West Germany

Printed in the United States of America

NOTICES

The Publishers have made an extensive effort to trace original copyright holders for permission to use borrowed material. If any has been overlooked, it will be corrected at the first reprint.

Library of Congress Cataloging in Publication Data

Zimmerman, Jack McKay.
  Hospice: complete care for the terminally ill.

  Includes bibliographies and index.
  1. Hospice care. 2. Hospices (Terminal care) I. Title. [DNLM:
1. Hospices. 2. Terminal Care. WX 28.61 Z72h]
  R726.8.Z55 1986   616'.029   859178
  ISBN 0-8067-2212-6

*Compositor:*Typesetting & Graphic Services, Inc.
Printer: Port City Press
Manuscript editor: Starr Belsky
Indexer: Mary Cahill
Production and design: Norman Och and Karen Babcock

ISBN 0-8067-2212-6 Baltimore
ISBN 3-541-72212-6 Munich

This book is dedicated to
Doris,
co-author of all that is best in my life

Contents

Contributors

Milton Buschman, M.D.
Chief of Psychiatry, Church Hospital

Gloria R. Cameron, M.H.A.
Vice President, Church Hospital

Paul S. Dawson
Director of Chaplaincy Services, Fairhaven, Sykesville, Maryland;
Former Chaplain, Church Hospital

Marjorie M. Lamb, R.N.,B.S.
Head Nurse, Hospice Inpatient Unit, Church Hospital

Yvonne M. Leacock, M.S.
Director of Bereavement Services, Hospice Program, Church Hospital

Maureen Mason
Senior Volunteer, Church Hospital

Lucy B. McBee
Director of Volunteer Services, Church Hospital

Kathleen A. Roche, R.N.,M.A.
Director of Home Health, Church Hospital
Administrative Coordinator, Hospice Program, Church Hospital

Frederick T. Wehr
Director of Public Relations and Development, Church Hospital

Jack McKay Zimmerman, M.D.
Chief of Surgery, Church Hospital;
Associate Professor of Surgery, Johns Hopkins University,
Baltimore, Maryland

Foreword

The present day hospice is a program rather than a place, an attitude expressed in a growing expertise that is being established in many different ways. It has developed out of the work of homes or hospices founded on both sides of the Atlantic at the turn of the century for patients with terminal cancer and tuberculosis. As the hospitals became more involved with acute care and turned these patients away to Poor Law or equivalent institutions, these turn-of-the-century hospices grew up.

Hospice therapeutics may be traced back to the classic *The Care of the Aged, the Dying and the Dead*, written by a family doctor for students of Harvard Medical School (Worcester 1935); but apart from a few articles from the homes and a Harveian Oration (Gavey 1952), little was written before 1960, when work developed at St. Joseph's Hospice began to be published (Saunders 1960). By this time advances in the treatment of malignant disease, which afflicted most hospice patients, had offered longer term control, better palliation, and sometimes cure to many patients, while for others it had greatly lengthened the time of ill health and dependence and led to mental as well as physical suffering. The trend for death to occur in the hospital rather than in the patient's own home isolated him from all that was familiar, often without the understanding or treatment appropriate for his or her special needs (Hinton 1963). The fear of a painful and isolated death was widespread.

The work in pain control that was observed at St. Luke's Hospital (an early hospice) from 1948 onwards was developed in St. Joseph's Hospice (founded in 1905) after 1958. By then it was possible to exploit the therapeutic advances of the 1950s: new psychotropic drugs, cancer chemotherapy, palliative radiotherapy, the techniques of the new pain clinics, and a greater knowledge of family responses to stress and bereavement in a new approach to the terminally ill. St. Christopher's opened in 1967 as the first research and teaching hospice. From the first it focused on the family as the unit of care and, where possible, as part of the caring team, as well as upon the nature of terminal pain, its better understanding, and therefore more effective treatment. Alongside this came a revival of the concept of the "good death, "attention to the achievements that a patient could still make in the face of physical deterioration, and awareness of the spiritual dimension of the patient's final search for meaning. Since then the work has spread in a wide variety of interpretations and has grown into the Hospice Movement.

A modern hospice, whether it is a separate unit or ward, a home care or hospital team, aims to enable a patient to live to the limit of his or her potential in physical strength, mental and emotional capacity, and social relationships. It offers an alternative form of treatment to the acute care of a general hospital, not in opposition but as a further resource for those for whom the usual acute hospital care is no longer appropriate. It is the alternative to the negative and socially dangerous suggestion that a patient with an incurable disease likely to cause suffering should have the legal option of actively hastened death, i.e., euthanasia.

For the present it appears that a limited number of research and teaching hospices will be needed to establish recognized techniques and standards of care that can be interpreted in the home as well as in other settings. A hospice aim from the start has been that such work should become part of general medical and nursing teaching, and this book is an important step in that direction. Perhaps the team or unit that is part of a hospital complex such as is here described has the greatest opportunity to integrate with and enrich general practice. The knowledge it contains will form a valuable reference for those working elsewhere in the field.

So far the American hospice has limited itself almost entirely to the dying cancer patient and his family. St. Christopher's, like St. Joseph's, has always had a mixed community of patients. Let us hope that the attitude of skilled attention and respect enshrined in this book will spread to include all those for whom the resources of acute medicine have become irrelevant, but who need help to complete their lives with a sense of personal worth to the end (Vanderpool 1978).

Dame Cicely Saunders

References

Gavey CJ: *The Management of the "Hopeless" Case.* Lewis, London, 1952.

Hinton JM: The physical and mental distress of the dying. *Quart J Med NS* 32:1, 1963.

Saunders C: *Care of the Dying.* Nursing Times Reprint, Macmillan, London, 1960.

Vanderpool HY: The ethics of terminal care. *JAMA* 239:850 – 852, 1978.

Worcester A: *The Care of the Aged, the Dying, and the Dead.* Thomas, Springfield, 1935; Blackwells, London, 1961.

Preface

Recently three articles in the same edition of the local morning paper caught the author's eye. The first dealt with a nurse who had been accused of the intravenous administration of a lethal dose of potassium to end a patient's pain. The second described the activities of the Hemlock Society, a group advocating "self-deliverance," in which "a good death" is chosen by the sufferer in preference to a prolonged and painful demise. The third article reported on the progress of the Natural Death Act in the state legislature.

Within the past few years, the old word "hospice," which used to refer to inns maintained by religious orders, has become the name for programs for the care of people who are dying and for whom no reasonable hope remains. A hospice program began to take shape at Church Hospital in Baltimore about ten years ago and has developed into an important component of the service that the hospital provides. The steady progress of that program was the product of careful planning based upon study of other hospices and an effort to learn from our own accumulating experience.

Like its first edition, this book is designed to be of assistance to those who are, in one way or another, concerned with the care of the terminally ill patient. Most particularly, it is directed at those who would like to know more about how the hospice concept may contribute to the comfort of the dying patient and his or her family.

Its primary purpose is to serve as a guide for all who are interested in, who are developing, or who are involved in the early stages of a hospice program. However, we hope that even those who have had some experience in hospice care may find something of value.

In the four to five years since the first edition of this book was published, our experience has grown, of course, and we have made some modifications in the program. In the environment around us there have been some significant changes. Among these are a heightened interest in cost containment in the health care delivery system, an increasing number of hospices, the availability of a Medicare hospice benefit, implementation of a national accreditation program, and the initiation of state legislation and regulations relating to hospice care. The goal of the current edition remains the same as that of the first but includes up-to-date information and recommendations with respect to the changes that have occurred in the interval. Also, we have expanded the sections dealing with certain aspects of hospice such as inpatient care, revised others such as those dealing with psychosocial issues, and added new chapters relating to ethical issues and to the relationship between hospice and the rest of medical care. The extension of the hospice concept to providing care for patients with nonmalignant terminal illnesses, such as irreversible neurological conditions, AIDS, and emphysema, is discussed in a new chapter.

My primary commitments are, of course, to the practice of surgery, to teaching, and to the administration of the surgical service at Church Hospital. As a surgeon I have had a long-standing interest in the role of surgery in the palliation of malignancy, particularly carcinoma of the esophagus, lung, and pancreas. From the inception of the hospice program at Church Hospital, I have served as chairman of the medical staff committee that oversees it and have been the attending physician for a portion of our hospice patients. I recognize that it is perhaps presumptuous and hazardous for one involved only part time with hospice care to undertake a description and analysis of that care. Nonetheless, it seemed worthwhile to distill and share our experiences with others. This was made possible by the generous provision of assistance from every member of our hospice care team, each of whom gave unselfishly of his or her knowledge and wisdom to make this book a reality.

Although much of it is written from a physician's viewpoint, this volume is intended to be useful to all who are involved in the care of the dying patient. This deserves particular emphasis because hospice care is, by its nature, multidisciplinary. It requires the active participation of nursing personnel, social workers, volunteers, administration, trustees, and others. In harmony with that fact, this edition has incorporated contributions from representatives of more fields than did the first edition. We have tried to take an orderly and logical approach in presentation of material, but each reader will doubtless find certain sections of more interest and value than others.

Although some effort has been directed at providing a comprehensive picture of hospice care for the terminally ill, our main thrust has been toward practical considerations in dealing successfully with the patient dying of cancer. To do this we have begun by identifying current problems in the management of the terminally ill and providing a brief overview of the way in which hospice care tries to respond to these problems. Consideration is then directed at the principles and practices of hospice care, including symptom control and meeting the emotional and psychosocial needs of the patient and family. Bereavement care is, of course, part of this. The composition and function of the hospice care team are reviewed, as are the cardinal features of both inpatient and outpatient care. Attention is then directed at the organization, financing, and staffing of a hospice care program and at the public relations aspects of such programs. The spiritual components of hospice are examined, not just as they relate to patient care, but in program design and function. We then move on to a description of bioethical issues in hospice care. Next, we examine the critical matter of the relationship between hospice care and medicine as a whole. A description of our experience in the Church Hospital hospice program provides a picture of one hospice; information from the first edition is not only updated but is compared with our current experience. The chapter on nonmalignant terminal illnesses is timely in part because of the increasing prevalence in the U.S. of AIDS, whose victims tend to be young and in need of the kind of care that hospice can provide. An attempt to answer some of the commonly asked questions about hospice care provides an opportunity to look back and to summarize what has gone before. We then take a brief look into the future. The book concludes with a list, organized by topics, of material that can provide additional information about the care of the terminally ill and about hospice.

No effort is made here to provide a detailed chronological history of hospice care or a definitive comparison between various types of hospices. This book is simply founded on the premise that our experience speaks to some of the issues in the care of the dying and that the results of that experience may help those who have some interest in or responsibility for treatment of terminally ill patients.

All of the contributing authors are or have been associated with the Church Hospital hospice program. As a result there is a natural consistency of philosophy and viewpoint, but this was not an imperative in selection of material. We therefore make no apology for differences of opinion nor for repetition. This is hospice looked at from different vantage points by different individuals. Both conformity and inconsistency flow naturally from this.

The reader will quickly perceive that we have written from the perspective of a hospice care program that is hospital based and that, for sound and practical reasons, has confined its initial commitment to patients with terminal malignancy. Those of us who have been involved with the Church Hospital hospice program believe in the value of hospital-based programs, while conceding that under some circumstances other models are appropriate. There are both advantages and disadvantages to restricting a developing program to the treatment of advanced malignancy.

For the most part, the approach we have taken is to provide basic information on the current status of hospice care. However, with respect to some of the controversies and uncertainties about hospice care, we have deliberately been provocative. It is often in response to this approach that the reader gains the clearest insights.

The approach here has been thorough in the sense of touching upon the important and practical matters in the care of the terminally ill. However, in the interest of being helpful, we have tried to be concise, and therefore our coverage is not exhaustive. Many of the topics dealt with here deserve deeper consideration than would be appropriate in a book such as this. Some are legitimately the topics of books themselves. This is, of course, the rationale for the concluding material.

The effort here is to provide only a framework upon which one may build. The current status of knowledge about the care of the terminally ill and the diversity of experience in hospice care thus far do not permit us to do more at present. Furthermore, there will always be the need to adapt to local circumstances. We have tried to provide a sound framework based upon a careful look at our own experience and that of others.

Let there be no misunderstanding: commitment to improve care for patients terminally ill from malignant disease in no way de-emphasizes the importance of efforts directed toward the prevention, early detection, and curative treatment of cancer or toward the rehabilitation of patients undergoing curative treatment. The same ethic applies to the nonmalignant terminally ill. A major thesis of this book is, in fact, the need for coordination, cooperation, and cross-fertilization between curative and palliative care.

There clearly is much about hospice that is international and catholic. However, certain things such as drug names, health care delivery organization and financing, and the like are peculiarly national. In these respects the book has an American bias.

Those of us providing care for the terminally ill today are immensely indebted to the hospice pioneers who went before us. There is still much to learn and to do. We can only hope that we also will lend a helping hand to those who follow.

Summer 1985   *Jack M. Zimmerman*

Acknowledgments

The preparation of this book has required the help of many people in many ways.

To Dame Cicely Saunders I shall always be deeply indebted, not just for her unique contribution to this field, but for her personal instruction and encouragement. From Dr. Thomas West I have learned much about how hospice care really works. The entire staff at St. Christopher's has, with good spirit, always been ready to help and give advice.

Dr. Eric Wilkes' delightful clarity of expression, graciousness, and imaginative approach have placed the stamp of St. Luke's in Sheffield upon the Church Hospital hospice program in Baltimore. My first visit to a hospice was to one that shunned the term; at St. Barnabas Home I received from the late Dr. F. R. Gusterson a superb and colorful introduction to hospice care. Dr. Balfour Mount's visit to Church Hospital in 1976 was a turning point for our entire program and for myself personally; he made it all seem possible and showed us a model that was applicable to our situation. Dr. Josephina Magno's leadership in hospice work nationally, and her kind assistance locally, have meant a great deal.

Hospice care exists at Church Hospital because Reverand Paul Dawson had both the vision and the perseverance to make it a reality. With her organizational skill Gloria Cameron made it possible to convert an idea into a functioning program. Kathleen Roche brought to us expertise in both home care and thanatology. Dr. Milton Buschman has demonstrated the numerous contributions a psychiatrist can make to a hospice program that did not have one at the beginning. Yvonne Leacock filled a gap in the services we initially provided through the development of bereavement care as an integral component of our program. Marge Lamb, who has been a friend since student days at Hopkins, typifies excellence in nursing practice and leadership. Fred Wehr has been our interface with much of the community and with the media; he has asked the probing questions and provided valuable advice. Zu McBee as our Director of Volunteers has been instrumental in the function of our program through her imaginative development of volunteer participation. Maureen Mason's tireless work as a volunteer and as an articulate spokeswoman for the program has been invaluable.

Maureen's husband George was also instrumental in the founding of Church Hospital's hospice program; as Vice President of the Hospital when the program was conceived, he guided its early steps. Without commitment from the hospital administration under the leadership of T.G. Whedbee as President and James Bobb as Executive Vice President and support from the governing board under the leadership of George Riepe, there would have been no hospice program at Church Hospital.

The late Helen Fowler was an inspiration to us all. She was part of Paul Dawson's original team and at the beginning was a one-woman home care program. Her devotion to her patients and her own valiant battle against cancer were a model of life as it should be lived.

At the beginning Dr. Bernard Yukna was our hospice physician. He brought to this work an understanding compassion that was critical to the success of the program. He was succeeded by Dr. Lydia Jumanoy, who contributed to the program her expertise in oncology, thus adding a dimension we had not had previously. Both quickly became among the most knowledgeable people in the world about symptom relief in the terminally ill. Bonnie Ray was until recently our clinical nurse practitioner; she not only made the program operate from day to day but made it do so vigorously and harmoniously. Chris Elder drew up the nursing standards of care for the hospice patient.

Miriam Wallace has been our inpatient social worker from the beginning; she has always had the interest of the patient and the program uppermost in her mind. Joyce O'Shea, Director of Nursing, and Marietta Friesner and Jan Bahner, nursing supervisors, have provided leadership in meeting the needs of the program and have given thoughtful help to the author. Each of the members of the hospice team, staff and volunteers, inpatient and home care, have been a key part of this book. They have done the work that we have written about.

Dorothy Eckels, our hospital librarian, has provided reference materials and has been of assistance in manuscript preparation. There would have been no book without the patience and indulgence of my secretaries. Carol Tracey gathered, reviewed, and organized material. Ruth Ann Rochlitz typed tirelessly for an author who was an unfortunate combination of compulsive and disorganized. What is truly remarkable is that both not only survived the first edition, but willingly pitched right in for the second.

Finally, a very special expression of thanks must go to our patients and their families. They have been the central characters in all of this and it is from them that we have learned the most.

Chapter 1

Hospice Care as a Response to the Problems of Terminal Illness

Jack M. Zimmerman

Problems in the Care of the Patient Dying from Cancer

Cancer is the most common disease with which hospice has dealt and serves as the best example of problems in the care of terminally ill patients. Medical science has achieved varying success over recent years with the prevention, early detection, and curative treatment of malignant disease. Though some encouraging and promising advances have been made, there are still many patients who, at the time they initially come to a physician's attention or subsequent to efforts at curative treatment, are incurable. It is the palliative care of such patients that is the subject of this book.

Malignant disease beyond the possibility of cure is not uncommon. Patients in this situation are part of the common experience not only of medical personnel but of most people. There are few of us whose lives have not been touched by someone dying of cancer.

Looked at from a statistical standpoint, cancer ranks second to diseases of the heart among the leading causes of death in the United States. The average death rate from cancer per 100,000 population per year is currently about 197, which means that there will be an estimated 462,000 deaths from cancer in the United States in 1985. Put differently, malignant disease accounts for more than 20% of all deaths. That percentage is likely to increase as the absolute number of cancer deaths increases but also as deaths from other causes decline.

Death from cancer occurs in all age groups; in 1981 15% of cancer deaths occurred in individuals under age 55. In fact, cancer is the leading disease killer in young adults between the ages of 15 and 34 (Silverberg 1982).

It is also part of our common experience that care for terminally ill patients is fraught with difficulties and is often less than an ideal. There is clearly room for improvement.

There are a multitude of interlocking factors that make the palliative care of patients with advanced malignancy very demanding. The reasons for and the nature of problems in the care of the dying patient have been well described by a number of authors including Mount (1976a) and Ryder and Ross (1977). Graphic and touching reports based on personal experience have been provided in books such as John

Gunther's *Death Be Not Proud* (1949), Stewart Alsop's *Stay of Execution* (1973), and the Ryans' *A Private Battle* (1979). Because the reader has doubtless already recognized these problems and perceived the need for improvement, we will not deal with this matter exhaustively but will only make a few observations.

The human situation of terminal illness may be looked at in a number of different dimensions. It is both *terminal* and *illness*. Impending death brings one face to face with his mortality and with the reality of practical preparation for permanent separation. However, the illness itself, entirely aside from the fact that it will be lethal has a profound impact upon those who are touched by it. Furthermore, sickness has both *medical* and *nonmedical* aspects. The disease process, its symptoms, and its ramifications are clearly medical matters. The effects of both the illness and impending death upon personal relationships and finances are not, strictly speaking, medical matters. Also, dying must be looked at as involving the patient *and* his family. Both are clearly involved in the dying process, and the long-range effect of the patient's death on the family may be considerable. Finally, terminal illness does not occur in isolation from the rest of life but is part of a continuum. *Preexisting problems*, anteceding the terminal illness, although not immediately related to illness or death, are thrown into sharper focus and sometimes require more definitive resolution because of the terminal illness.

When each of the dimensions of terminal illness is examined separately, the origin and nature of the problems relating to it become clearer and perhaps a bit easier to comprehend, if not to accept.

Looked at from a medical standpoint, it is clear that terminal illness from cancer is the consequence of a serious and advanced disease. By definition the disease process cannot be reversed, and thus the overall course is one of inevitable functional decline that is disheartening to the patient, loved ones, and caregivers. The tumor itself produces a variety of troublesome symptoms such as pain, weakness, and anorexia for which there are often no simple measures of relief. All forms of anti-tumor therapy (as described in Chapter 14) may also produce distressing and difficult-to-manage symptoms such as malaise, nausea, and hair loss. Even palliative measures designed to make the patient more comfortable have undesirable side effects. Potent narcotics, for example, produce constipation. Thus, the tangle of physical symptoms in the terminally ill patient can pose some very difficult medical problems.

Patients, family members, and caregivers bring to the situation of terminal illness not only their individual values and prior experiences, but also differing expectations with respect to the course of the illness and to the results and side effects of treatment. In the distressing and tense environment of fatal illness, communication can be limited, so that information about these differing values and expectations may not be shared.

Serious illnesses of all kinds bring with them difficult psychosocial problems. Feelings of fear, depression, loneliness, and loss of control are almost universal among the sick. The normal family and social relationships are disrupted. Financial considerations can be significant if not overwhelming. Self-image is changed.

These matters relate to the seriously ill patient and his or her family whether or not death is impending. The fact of imminent death introduces the whole panorama of problems related to death, separation, and loss. Superimposed now on the fear of pain and discomfort arising from illness are fears about dying and death. For the patient this includes fear of loss of dignity, autonomy, identity, and personhood. Caregivers also must come face to face with their concept of death. For family members these problems do not end with the death of the patient. No matter how long and careful the period of preparation, much grieving must be done after the patient has died. The period of bereavement has its own set of physical, psychological, and social difficulties.

It is important to note that the above problems are timeless. There has been a tendency, perhaps, to romanticize dying "in the old days" and to blame modern society for the trauma of terminal illness. This simply does not conform to the facts. However, some of the patterns of contemporary life *have* magnified the above problems and *have* impaired our capacity to deal with them.

The immense technological advances of recent years have improved the potential for cure of many previously disabling or lethal conditions. It is natural that our system of health care delivery has responded by organizing itself to facilitate such cure. This is not only natural, but fortunate and commendable. There has, however, been an unfortunate by-product: the provision of supportive palliative care for the incurable has suffered in a number of ways. As medical care has become increasingly technologically sophisticated, the most advanced care has become institutionally based. As a consequence there is a tendency to place all severely ill patients in the hospital rather than at home. Hospitals tend to be threatening, restrictive, and impersonal. Furthermore, in the hospital setting the availability of a vast panorama of medications and other therapeutic techniques can make it difficult to withhold treatment measures. Also, the inroads that curative techniques are making against malignant disease make it difficult for physicians to determine definitively whether or not the patient has passed beyond the point of cure. Increasing specialization, itself a by-product of expanding technology, has led, through fragmentation, to less continuity of care. In subtle but definite ways, probably only in part related to technological advance, the interpersonal relationships between those providing care and the patients have deteriorated. This development hampers relief of symptoms, which depends upon communication between patient and caregiver. Furthermore, in recent decades, clinical scientists have directed less attention to symptom relief than to disease control. All of these factors have combined to impede the provision of optimal palliative care to patients beyond the hope of cure.

There are still many physicians and nurses who believe that the emotional, social, and psychological ramifications of illnesses deserve their attention. Their interest in the whole patient and all of his problems keeps faith with the finest traditions of medicine. However, the ability of professional caregivers in this respect varies immensely from individual to individual. In and out of the hospital there are many support systems available for dealing with psychological and social problems that were not available in the past. There are social work departments, discharge planners, counselling services, and financial assistance organizations of various types. However, a number of factors have tended to make institutions and individuals less willing and able to attend to the emotional, psychological, and social problems of seriously ill patients and their families.

Not only changes in medicine, but transitions in society as a whole have adversely affected the care of the dying patient. Modifications in family structure with greater mobility and less stability have had a negative influence on the care of the chronically ill. Attitudes toward the elderly have not had a positive influence. Ours has been characterized as a death-denying and a youth-oriented society; in large measure these charges are doubtless true. Ours is an urbanized society that has lost touch with the cycles of nature and has come to expect medical science to conquer all disease. These attitudes toward death have unquestionably helped shape both personal reaction and public policy toward death. The way in which society deals with the economics of health care affects the care of the terminally ill. Medical insurance grew up in the United States not as *health care* insurance but as *hospitalization* insurance. From the 1930s into the 1970s much of medical care was covered by insurance only if the patient was hospitalized. Patients, families, and caregivers thus developed a bias toward hospitalization. In addition, there was a concomitant tendency for insurance plans to reimburse providers more generously for *procedures* than for other types of care. There was inevitable accentuation of the move toward more technology and less concern with emotional support in the care of patients. The current thrust in the economics of health care is, of course, cost containment. Precisely where this will lead is presently uncertain, but the threat to the psychosocial dimensions of patient care and to concerns with patient comfort and support of family must be recognized.

Compounding all of the above is the fact that the medical and psychosocial problems to which the patient and family are subjected do not arise in isolation. They occur against the background of earlier existence. Intercurrent diseases such as heart trouble and emphysema not only continue but may be aggravated by malignancy and its treatment. Irritating personality traits, tensions in family relationships, and economic difficulties persist and may be accentuated. Problems related to drug addiction and alcoholism do not dissolve because the patient is dying.

It is not surprising therefore that the care of the terminally ill can be difficult and frustrating.

In recent years there has been increasing attention to death and dying that, one hopes, will ultimately provide some practical results in the way in which people approach death. The seminal work of Elizabeth Kübler-Ross (1969) sharpened the focus on the process of dying, a concern characteristic of the 1970s. Brim (1970) and Horan and Mall (1977) have viewed from a broad perspective the matter of dealing with the dying. Ramsey (1970) and others have explored the ethical issues related to our attitudes toward death. Noyes (1971), Dunphy (1976), and Wiles (1984) have looked critically at the clinical aspects of the care of the dying. There has been recognition within medical schools that medical students should be taught about death and dying (Barton et al. 1972; Dickinson 1981).

Nonetheless, there remain factors that interfere with making the dying process as comfortable as possible. These problems are as real as they are obvious; their effects can be seen daily in graphic, personal terms. For example, they lead often to one of two medical approaches to the terminally ill patient that although different, are not necessarily mutually exclusive. At one extreme there may be a "nothing further can be done" approach in which semantic confusion occurs between being able to do nothing further *about the tumor* and being able to do nothing further *for the patient*; these are two very different things. At the other extreme, there is the frantic utilization of multiple modalities of antitumor therapy and aggressive life-support systems in a vain effort to "do something"; there is a confusion between what *can* be done and what *should* be done.

Similarly, professional caregivers and families alike, because of difficulties related to the acceptance of impending death, find themselves with no meaningful way in which to relate to the patient and to each other. A number of unhappy scenarios may result. The most common is probably the closing of all lines of communication so that the patient and family see the caregivers as cold and heartless, and the caregivers see the patient's family as unconcerned. Another pattern is that in which the caregivers feel helpless but see the patient's family as demanding and guilt ridden. In summary, the criticisms of terminal care that we hear most frequently from dying patients and their families are the unnecessary prolongation of life, ineffective control of symptoms, lack of emotional support, and fragmentation of caregiving responsibility.

Before approaching the matter of methods for dealing with these problems of terminal illness, we must establish an operational definition. In a sense, each of us is dying from the day he is born. However, Silver (1980) has, quite correctly, described this concept as "excessively lugubrious and . . . not workable." Dictionary definitions of the term focus on the *time* element by using phrases such as "about to die" and "drawing close to death." Wilkes (1982) emphasizes, rather, that death is *expected* by those attending the patient. Bayer (1983) proposes the following definition: "an illness in which, on the basis of the best available diagnostic criteria and in the light of available therapies, a reasonable estimation can be made prospectively and with a high probability that a person will die within a relatively short time." For cancer patients, terminal illness can be defined as the existence of a malignant tumor for which antitumor therapy does not offer a reasonable possibility of cure.

This is a relatively precise definition because for most types of tumors, duration of life expectancy is quite limited once the patient has reached this point. Even among malignant tumors there is, however, considerable variability and unpredictability. The natural history of a particular tumor can be anticipated imperfectly, and palliative antitumor therapy can influence the course of tumor progression in ways that are difficult to determine in advance. Thus, within the restricted area of malignant tumors, it is difficult to quantitate life expectancy for patients who are terminally ill. For example, breast cancer with distant metastases is incurable, but the natural history of the disease combined with response to antitumor therapy may result in relatively lengthy survival. Conversely, in other types of malignant disease, the interval from diagnosis to death may be quite short.

When one takes into consideration terminal illness from disorders other than cancer — for example, emphysema or kidney disease — the matter of duration of life expectancy becomes even more complex.

It is important to note, therefore, that our operational definition of terminal illness does not encompass a prediction of life expectancy. Likewise, it does not include mention of whether or not the patient is symptomatic. Under this definition terminal illness is not incompatible with the absence of symptoms and a relatively long life expectancy. The practical implications of these matters of definition for the care of the terminally ill must be recognized and are dealt with in several places in this book.

It is evident that all of the previously identified problems in dealing with terminal illness are compounded by the fact that, as defined, the terminally ill are a heterogeneous group. Each patient brings to his or her terminal illness a tumor of specific type and extent, individual manifestations of the tumor, and individual attitudes toward the disease, family members, and impending death.

Furthermore, all of these factors are dynamic, not static; they are in constant flux. It is not surprising, therefore, that the provision of optimal care for the dying patient is difficult and is deserving of our most thoughtful attention and strenuous effort.

Objectives in the Care of Terminal Illness

The logical place to begin in the design of a program for the care of the terminally ill is with the objectives of such a program. What is it we would like to accomplish in the care of the dying patient?

The articulation of practical, helpful objectives in the care of terminal illness is not a simple task. Differences of opinion regarding definitions and substantive matters create difficulty. It is very easy to become entangled in a web of controversy while simply trying to identify the principal purposes of a program.

Considerable disagreement has occurred over the phrase "death with dignity" as a goal of programs for the care of the terminal illness (e.g., Vanderpool 1978). The term "graceful" has been suggested as a more appropriate description than "dignified" as the way in which most of us wish to die. Although the distinction may seem trivial, the controversy itself perhaps suggests some deep differences in the way in which people think about optimal handling of the dying process. As a physician the author's bias has always been toward "comfort," and the phrase we use at Church Hospital is "toward a gentler dying."

In examining the objectives of good palliative care for the terminally ill, attention must obviously be directed to both the *quantity* of life and the *quality* of life. Because both are important, the two must be balanced. It is the thesis of this book that there are presently available techniques that can help achieve this balance and thus make terminal illness a more comfortable experience for the patient and family. Yet we must recognize that there are very real problems in approaching both quantity and quality of life. In the patient with advanced cancer, quantity can be measured easily in terms of days, weeks, or months, but often we simply do not have available the information that will tell us how various options in treatment will affect the quantity of life. Furthermore, predictions of quantity of life without therapy are at best crude. Quality of life presents the problem of not being easily measurable. Factors influencing the quality of life are not only highly individual for each patient but are extremely subjective.

It is simple to set the provision of a maximum quantity and quality of life with an appropriate balance of the two as an overall goal in the care of the terminally ill. However, we would deceive ourselves if we did not recognize that for a particular patient with disseminated breast cancer, for example, we cannot predict with accuracy what effect the administration of a given program of chemotherapy will have on her life expectancy, nor can we determine in advance the degree of discomfort she will perceive. We certainly cannot determine for her whether she would prefer three months of uncomfortable life to an earlier, more comfortable death. Even the patient may have difficulty assigning priorities to the relief and avoidance of various symptoms of her disease and its therapy. Such are the vagaries of advanced malignant disease and its handling, but in any program for the care of the terminally ill we, with the help of the patient and family, are going to have to make these decisions.

With these reservations in mind, the following are suggested objectives for a program for the care of the terminally ill:

1. *Provide the finest available medical care for the patient's medical problems.* This means treatment directed both at control of the patient's disease and optimal relief of the symptoms. Treatment of the underlying disease must be undertaken with the recognition that, by definition, cure is not possible but that control of the disease may contribute materially to palliation.
2. *Provide for the patient and his or her family appropriate understanding of the nature of the patient's situation and psychological support to both in dealing with the illness and impending death.* What constitutes "appropriate" understanding will be highly individual for each patient.

3. *Provide appropriate spiritual support to the patient and family in dealing with the philosophical and religious aspects of the illness and impending death.*

4. *Provide assistance to the patient and family in dealing with interpersonal, social, and financial problems.*

5. *Render patient care in the optimal setting for the particular circumstances.* For some patients all care will be in an institution, for others all care can best be rendered at home, and for the remainder a combination of the two will be necessary.

6. *Provide certain valuable program characteristics such as continuity, comprehensiveness, and adaptability to individual circumstances.* There are many facets of this objective. Care of the seriously ill tends, because of technology and specialization, to be fragmented; this fragmentation has a number of negative consequences. A corollary of the need for continuity is the need for 24-hour availability of personnel. "Programs" by their very nature tend to be somewhat inflexible, and special attention needs to be devoted to adaptability to individual circumstances.

7. *Provide a setting for research into the care of the terminally ill.* We have much to learn if we are going to do things better.

8. *Provide for ongoing education in the care of the terminally ill.* This means education both for those whose primary concern is dealing with the dying patient and for others who may at one time or another be involved with the care of the terminally ill.

9. *Have a positive impact on the remainder of the health care system.* As noted, some of the problems plaguing the terminally ill and their families are also very real problems for other patients and their families. One hopes that as we learn more about the proper handling of terminal illness, we will learn things that can be applied in general medical care. Even failing this objective, programs for the care of the terminally ill should not disrupt the remainder of health care system and should integrate well with it.

10. *Be financially feasible.* All of these objectives may not be equally vital and achievable, and they are not listed in order of importance. As with the other objectives, there are problems of definition (Is it cost effective?) and substantive problems (How do you get reimbursed for it?), but we would be unrealistic if we did not include this as an objective of a program for the care of the terminally ill.

There is one special caution regarding these objectives. They are targets toward which we must aim as we develop programs for the terminally ill. No program will reach every objective at its inception; one who waits for a perfect program will have no program at all.

There is one final concern before beginning to look at the hospice concept as a response to the needs of the dying patient. As individuals and programs emerge to deal with problems, there is often a tendency for others to let up a little in the belief that the burden has now been fully and safely taken up. It is important to remember that palliative care is a responsibility, not just of those who are directly involved in its delivery, but also of the clinician whose primary responsibility is the provision of curative treatment to cancer patients. It is this physician who must make the often difficult decision that there is no longer a reasonable hope of cure and thus commit the patient to a program of palliative care. However, responsibility begins even before this. In certain forms of malignancy (for example, esophageal and pancreatic cancer), the potential for cure is often extremely limited even when the patient is seen early in the course of the disease. In the clinical planning of treatment for such patients, the prudent clinician is careful that in providing a slim chance of cure, he or she does not materially compromise the potential for adequate palliation. The consequences of an unwise choice of curative therapy can sometimes be a greater barrier to "a gentler dying" than is the underlying malignancy.

Hospice Care as a Response

For a number of reasons, hospice care is somewhat difficult to define. This is in part because the term "hospice" dates back to the Middle Ages and over the years has had different meanings. Furthermore, present day hospice care is characterized by its diversity. Nonetheless, the modern hospice has certain distinctive features. The medical dictionary definition of hospice is "an institution that provides a centralized program of palliative and supportive services to dying persons and their families, in the form of physical, psychological, social, and spiritual care. Such services are provided by an interdisciplinary team of professionals and volunteers who are available at home and in inpatient settings." (*Stedman's Medical Dictionary* 1982).

Hospice care is a comprehensive program of management that offers an opportunity to provide palliative care for terminally ill patients. Its multidisciplinary approach is designed to relieve the patient's symptoms and to provide support to both the patient and family. It is care that can be rendered in any one of a number of settings: the patient's home, a nursing home, a free-standing hospice unit, or a hospital. Although most hospice programs have focused primarily upon terminal illness from malignant disease, many have provided care to other types of patients, such as those with progressive neurological diseases, including multiple sclerosis and amyotrophic lateral sclerosis. Some programs are addressing the problems of patients with acquired immune deficiency syndrome (AIDS).

In medieval times a hospice was a way station for travelers; in this sense, the adoption of the term for a program for the care of the terminally ill is quite fitting. However, there are obviously some problems with its use. Before the term was adopted by programs for the dying, it had already been used by other types of institutions such as convalescent homes and facilities for the care of the mentally ill. In addition, the term possesses a religious connotation to which some have taken exception. Some programs that clearly are hospices in the functional sense have for these reasons adopted other names, such as "palliative care unit" or "home." Although the term may lack clarity, its use is widely accepted, and there does not appear to be an alternative that is both simple and accurate.

The lack of precision in the term "hospice" has created some practical problems. It is not reasonable to seek a copyright on the term; in turn, this creates difficulties in certification and accreditation, as there can be no restriction on the use of the word.

At this point it would be well to observe that the word "hospice" is presently used as both a noun and adjective. The noun "hospice" possesses different meanings. It is used as part of the title of certain convalescent and residential homes that are only incidently involved in the care of the terminally ill. These institutions have usually possessed the name hospice for many years and, except coincidently, are not involved in the use of current hospice principles in palliative care. For example, Stella Maris Hospice near Baltimore has for years provided residential and nursing care but has now instituted a hospice program specifically designed for the care of the terminally ill. "Hospice" is also used as a noun to describe the type of care for the terminally ill that is the subject of this book. But even here it has several meanings. Sometimes it is used to describe a place or physical facility, such as Hospice, Inc., of Connecticut. Sometimes it is used to describe a program that has little or no exclusive location, such as the Church Hospital hospice. Sometimes it is used to encompass the entire approach to terminal illness that is based upon the principles of hospice care, as in "hospice is an idea whose time has come." As an adjective used to modify nouns such as care, program, concept, movement, and approach, hospice almost invariably denotes management of terminal illness.

In tracing the history of hospice care, it is difficult to know precisely where to begin. One might start with medieval institutions that were termed hospices or with institutions devoted to the care of the terminally ill, whether designated as hospices or not. Alternatively, one might consider the initial hospices to be individuals, institutions, or programs that used some of the principles associated with present hospice care. The early history of hospice is intertwined in part with that of hospitals, for the latter were at one time largely places for the dying poor. Goldin (1981) has traced the evolution of modern hospices for the care of the terminally ill in relation to the origin and history of the word "hospice." Koff (1980) described the relationship between hospice as we know it today and several institutions formed in the late nineteenth century for the care of the dying, which he describes as the ancestors of current hospices. The modern hospice program really began when the specialization and attention those institutions provided were combined with mid-twentieth century techniques of symptom relief through the pioneering work of Dame Cicely Saunders, who opened St. Christopher's Hospice in Syndenham, England, in 1967. The concept spread rapidly throughout England, with the opening of many hospices. These were almost exclusively free-standing units separate from hospitals.

Hospice care came to North America in January 1975 with the opening of the Palliative Care Unit at the Royal Victoria Hospital in Montreal under the direction of Dr. Balfour Mount (Mount 1976b). This very successful prototype program is a hospital-based unit. At about the same time an imaginative, industrious, and pioneering group at New Haven was founding Hospice Incorporated of Connecticut (Lack and Buckingham 1978); this was a free-standing unit that began with home care before it possessed a physical facility. As in England the hospice concept has caught on in North America; there are now many hospices in various stages of operation and planning throughout the United States and Canada. Because of the problems with definition and data gathering and because the stiuation is dynamic, it is difficult to say precisely how many hospice programs are in existence at any given moment. The Comptroller General of the United States (1979) reported that in November 1978 there were 59 operating hospices in the United States. Cohen (1979) listed more than 200 hospices in different stages of development in this country. In 1984 the National Hospice Organization (NHO) reported the existence of 1345 programs in the United States, 935 of which were fully operational and the remainder being in various stages of development. Six hundred were provider members of the organization (*Hospice News* 1985). The NHO has published a directory of hospices in the United States (Corless 1984).

The transplantation of hospice care from the United Kingdom to the United States has required some modification in hospice organization. In addition to obvious general social and cultural differences between the two countries, there are some very important differences in the medical care systems. England, of course, has a compulsory national health insurance system that the United States does not. An even more important difference, however, relates to the way in which physicians are organized to deliver health care in the two countries. In England there are two categories of physicians: there are general practitioners who work strictly on an outpatient basis and specialists (consultants) who work strictly within hospitals. Every citizen is not only assigned to a general practitioner but also has a district nurse. This health care delivery system is vastly different from that of the United States, and this difference has had an impact as hospice care has come to America.

There has been concomitant development of hospice programs around the world. In June 1980 the author was privileged to attend the International Hospice Conference in London. At that celebration of St. Christopher's "bar mitzvah," there were representatives of hospices in 17 countries, including three representatives from behind the Iron Curtain.

The term hospice, which has its origins in the Latin root having to do with guests and hosts has appeared in general dictionaries for many years. *Webster's New World Dictionary* in 1972 defined a hospice as "1) a place of shelter for travellers, especially such a shelter maintained by monks, 2) a home for the sick or poor." The term's appearance in *medical* dictionaries has been, however, much more recent.

Dorland's Medical Dictionary in 1981 did not include the word, but it was defined in the 24th edition of *Stedman's Medical Dictionary* in 1982. The 15th edition of *Cecil's Textbook of Medicine* published in 1979 did not index "hospice," but the next in 1982 (Wyngaarden and Smith 1982) included brief mention, which was indexed. The 17th edition, published in 1985 (Lack 1985), contained a section on hospice written by Sylvia Lack.

Cohen (1979) traces the origin and development of hospice programs. Stoddard (1978) also provides a colorful look at the history of hospices and many of the personalities who have been important in its development.

Although all are committed to providing palliative care for the terminally ill, hospices throughout the United States have taken various forms and have had various criteria for the admission of patients. Basically, they have been of several organizational types:

1. home care only
2. free-standing hospice unit, usually with provision of home care
3. hospital-based program, usually with provision of home care
   a. discrete unit within the hospital
   b. no discrete unit within the hospital.
   Within this subcategory, several different approaches have been employed. Some programs have utilized "swing beds" on one nursing unit and others have used a "scatter bed" approach throughout the hospital. Both of these systems in effect utilize a symptom control team, which may either serve in a consultant capacity to the attending physician or take primary responsibility for the care of the patient.

It must be emphasized that the distinction between these several organizational types is not always clear cut. There are numerous variations in the types listed. For example, there are some free-standing units that are hospital affiliated; in other words, the physical facility for care of the terminally ill is outside of the hospital, but the program there is in some measure coordinated with in-hospital care. Erle (1982) has briefly described various features of the different types of hospices. Although it is not absolute and does not address the matter of funding, the classification used here is useful in beginning our look at hospice care.

The diversity of hospice care is evident; although it has created some problems, unquestionably, it has also been one of the strengths of hospice care. It has permitted the development of hospices under circumstances in which a more standardized format would have been stifling. In addition, it has encouraged the type of innovation that is essential to growth.

Furthermore, although diverse, hospices have many things in common. Their orientation is humanistic in their concern for the well-being of the patient and his family. They are holistic in directing attention to "the whole patient" and drawing upon the whole armamentarium of medical care through the use of a multidisciplinary team. Their focus is upon life and living rather than upon death and dying. They view death as a natural part of life, but as one that, like birth, can be made easier by the provision of some help.

These shared characteristics, together with some common approaches and techniques, are what is included under the term "hospice" as it is applied to the care of the terminally ill patients and their families.

The National Hospice Organization was formed in 1977 and is incorporated in Washington, D.C. It is composed of various categories of institutional and individual members and is governed by a Board of Directors. Membership is open to individuals and institutions interested in hospice care, but voting membership is restricted to incorporated providers of hospice care and regional and state-wide hospice organizations. The purposes of the NHO include exchange of information between hospice groups, provision of information about hospice care to the public, and establishment and maintenance of standards for hospice care.

In various ways government at different levels and locales has recognized the existence of hospice care. In 1979 and 1980 the Department of Health and Human Services designated certain hospice programs as pilot projects for the purpose of studying mechanisms of reimbursement for hospice care. The Tax Equity and Fiscal Responsibility Act of 1982 included a Medicare hospice benefit that offered hospice care providers an alternative payment method (see Chapter 10). State legislatures have passed bills and resolutions of various types dealing with care of the terminally ill generally and hospice care specifically. In Maryland, for example, the Hospice Care Reimbursement Study Commission, of which the author was a member, made recommendations for legislation mandating the availability of provisions for hospital services in insurance coverage. The resultant hospice reimbursement legislation was passed and signed by the governor in 1982. That commission also studied the availability of services beneficial to the terminally ill and their families and ways in which the insurance industry and the state medical assistance program could approach the provision of needed forms of insurance coverage. Actions taken in other states have ranged from establishment of hospice pilot projects to acts defining hospice care and including hospices in the state's certificate of need and facility licensing regulations.

The Joint Commission on Accreditation of Hospitals, in cooperation with the NHO, has developed a voluntary accreditation program. Torrens (1985) defines the terms *certification, accreditation, licensure,* and *deemed status* and reviews their current application to hospices.

Private insurers, including Blue Cross, have carefully monitored the experience of hospice programs and their impact on health care costs. A national survey has recently revealed that 44% of employers offer a hospice care benefit to their employees (*Hospice News* 1985).

As hospice programs have become an increasingly visible part of the fabric of society, there has been increasing interest in study of their value. Although such
studies are unquestionably needed, their proper performance poses some difficult
methodological and other problems. Although some have confirmed the benefits of
various aspects of hospice care (e.g., Gold 1983; Hinton 1979; Kane 1984), there have
been two major research projects that have failed to find differences in the quality of
care between hospice and nonhospice patients. The results of the study carried out
at UCLA Veterans Administration Hospital have been published (Kane et al. 1984).
The final report of the other, conducted at Brown University, has not yet been published. A monograph, published by the NHO, provides an informative critique of
these two research projects (Cassileth 1984).

There are some additional matters related to hospices in general which deserve
comment at this point. As has been pointed out, the word hospice has been used as
an adjective before a number of nouns, including movement, concept, and
philosophy. In a sense there are and have been all of these things, although as a surgeon the author finds the phrase "hospice movement" somewhat awkward and con-
fusing. We have reached the point where hospice programs are just as much a reality
as are open-heart surgery programs. Granting the obvious differences, the latter
also developed without an "open-heart surgery movement." Perhaps the term
"movement" reflects the relatively greater involvement of individuals outside the
medical field in the development of hospice programs. This initiative and support is
welcome and essential. However, there is an aspect of this issue that raises some
concern. Although hospice care depends upon a multidisciplinary approach,
utilizes families and volunteers in imaginative ways, and requires support from outside the health care team, hospice care in particular and medical care in general will
suffer if hospice care becomes separated from medical care. To meet its full potential, hospice care must be a medical program.

To the extent that a hospice movement stimulates and supports a medical program of hospice care for the terminally ill, our society will be enriched. However, a
movement growing outside of the medical care system can pose serious dangers.
The ways in which hospice care can be interlocked into our health care system are
multiple and can be adapted to local circumstances. It would be regrettable if medical and nonmedical people failed to cooperate in providing optimal care for the terminally ill.

It has been argued that hospice care is not a new development, but rather a return
to old values. There is little to be gained from exploration of this argument. Surely
hospice care is founded upon the finest traditions of medical care and man's concern
for his fellow man. Clearly it utilizes some techniques that date back many years.
However, as is often the case with worthwhile advances, it represents some new applications of old knowledge. The successful use of a broad-based multidisciplinary
team is not unique to hospice care, but no one can deny that this approach has immensely enlarged the scope of our capacity to deal with the terminally ill.

It is important to point out that hospice care programs have not provided all of the answers to the problems of caring for the terminally ill. As with many worthwhile endeavors, hospice care has raised more questions than it has answered. However, pertinent questions lead to progress. This may seem trite and pedantic, but its practical importance to hospice programs cannot be overemphasized. Unrealistic expectations on the part of patients, families, and hospice workers have probably led to more unhappy consequences than any other single factor in hospice care. It is important to recognize and accept the fact that the best of hospice care is not going to make every death beautiful and easy. The zeal of hospice workers and the enthusiasm of surviving family members have contributed immensely to the success of hospice care, but they must be tempered by an understanding that serious illness and death have unpleasant features that cannot be overcome by any program designed and operated by human beings.

References

Alsop S: *Stay of Execution.* JB Lippincott, Philadelphia, 1973.

Barton D, Flexner JM, van Eys J, Scott CE: Death and dying: A course for medical students. *J Med Educ* 47:945, 1972.

Bayer R et al.:The care of the terminally ill: Morality and economics. *N Engl J Med* 309: 1409, 1983.

Brim OG: *The Dying Patient.* Russell Sage Foundation, New York, 1970.

Cassileth BR: *Major Hospice Research Projects: Research and Evaluation.* National Hospice Organization, Arlington VA, 1984.

Cohen KP: *Hospice: Prescription for Terminal Care.* Aspen Press, Germantown MD, 1979.

Comptroller General: *Report to the Congress of the United States.* HRD 79–50, March 6, 1979.

Corless IR, et al.: *Guide to the Nation's Hospices.* National Hospice Organization, Arlington VA, 1984.

Dickinson GE: Death education in U.S. medical schools: 1975–1980. *J Med Educ* 56:111, 1981.

Dorland's Medical Dictionary ed 26. WB Saunders, Philadelphia, 1981.

Dunphy JE: Annual discourse — on caring for the patient with cancer. *N Engl J Med* 295:313, 1976.

Erle HR: Terminal care. The national scene and the individual patient. *Med Clin North Am* 66:1161, 1982.

Gold M: *Life Support: What Families Say*

About Hospitals, Hospice and Home Care for the Fatally Ill. Consumer Union Foundation, Mount Vernon NY, 1983.

Goldin G:A protohospice at the century: St. Luke's House, London, from 1843 to 1921. *J Hist Med Allied Sci* 36:383, 1981.

Gunther J: *Death Be Not Proud.* Harper Brothers, New York, 1949.

Hinton J: Comparisons of places and policies for terminal care. *Lancet* 1:29, 1979.

Horan JD, Mall D: *Death, Dying and Euthanasia.* University Publications of America, Washington DC, 1977.

Hospice News 3:2, January 1985.

Kane RL, et al.: A randomized, controlled trial of hospice care. *Lancet* 1:890 ,1984.

Koff TH: *Hospice — A Caring Community.* Winthrop Publishers, Cambridge MA, 1980.

Kübler-Ross E: *On Death and Dying.* Macmillan, New York, 1969.

Lack SA, Buckingham RW: *First American Hospice.* Hospice Inc, New Haven CT, 1978.

Lack SA: Care of dying patients and their families. In: *Cecil's Textbook of Medicine,* ed 17. WB Saunders, Philadelphia, 1985.

Mount BW: The problem of caring for the dying in a general hospital: The palliative care unit as a possible solution. *Can Med Assoc J* 115:119, 1976a.

Mount BM: *Palliative Care Service: October 1976 Report.* Royal Victoria Hospital,

McGill University, Montreal, 1976b.

Noyes R: The care and management of the dying. *Arch Intern Med* 128:299, 1971.

Ramsey P:*The Patient as a Person*. Yale University Press, New Haven CT, 1970.

Ryan C, Ryan KM: *A Private Battle*. Simon and Schuster, New York, 1979.

Ryder CF, Ross DM: Terminal care — Issues and alternatives. *Public Health Rep* 29:20, 1977.

Silver RT: The dying patient: A clinician's view. *Am J Med* 68:473, 1980.

Silverberg E: Cancer in young adults. *CA* 32:32 1982.

Stedman's Medical Dictionary, ed 24. Williams and Wilkins, Baltimore, 1982.

Stoddard S: *The Hospice Movement*. Stein and Day, Briarcliff Manor NY, 1978.

Torrens PR: *Hospice Programs and Public Policy*. American Hospital Publishing, Chicago, 1985.

Vanderpool HY: The ethics of terminal care. *JAMA* 239:850, 1978.

Wyngaarden JB, Smith LH, eds: *Cecil's Textbook of Medicine*, ed 16. WB Saunders, Philadelphia, 1982.

Webster's New World Dictionary, college ed 2. New World Publishing, New York, 1972.

Wilkes E: *The Dying Patient — The Medical Management of Incurable and Terminal Illness*. George A Bogden and Sons, Ridgewood NJ, 1982.

Wilkes E: Dying now. *Lancet* 1:950, 1984.

Chapter 2

General Features of Hospice Care

Jack M. Zimmerman

Although one of the most prominent aspects of hospice care is its *diversity* as delivered by different groups, there are common threads that weave through hospice care programs. Certain measures have proved so consistently helpful that they appear to be fundamental to the hospice care approach. It is to these characteristics that we will direct some attention in this chapter. A few of them requiring amplification are covered in more detail in subsequent chapters.

Definitions of Hospice

Although definition is certainly important in a number of respects, including communication, accreditation, quality assurance, and reimbursement, the term "hospice" has been variously defined. In the past the term has been used in a variety of ways, and until recently the word has had no medical meaning. In Chapter 1 we traced general and medical dictionary definitions of hospice. *Webster's New World Dictionary* (1972) defined a hospice as an inn for travelers, especially one kept by a religious order, and secondarily as a home for the sick or the poor. *Stedman's Medical Dictionary* (1982) defines hospice as

> an institution that provides a centralized program of palliative and supportive services to dying persons and their families, in the form of physical, psychological, social, and spiritual care. Such services are provided by an interdisciplinary team of professionals and volunteers who are available at home and in inpatient settings.

In 1978 the National Hospice Organization (NHO) adopted the following definition:

> Hospice is a medically directed, nurse coordinated program providing a continuum of home and inpatient care for the terminally ill patient and family. It employs an interdisciplinary team acting under the direction of an autonomous hospice administration. The program provides palliative and supportive care to meet the special needs arising out of the physical, emotional, spiritual, social and economic stresses which are experienced during the final stages of illness and during dying and bereavement.[1]

---

1. Background materials provided to the author by the staff of the Maryland Hospice Reimbursement Commission, 1981.

For the purposes of participation in the Medicare hospice benefit program, the Health Care Financing Administration has listed an elaborate set of requirements that an organization must meet to qualify as a hospice (Department of Health and Human Services 1983). Legislation in various states defines and describes *hospice* in different ways. In Maryland the law (*Annotated Code* 1981) specifies that

the term hospice describes a humane approach to care for the terminally ill patient, distinguishing it from traditional health care in the following four ways:

1. The patient and his family are considered as a unit;
2. An interdisciplinary team is used to assess the medical and social needs of the patient, develop an overall plan of care, and provide coordinated care;
3. The patient receives palliative rather than curative types of treatment;
4. Bereavement follow-up is provided to the family.

In Nevada the annotated code specifies that

hospice means an establishment which is staffed and equipped to :

1. Provide care, either in the home or in a facility, or both, for persons who are terminally ill and do not require full services of a hospital or skilled nursing facility;
2. offer medical service under the direction of a physician and a 24 hour professional nursing staff;
3. Provide directly or by arrangement, social, psychological, or spritual services for the patient and his family." (See footnote 1).

In California

hospice is a program which provides palliative care for terminally ill patients and their families either directly or on a consulting basis, with the patient's physician or a community agency, such as a Visiting Nurses Association. The whole family is considered the unit of care, and care extends through the mourning period. A full scope of health services are provided by an organized interdisciplinary team available whenever necessary." (See footnote 1).

Naturally, in all states having legislation covering hospice care, that legislation includes some definition of hospice, and as can be seen, there are differences among these definitions, some potentially important. Some states have adopted variations of the NHO definition.

Cardinal Principles of Hospice Care

Hospice care strives to be comprehensively effective in every dimension. Because it is palliative care, it is directed at symptoms; however, symptoms are defined in the broadest sense to include not only physical but also emotional, spiritual, and social concerns. The interrelationship between the physiological and the psychological is recognized. Just as the objective of hospice care, the relief of all symptoms, is comprehensive, so its techniques are comprehensive in length, breadth, and depth. In length it provides continuity of care as the status of the patient's disease changes over time and necessitates various types of care. In breadth hospice care encompasses not just the patient, but his family as well. In depth it provides a multidiscipli-nary team to cope with problems at all levels.

As with all endeavors that are comprehensive, integration of the parts is essential if continuity is to be achieved and fragmentation avoided. Although the various parts of hospice care are considered separately here for purposes of clarity, the com-munication, coordination, and interrelationships between them is essential to the successful implementation of hospice care.

The following five items are the cardinal principles of hospice care. The first de-lineates the *territory* within which hospice functions, the second defines its *objec-tives*, and the remaining three describe its *methods*.

Toward a Gentler Dying

The scope of hospice care is terminal illness. Chapter 1 dealt with some of the prob-lems in defining terms such as *terminally ill* and *dying* . As a practical matter hospice addresses itself to the care of those for whom the determination has been made that cure is not possible, that the disease will lead to the patient's death, and that efforts must be directed primarily at palliation. As has been noted, there may at times be disagreement with respect to a particular patient as to whether or not the patient falls in this category. In such instances a difficult decision must be made. Insofar as pos-sible the patient and his or her family should not only be informed about but should be participants in the decision. Although resolution of this matter can be trying and even heart wrenching, failure to deal with it appropriately can lead to most unfortu-nate consequences. The very availability of hospice, the thrust of which is to pro-vide as much quantity and quality of life as possible for patients placed in this cate-gory, makes the decision a little easier.

Symptom Control

Key feature of hospice care is that it is directed primarily at symptom control rather than at disease control. This does not mean that there is no place for antitumor therapy, for example, in such a program but simply that it plays a secondary role in that it is utilized only to the extent that it contributes to symptom control.

The details of methods employed in control of physical symptoms in terminally ill patients are the subject of the next chapter. It will be seen that in many respects the techniques used for control of symptoms in the terminally ill are similar to those employed in other patients, although in some instances there are sharp departures from conventional care. As would be anticipated, there are differences in methods utilized by different hospice programs. What is common to all of them, however, is primary concern with relief of symptoms.

In all medical care attention should be paid to symptom relief, but in most situa-tions in which a choice must be made between symptom control and disease control, the latter takes priority. Except for self-limiting diseases for which there are no satisfactory treatments (e.g., the common cold), there are few circumstances other than terminal illness in which attention must be directed predominantly at the relief of symptoms. It is this simple, but basic change in approach that so many physicians and others find an impediment to good palliative care.

In hospice care symptom control is accomplished with the use of a minimum of diagnostic studies and invasive therapeutic measures. Furthermore, symptoms are considered to include psychosocial problems as well as physical complaints (Schoenberg et al 1972; Garland 1978). As a result hospice patients receive relatively little technological, but a great deal of personal attention.

Chapter 3 describes techniques that have been used in the relief of physical symptoms. Chapter 4 deals with meeting the psychosocial needs of the patient and family.

As will be noted subsequently, for some cancer patients it is extremely difficult to predict whether antitumor therapy in the form of surgery, radiation, chemotherapy, endocrine manipulation, or bone marrow transplant will or will not contribute to palliation. As practical matter, however this problem arises relatively infrequently; in the instances in which it does occur, the responsible physician must, as in so many other circumstances, make the best possible decision in the face of inadequate information.

Palliative Care in Multiple Settings

For optimal management of terminal illness, the patient must be in the setting most appropriate to his or her needs at the time, and there must be continuity of care as the patient shifts from one setting to another. Successful hospice care therefore requires a mechanism that will permit a comprehensive approach to the patient, whether the individual is located at home, in the hospital, or in an intermediate facility of some type. In other words, hospice care must be deliverable on an inpatient or an outpatient basis in order to meet its full potential.

The most suitable setting for a particular patient at a particular time obviously depends upon a number of factors, including the patient's physical condition, home situation, and attitudes toward the illness and his or her family. The input of members of the multidisciplinary team is important in making decisions about where the patient can best receive care.

It has been our experience that most patients and their families prefer to have the patient at home for as much of the terminal illness as possible. Although there are exceptions to this preference, the ability to be surrounded by familiar things, the freedom from institutional restrictions, and the ready access to family and friends usually make the home setting a more comfortable environment for the patient. There are also obvious economic advantages to having the patient at home.

There are some considerations with respect to where the patient is located at the time of death. Patients and family who, for one reason or another, may have preferred home or hospital for much of the terminal illness may reverse this preference for the site of death. Mor and Hiris (1983) have studied factors that determine the site of death among cancer patients.

It is in providing hospice care in all possible settings that many hospice programs have encountered difficulty. Programs that provide home care only may have little influence on care once institutionalization is necessary. Most free-standing hospices with home care programs are handicapped when acute hospital care is necessary. Like most hospital-based programs, the experience of the Church Hospital program has been almost entirely with hospital and home care. Ideally, there should be facilities available for an intermediate level of care in a nursing home arrangement. This is particularly useful for patients who do not have willing and able caregivers in the home or for that small group whose requirements for care are a little more than can be provided in the home but a little less than necessitate hospitalization. We have dealt with this problem by attempting to make our selection of patients in such a way as to take only those who can be managed at home when they do not require acute general care. In addition to excluding a few patients who would otherwise be accepted in the program, this approach has the disadvantage that one cannot always determine in advance which patients will profit from time in an intermediate care facility.

To the extent that hospice care programs are able to provide service in a variety of settings, they make it possible for the patient to enter the program without the need to change his or her current setting unless there is a medical necessity to do so. In other words, patients can enter the program while hospitalized or while at home and can, without loss of continuity, shift back and forth between settings as necessary.

In addition to providing hospice services at varying levels of care, it is important that hospice care be available 24 hours a day. Problems arise unexpectedly at all hours of the night; the capacity for prompt response to the needs of the patient can contribute immensely to palliative care. Chapters 8 and 9 discuss care in the home setting and hospital, respectively.

The Patient and Family as the Unit of Care

In hospice care programs, the unit of care is not just the patient, but the patient and his or her family. It can be argued that to some extent this should be true of all medical care, but it cannot be denied that it has special importance in the care of the terminally ill. Naturally, the close relatives of the dying patient face problems that seem insurmountable to them. Some of these are problems growing out of their impending loss. Some are practical problems such as financial and living arrangements. Others are psychological problems related to understanding and accepting their altered circumstances in life.

The logical first step in dealing with the patient's family is to identify the family members and gain some insight into their relationships with the patient and with each other. This is not always an easy matter and in actual practice seldom can be done as a first step. Hospice care team members must begin to cope with the family's needs before intrafamily relationships have been clarified. Thus dealing with the family can be extremely demanding.

It should be understood that the term "family" is used here in its very broadest sense. In spite of trends to the contrary in society today, the family is most frequently composed of those immediately related to the patient by blood and marriage: husband, wife, children, parents, etc. Some patients obviously have fragmented families, combined families, or extended families. The closest interpersonal relationships of some patients are obviously with individuals who are not related by blood or marriage. Even with the nuclear family it can be difficult sometimes to gain insight into the relationships within the family.

As family members are identified and their relationships with the patient are clarified, efforts are made to provide them with understanding of the patient's illness and prognosis. This can be more complicated than it seems. Families begin at different levels of understanding and acceptance, and within each family there may be significant differences. Preconceptions on the part of family members, intrafamily antagonisms, and uncertainty even among hospice personnel regarding the nature of the patient's illness and prognosis can all serve as barriers to understanding of the situation by family members.

As family members gain a comprehension of the nature of the situation, their individual problems and needs begin to crystalize and the hospice care team can start to deal with them appropriately. Necessary practical and psychological support can be provided using the whole arsenal of weapons available to the multidisciplinary hospice care team.

As family understanding and acceptance grows, it becomes possible to use the family as part of the therapeutic team. This capacity to employ family members to provide the patient with physical and emotional assistance has been one of the most gratifying results of our hospice program. The benefit to both the patient and family members that comes from loved ones participating in the care of the patient can be immense.

Hospice care involvement with the family does not end with death. Bereavement follow-up is important and is discussed in Chapter 5. No matter how much anticipatory grief close family members experience before the patient's death, the feelings after death are deep and intense. Furthermore, there is evidence that bereaved individuals are prone to develop serious illness (Reese and Lutkins 1967). Much has been learned in recent years about coping with grief, and this knowledge can be brought to bear in dealing with families after the patient's death (Parkes 1980).

A Multidisciplinary Approach

Hospice care is a genuinely multidisciplinary undertaking. Physicians, nurses, clinical nurse practitioners, social workers, physical therapists, chaplains, and volunteers are all important components of a hospice care program. Speech therapy, art therapy, and music therapy all may have critical roles to play in the care of some terminally ill patients. Symptoms can come from a variety of sources: physical, psychological, social, financial, legal, and so on. A team approach is best suited to this situation. As important as is the presence and availability of each of the disciplines, their proper coordination is equally important. The function of the individual components of the multidisciplinary team and their integration into a functioning unit is dealt with in detail in Chapters 6 and 7.

Other Basic Considerations

Although a multidisciplinary approach is fundamental to hospice care, to reach its full potential a hospice program must, in the final analysis, be a *medical* program. The sick and dying patient is at the center of the program's focus, and the medical care of the patient cannot be placed on the periphery. From its inception a hospice program must have not only physician support, but the enthusiastic involvement of physicians. In the operation of the program, physician participation must be available and visible. Physician leadership in day-to-day care of patients and in the administrative management of the program is essential. Physician participants must indeed be prepared to function as team members and to share responsibility. To attempt to operate a hospice care program without active physician involvement either results in failure or the development of a program that exists outside of the conventional care system, leading to further fragmentation and, inevitably, poorer patient care.

In addition to tracing the historical development of hospice programs, Stoddard (1978) and Cohen (1979) review some of the elements of hospice care in various institutions. Buckingham and Lupu (1982) have studied hospice services available in the United States. Lack and Buckingham (1978), Mount (1976b), Saunders (1978), and Walter (1979) provide excellent descriptions of experience with the development of individual hospice programs in various settings. Lamerton (1973), Rossman (1977), Davidson (1978), Koff (1980), Hamilton and Reid (1980), and the Maryland Hospital Education Institute (1980) provide reviews of fundamental principles in hospice care.

As a palliative care program develops, all associated with it must be constantly on guard to be certain that potentially curable patients are not deprived of a chance for cure and that incurable patients are not denied a chance of prolonged survival through the use of antitumor therapy (in the case of cancer patients). In other words, hospice personnel must guard against an overreaction to the overtreatment that they have sometimes seen terminally ill patients receive. To the extent that there is physician involvement in hospice care, the potential for this overreaction is diminished. However, even hospice physicians must be careful that in their zeal to provide good palliation, they do not become therapeutic nihilists with respect to dealing with the tumor itself. Fear of this reaction has been expressed by responsible observers (Krakoff 1979; Potter 1980).

Obviously, the decision whether to direct management toward potential cure or palliation and the decision whether or not to utilize antitumor therapy for palliative purposes are ones clinicians must make all the time, whether or not hospice care is available. In fact, the availability of hospice care probably is helpful in making these decisions. In the first place it may force the patient's physician to crystallize his or her thinking, rather than to muddle through in a state of indecision. Unsatisfactory care is the result when those who are responsible fail to make the decision for either cure or palliation clear. In this situation they remain uncertain in their approach to the patient, making it impossible for others involved in the patient's management to know whether or not an effort is being directed at cure. The availability of hospice care can also assist in making these decisions by providing an alternative to futile antitumor therapy for those who would like to do something for the patient with cancer.

Krakoff (1979) decries "the development of a death and dying cult that is anti-therapy and anti-therapist." One of the important reasons for physician involvement in hospice care is the avoidance of this excess. Good palliative care for the patient for whom there is no hope of cure should be a part of the continuum of the patient's medical care. We must be willing to recognize that we will not be absolutely correct in every decision regarding every patient; however, we must face decisions realistically and make them forthrightly on the basis of the best available evidence. If we create a system in which patients can be shifted back and forth between curative and palliative systems as circumstances change or errors are recognized, we will have contributed immensely to the care of patients with terminal illness.

It is the author's conviction that it is easier for a hospice program to achieve optimal integration of curative and palliative care in an acute care hospital than in a freestanding unit. The use of a tumor board approach is also helpful in troublesome cancer cases. One of the interesting things about our tumor board experience is that it has demonstrated the difficulty of decisions regarding curative versus palliative care or the use of antitumor therapy for palliation. It has shown that in a number of instances, there simply is irreconcilable disagreement between physicians. Nonetheless, we feel that it is far better for this type of decision to be made in the context of the availability of hospice care in addition to other forms of therapy.

In caring for the dying patient, the issue of achieving the proper balance between quantity and quality of life can be extremely challenging. As options in management present themselves, difficult choices must be made. Eisman (1981) has pointed out that "life has meaning in depth as well as length; quality of life is its second dimension." He emphasizes that the second dimension is frequently ignored because it is difficult to measure and proposes the use of a "vitagram" to display the quality and quantity of life as coordinates on a graph. Tools such as this can be useful in making decisions regarding options in care.

Another vexing problem in terminal cancer care is the presence of metastases from an unknown primary tumor (Didolkar et al. 1977; Gaber et al. 1983). Such metastases may show up in a number of ways, such as a lymph node in the neck, a lesion seen on chest x-ray, or a skin nodule. They may or may not be symptomatic. The critical question that arises, of course, is the amount of time and effort that should be expended in searching for the location of the primary tumor. This is a matter in which several informed opinions and the use of good sense can vastly improve care. Neither a completely defeatist approach nor a relentless and senseless search for the primary tumor is in the patient's best interests. Generally speaking, we feel that a reasonable search should be made for any likely primary tumor for which treatment could contribute materially to palliation in terms of quantity or quality of life. There is no point, however, in exhausting the patient and using valuable time to find a primary tumor for which no treatment is feasible. For example, when metastatic adenocarcinoma is diagnosed, search beyond the thyroid, breasts, and ovaries is unlikely to turn up an asymptomatic primary for which antitumor therapy is likely to be helpful. Although the attending physician is the one who must make the critical decision, the use of consultations and the knowledge of tumor board members can be of enormous assistance in dealing with the troublesome problem of metastasis from an unknown primary tumor. This selective approach requires careful thought in each individual case rather than the rote performance of a standard battery of tests.

As hospices have developed throughout the United States, increasing attention has naturally been directed to the matter of standards and accreditation. This has produced a great deal of controversy and will doubtless continue to do so for some time. There are a number of problems. Few would deny that there is a need for the establishment of standards for the palliative care of the terminally ill. On the other hand, hospices have been characterized by their diversity and this diversity has contributed to their strength. There is still a great deal to be learned about how to organize and operate hospice care programs and about the proper means of caring for the terminally ill. It is only by encouraging innovation and permitting flexibility that this will be possible. But therein lies a dilemma for standard setters and accreditors.

Furthermore, it would be unrealistic to ignore the fact that hospice care lends itself to abuse. All forms of therapy do, but there are perhaps certain features of hospice care that make it particularly prone to such problems. For example, there is the potential for it to become a quasi-medical or cultlike movement. In addition, as hospice care becomes increasingly recognized as beneficial, such services will increasingly be reimbursed by third-party payors. As this happens, unless there are reasonably firm standards, it will be possible for profit-seeking but unqualified entrepreneurs to exploit hospice care.

These problems are compounded by the selection of the term "hospice" to designate this system of palliative care. The term is old and has been used in a variety of connections. There does not seem to be any reasonable way in which to stop anyone who wishes to from operating anything from a motel to a brothel and calling it a "hospice."

Finally, there is a jurisdictional controversy with respect to standard setting and accreditation. Two organizations with an interest in this area come immediately to mind: the National Hospice Organization (NHO) and the Joint Commission on Accreditation of Hospitals (JCAH). Both are, of course, nongovernmental bodies. It will not be surprising, however, if other agencies, particularly governmental ones, express an interest in having a role in standard setting and accreditation.

The NHO is representative of existing hospices and is clearly knowledgeable and responsible. At present it does not possess the mechanics, expertise, or experience to survey and accredit hospices. Furthermore, although it serves both free-standing and hospital-based units, its early emphasis has been toward the former; this creates problems regarding accreditation of hospital-based units. The JCAH, on the other hand, possesses the mechanics for hospital survey and accreditation but has had limited expertise in hospice care and none with respect to free-standing hospice units. In 1983 the JCAH and NHO approved the establishment of an accreditation program for hospice care designed for independent hospices and for hospice programs based in hospitals, home health agencies, long-term care facilities, and psychiatric facilities (JCAH 1983).

As noted, it is important that standards foster excellence in practice while still permitting innovation and adaptation to local circumstances. For the most part, these dual objectives seem to have been met by the JCAH accreditation program for hospices. Many of us hope that in view of the nature of hospice care, the standards will be comprehensively reviewed after they have been implemented and some survey experience employing them has been accumulated by the JCAH.

There are certain elements of the standards that may be excessively restrictive or cumbersome. For example, in a number of places the possession of academic degrees is required "or the documented equivalent in education, training and/or experience" (JCAH 1983). Much has been said and written on this general issue, but one could certainly argue that in standards for hospice care such an approach is inappropriate. The standards also require documentation of the ongoing communication between attending physician and other members of the interdisciplinary team. Such communication is essential, but one could certainly argue that not all of it needs to be documented. As in all medical care, it is critically important that precious time be spent predominantly in contact with patients rather than in paper work. One would hope, furthermore, that the requirement for a stated policy with respect to cardiopulmonary resuscitation, chemotherapy, and intravenous fluids will be defined in such a way that many different types of statements will be acceptable.

The best prospect for the continuing development of sound and workable standards is continuing cooperation between the NHO and JCAH in standard setting, survey methods, and accreditation mechanisms. It is imperative that standard development, inspection, and certification be cooperative functions of responsible hospice providers rather than of governmental agencies and professional regulators. So much of what is fine and true and noble in hospice care could be lost in a maze of bureaucracy.

With the development of federal and state legislation relating to hospice, governmental involvement has of course begun. Much attention has focused on the Medicare hospice benefits enacted under Section 122 of Public Law 97-248, The Tax Equity and Fiscal Responsibility Act of 1982. The implications of the Health Care Financial Administration regulations governing hospice care under this act are discussed in Chapter 10, "Administration of a Hospice Program." The provisions of the legislation itself and of those regulations were the result of considerable study, discussion, and debate (Bayer and Feldman 1982). Several components of the hospice benefit package pose problems for hospices and hospitals and their medical staffs (Pryga 1983). Of course some of the difficulty has arisen simply from the fact that regulations must by nature delineate, define, and stipulate, processes that create problems for an activity as diverse and innovative as hospice. In addition, the regulations grew up in an atmosphere of emphasis upon cost containment, and thus the assurance of economy achieved a higher priority than had been intended by the initial supporters of the legislation. It is not surprising, therefore, that a limited number of hospices have sought certification under the program. A survey by the Health and Human Services Inspector General six months after the program began revealed that only about 20% of hospices would be Medicare certified by April 1984. Hospital-based hospices were particularly unlikely to seek certification. The reasons for electing nonparticipation were in part fiscal and in part organizational and philosophical (American Hospital Association 1984).

In addition to this federal legislation, state legislative and regulatory requirements are beginning to affect hospices. In April 1984 the NHO reported that 17 states currently had licensure laws and that five were in the process of developing legislation. The NHO has provided some guidelines for the implementation of state licensure (National Health Organization 1984). One hopes that the aim of licensure, wherever it is undertaken, will be to assure excellence rather than to be restrictive. It is imperative that the terminally ill be assured that the care provided them, in and out of hospice programs, is of the highest possible caliber. Quality-assurance techniques developed for other aspects of health care should be applied, insofar as possible, to hospice programs. Rolka (1983) has explored some of the issues in quality assurance for the terminally ill.

It is important for those developing and operating hospice care programs to remember that competence and compassion are not mutually exclusive. We tend sometimes to think in dichotomies. We envision, on the one hand, the technically efficient superspecialist expert whose affect is sterile, whose heart is cold, and who rushes quickly in and out of the patient's room, pausing only long enough to check easily measurable parameters of the patient's status. We think, on the other hand, of the bumbling, bottom-of-the-class, kindly but inept soul who will spend hours listening and providing sympathy. Dr. Cicely Saunders and Dr. Frank C. Spencer (1979) are among the capable clinicians who remind us (both in their writing and in their work) that excellence does not preclude kindness. What we must demand in hospice care is compassion with no sacrifice of competence.

Although there are limitations to the "power of positive thinking" approach, one of the items most needed by a group establishing a hospice care program is a "can do" philosophy. It is a temptation to look at all the impediments and permit negative thinking to prevail. If one begins with a perception of the need, a firm desire to meet that need, and a willingness to do what can be done and to compromise on what cannot be done, it is not a complex matter to establish a hospice care program. Most of us associated with Church Hospital do recognize that its tradition of concern makes it a special place. It is a hospital that for years has been recognized locally for the excellent quality of its nursing care. But actually it is not terribly different in most respects from most hospitals of similar size. The key ingredient is *commitment*.

As a hospice program develops, it is important that it avoid offering more than it can deliver. This is true with respect to the specifics of the program itself and to terminal illness in general. At the outset those responsible for the program must determine its assets and capabilities and deploy these in the wisest possible way. However, they must concomitantly recognize the limitations within which they must function and be realistic and honest in what they offer. No program can make having terminal cancer pleasant, nor can it make death easy for the patient and family. Pictures of smiling and relaxed hospice patients are very real, very honest, and a source of much satisfaction to those of us involved in palliative care of the terminally ill. However, they can be deceptive; that deception may result in bitter disappointment, which creates serious problems for patients, families, and hospice care staff.

Dying children and adolescents present some special consideration. The child, of course, possesses few sophisticated defense mechanisms to deal with impending death. Parents of children and adolescents, by the very nature of the child-parent relationship, present problems different from those posed by family members of a terminally ill adult. Caregivers also have difficulty coping with the reality of the death of a young person. Grant Taylor (1981) has suggested some guidelines for helping families to cope when a child has cancer and he has reviewed some of the literature on this subject. Other resources are available on the topic (Corr and Corr, 1985; Gyulay 1978; Mott 1982). For example, the Children's Hospital Medical Center of Akron, Ohio sponsored a seminar on children and death in November, 1984.

Because Church Hospital does not have a pediatric service and death from malignancy among adolescents is relatively uncommon, we have had no experience with children and very little with adolescents. Most other hospice programs also have had limited experience with these age groups. However, there have been a number of hospice programs that have been designed exclusively for children, placing a heavy emphasis on the pediatric age group (Burne 1982, 1984). Thus far the avenue apparently most productive in the United States is the establishment of first-rate home care programs similar to that established in Minneapolis-St. Paul, Minnesota, by Martinson (1976), who has been a pioneer in the development of programs for the care of the dying child. Similar programs have been established in Los Angeles and Seattle. It would appear at this point that there is a limited need for inpatient facilities for dying children; most can be cared for at home throughout much of their terminal illness. There is a need for the development of new knowledge in the care of dying children and adolescents, for the wider dissemination of existing knowledge in this important matter, and for the development of high-quality home care programs for terminally ill young people.

Developing hospice programs must be conscious of their interface with the community, as discussed in Chapter 11. Acceptance and support by the community are essential in a number of respects. The preparation of some explanatory printed material such as brochures can be very helpful. As community recognition develops, some thought should be given to the coordination of public education about the program. This often can be done best by designating a spokesperson to whom public inquiries will be directed and who may also take the initiative in dissemination of appropriate information to the public. In addition, the spokesperson may serve as the interface with other hospice programs.

Admission to the Program

One of the most important decisions that will be made by a hospice patient is, of course, the decision to enter the program. It must be a joint determination on the part of the physician or physicians responsible for the patient, the patient him or herself, and the family.

Admission Criteria

Each hospice program must establish a set of criteria or guidelines for admission. This is a highly individual matter that obviously involves local philosophical and practical considerations. Criteria for admission to the Church Hospital hospice program are described and briefly commented upon in Chapter 15. Before criteria can be established, the program leaders obviously must agree upon the objectives and capabilities of their program. For example, it must be determined whether or not the program will be restricted to patients with malignant or other diseases. A decision must be made with respect to geographic area to be covered and other eligibility criteria. For the foreseeable future the demand for hospice care will exceed the available supply, and this fact must be taken into account as criteria are developed.

A life-expectancy criterion is a matter demanding some attention because the way in which this is handled will shape a number of the program's characteristics. Prediction of life expectancy in all terminal illness (as in all circumstances of life) is subject to much inaccuracy and is the source of much misunderstanding. As a surgeon the author has made it a policy to avoid specific predictions of life expectancy for individual patients—a policy he seldom relaxes.

Nonetheless, in designing a hospice care program, one must determine whether or not one wishes to provide hospice services to long-term patients. If not, the progressive neurological disorders must obviously be excluded. There are advantages and disadvantages to the inclusion of long-term patients in a program. In programs that have accepted such patients, such as the one at St. Christopher's, they are thought to have enriched the experience of other participants. However, their physical and psychosocial needs may be quite different from those of patients with a shorter life expectancy, and not all programs are in a position to provide such care. Because the mix of patients will shape the demands upon a program and determine in some measure the facilities required, it is a matter that deserves careful attention in program planning.

The Church Hospital hospice program has been designed for patients with less than a five or six month life expectancy. Therefore, the referring physician is required to make a broad estimate of the patient's life expectancy. The uncertainties in this area are recognized, and the physician is not necessarily expected to share such predictions with the patient or the family.

Most patients who are terminally ill from malignant disease and have a life expectancy of more than six months are at a stage in which little care is required. Therefore, entry into the program can be deferred for a time. Conversely, it can be argued that both patient and family might profit from admission to the program as soon as it is recognized that the patient is incurable. The leaders of each program must decide how to utilize their available facilities.

Patients with an extremely short life expectancy also present a problem. The patient who dies within a day or so of entering the program almost invariably gains little or nothing from participation while using some of the limited resources of the program. Obviously, in some instances there is gain to the family. Nonetheless, we have felt it prudent to take patients with life expectancy of a few days or less only under unusual circumstances.

Admission Procedure

Once admission criteria have been agreed upon, an admission procedure through which these criteria can be implemented must be established. Again, the particular procedure utilized will depend upon local factors and will be highly individual for each program. It may even change as personnel change. In any event, it should aim to be relatively simple and enable rapid action. Like the criteria it should be understood by all involved. The admission procedure should ensure that all eligible patients who can be satisfactorily handled are admitted and that all patients who do not meet the criteria or for whom the program presently does not have capacity will be excluded.

The difficulties and advantages of making a categorical decision as to whether a particular patient should be provided with only palliative care have been discussed above. The procedure employed for making this decision should maximize the chance that the best decision will be made for the patient and his or her family. For patients with cancer, consultation and the use of a binding or nonbinding tumor board decision can be employed for particularly difficult cases, but they are obviously not necessary in many instances. However, even in the "obvious" case extreme care should be exercised to confirm that the diagnosis is correct; review of patient records, including operative notes, pathology reports and results of diagnostic studies, should be *routine*. Failure to do this can lead to lethal errors.

In the implementation of the admission procedure, patient and family understanding and acceptance requires the closest attention. In subsequent sections and chapters we will deal in greater detail with the issue of patient and family understanding and what to tell the patient. These are dynamic, ongoing concerns throughout the patient's terminal illness, rather than static one-time propositions. They are also complex issues, highly individual to each case. However, when the patient's physician makes the decision that hospice care would be appropriate, the patient and family must also understand and agree. This can be a critical time in many respects. Various aspects of this matter are discussed in Chapter 14.

Again this has to be handled on a strictly individual basis. Patients and families come to this momentous personal occasion with widely varying perceptions of the disease the patient has, the options in care, and what a hospice is. An infinite number of possible combinations exists. Patient and family may both have a crystal clear comprehension of the nature of the disease and the alternatives in treatment; they may all be familiar, through previous contacts, with the hospice care program. Unfortunately, it is more usual that the family understands something of the disease but knows little about the alternatives of treatment, the patient knows very little about either, and both are totally unfamilair with hospice care.

During the discussions that provide the patient and family with the understanding necessary to make an informed decision, the issue of initiation or continuation of antitumor therapy often arises. Health care professionals sometimes fail to realize that the expectations of the patient and family regarding prognosis may be vastly different from that of the physician. The impact upon prognosis of certain events that physicians and nurses easily recognize may not be evident to laymen. For example, local recurrence of breast carcinoma or the development of a distant metastasis several months after resection of colonic carcinoma may be viewed very differently by the nonprofessional and the professional. This must be remembered, otherwise the professional may make incorrect assumptions about the patient's view of his or her status. Therefore, as a decision is being made about whether or not the patient's disease is incurable, a decision also must be made as to when this information is to be shared with the patient and family.

In each case the hospice staff members who are charged with that responsibility through the admission procedure must achieve sufficient understanding on the part of the patient and family so that a meaningful choice can be made by them. This requires a combination of knowledge, patience, perseverance, diplomacy, and luck. It is expecting too much in most instances to require full insight from the patient and family at the time of first contact. Nonetheless, a basic or serious misunderstanding at this point can lead to profound difficulties subsequently. Again, individual circumstances dictate what is best in a particular situation, but the patient and family should understand in most instances that further care will be strictly of a palliative nature. They should be assured that many symptoms, including pain, can be relieved and avoided, but unrealistic promises must not be made.

It is after these matters have been discussed with the patient and family that they will make the decision for or against entering the program. Every hospice program has encountered a number of patients who simply are not ready to accept strictly palliative care when hospice care is first explained to them; many of these ultimately enter the program.

Most hospice programs do not have a firm proscription against the use of antitumor therapy for cancer patients in the program. Such therapy may contribute to symptom relief, prevent the development of symptoms, or increase the patient's life expectancy. However, we have tried to avoid accepting patients for whom antitumor therapy was still being utilized under the thin guise of these reasons while in reality its sole purpose was to appease the patient's desire for a continued effort at cure. We have felt that generally this was a poor mental setting in which to begin hospice care. Nonetheless, individuality, flexibility, and adaptability are trademarks of hospice care, and in special circumstances where the antitumor therapy was free of significant side effects, we have accepted some such patients.

Slightly different, but similar conditions prevail when the patient wishes to embark upon unapproved or unaccepted therapies. The most widely publicized of such methods is, of course, Laetrile, although there are innumerable other similar medications and approaches. Not infrequently it is confrontation with hospice staff regarding admission that first makes it totally clear to the patient that he or she has an incurable tumor. It is therefore not surprising that at this point a number of patients turn to nonmedical methods for control of their disease. By and large we have felt that, although understandable, such efforts by the patient reflect a mental set that makes the provision of hospice care impractical. Furthermore, some of these non-medical methods take the patient out of the country for a protracted period of time or involve time-consuming "treatments" that would seriously conflict with hospice care.

Resolution of this matter of patient and family understanding in one way or another brings one to the issue of consent forms for those patients who are accepted and elect to enter the program. This is the *legal* dimension of patient and family comprehension and acceptance of hospice care. Informed consent for hospice care is subject to all the uncertainties and disputes attending its application anywhere. In addition, however, there are things about terminal illness that magnify the problems of such consent. Denial of illness and death, mental impairment by the disease process, the role of the family in hospice care, and a number of other factors complicate this already complex issue.

As discussed earlier, there is uniform agreement that the patient and the family should generally have a clear understanding of the nature of the problem, of what hospice care does and does not offer, and of the alternatives to hospice care. Patients should be accepted into the program only after giving their informed consent. Potter (1980) and Brooks (1980), in remarkably similar passages, seem to go beyond what we have designated above as understanding: they draw an analogy with patients entering formal clinical trials. The analogy, of course, does not hold up in all regards.

As a practical matter, it is applying the principle of informed consent in specific situations and converting this informed consent to a written document that create the greatest problems. Although a major thrust of hospice care is usually to foster patient understanding and acceptance of his or her situation, we must recognize that this may not be possible or desirable at the outset in every instance. There may be patients with a high level of denial who will profit immensely from hospice care. It may not be possible—or kind and wise—to break through that denial in order to obtain informed consent. Patients themselves sometimes benefit most from hospice care if they enter at a stage at which their level of acceptance of their terminal illness is such that they cannot engage in the kind of candid interchange necessary for true informed consent. Furthermore, both the patient and family benefit from the hospice care program. Should the family of an irrational terminally ill patient be denied the benefits of hospice care because truly informed consent cannot be procured from the patient?

Even more difficult than the issue of being certain in one's own mind that genuinely informed consent has been procured is the matter of whether or not to have the patient sign special forms. It is really impossible to make a definitive and comprehensive comment regarding consent forms for hospice care. So much depends upon location and time: different areas of the country (to say nothing of the world) take different views of informed consent, and the legal system's handling of informed consent is still evolving.

For what it is worth, patients entering the Church Hospital hospice care program do not sign any special form for hospice care. They sign forms only if they enter the hospital as inpatients. In this case hospice patients sign the general consent form signed by all patients being admitted, and specific permits for individual diagnostic and therapeutic procedures, of which there will be very few. To be crudely devious is the antithesis of the hospice philosophy. In keeping with that philosophy, however, we do not feel that it is possible or prudent to reduce the complex, dynamic, highly individual matter of patient and family understanding and acceptance to a signed form.

Patient Management in the Program

Overall Features

In spite of careful admission procedures, an occasional patient whose diagnosis or prognosis is incorrect will be admitted to the program. There are a number of circumstances under which this can occur, but the important point is that the error be recognized so that appropriate steps may be taken promptly. For example, we had a severely debilitated patient with limited comprehension of English who was admitted to the program from another hospital; his clinical and x-ray picture strongly suggested advanced incurable bronchogenic carcinoma. To expedite his care, he was taken into the program quickly, although we recognized that a histological diagnosis had not been established. Not long after admission we secured old records from a third hospital, revealing that six years earlier the x-ray picture had been the same and the abnormal x-ray appearance had been demonstrated as due to vascular abnormality. Further investigation revealed that his debility was related to severe depressive reaction. He was dropped from the hospice care program and treated appropriately.

In our experience true errors regarding curability have been extremely unusual. It is rare that a patient thought to be incurable at the time of entry into the program has subsequently been found to have a curable disease, although in hospice programs not restricted to terminal malignant disease an increased percentage might be expected. It is certainly not beyound the realm of possibility for advances in antitumor therapy to transform a particular cancer patient from incurable to curable. This points up the need for those involved in hospice care to have a mechanism for remaining abreast of other developments in the field of oncology.

Protracted spontaneous or therapeutically induced remissions are not at all uncommon and are one of the factors making prediction of life expectancy so difficult. They are particularly common, although still relatively unpredictable, with certain forms of tumors such as breast and prostatic cancer and various types of lymphoma. When such periods of remission are symptom free and prolonged, a patient can be placed on inactive status in the hospice care program, requiring only periodic check and having reactivation available when the situation changes.

As has been repeatedly stressed, those who provide hospice care must be adaptable and flexible. While recognizing fundamental standards of excellence and cardinal principles, one must be prepared to adjust to particular circumstances if the unique needs of the individual patient are to be met. Similarly, hospice care programs must be ready to reevaluate and revise policies as conditions and personnel change. It also may be necessary to attempt to implement change in the community.

The use of mithramycin in the treatment of hypercalcemia is illustrative. Mithramycin has been shown quite effective in treating hypercalcemia in patients with advanced malignancy; it produces dramatic symptomatic response without serious toxic side effect. In an effective dosage range no monitoring is necessary. However, it is often best given intravenously about two times per week. There are a number of terminally ill patients for whom hypercalcemia is a principal source of symptoms. For these patients, the capacity to treat hypercalcemia at home is an immense advantage. However, up to this time we have not used *bolus* intravenous medication on an ongoing basis in our home care program nor have many other home care providers. It would be a shame to keep a patient with hypercalcemia hospitalized only for treatment with intravenous mithramycin two times per week or to require semiweekly clinic visits for this purpose. Changes in policy and procedure to permit its administration at home are necessary in order to make available the full benefits of this form of therapy.

In hospice care one must be prepared to meet the various fears, concerns, and reactions of the patient and the family. Sometimes fears are expressed, but often they must be sensed by the hospice staff. Most people facing death from cancer are in fear of pain and discomfort. In the minds of many in our society, cancer seems to equal a painful death. Reasurance that pain and discomfort can be minimized is an important early component of hospice care. Most patients and their families have a fear of dying and death. The way in which this is best allayed will depend upon the individual circumstances. The author's experience is similar to that of Lewis Thomas (1974) who writes that agony in the final moments of terminal illness is extremely unusual. He points out that patients seem to be showing us all the time that "dying is not such a bad thing to do after all." This can and should be conveyed to patients and their families.

An often unexpressed fear on the part of the family has to do with contagion and heritability of cancer. One need only recognize the fear of cancer as a communicable disease in order to provide reasurance on this point. The matter of heredity may be a bit more complicated, but it does constitute a part of the care of the family. For certain forms of malignancy, the complete absence of any hereditary tendency can be described with confidence to the family. For other forms a different approach is necessary. The female members of the family of a breast cancer patient must be told at some point that they have a somewhat increased risk of developing breast cancer. The net effect of this advice must be heightened alertness on their part without the creation of an overwhelming fear.

The family, like the patient, passes through stages in the course of terminal illness. Among these stages is anger. This may be diffuse and directed at the professional caregiver. Recognition of this fact can prevent bruised feelings. In dealing with angry family members, it is usually prudent to explore the causes of the anger. Anger may arise from correctable problems in the patient's situation. As family members pass through various stages, explanations and discussions with them should continue. The door must be *kept* open.

Despite the spectrum of talents provided by a hospice multidisciplinary team, such a team, in and of itself, cannot meet the manifold needs of the terminally ill patient and his or her family. What the multidisciplinary team does bring to hospice care is ready access to the various community resources available. One resource in many communities and of particular help to cancer patients and their families is the local chapter of Make Today Count. This is an organization that tries to bring together persons with serious illness and their families to help them cope with problems of cancer, death, and dying.

It is all too easy to look at the care of the terminally ill as a grim and humorless affair. There are, to be sure, overwhelmingly sad and depressing aspects to it. However, the emphasis of hospice care is indeed upon *living*. Humor is a vital part of life and terminal care is no exception. The gentle and appropriate use of humor can do things no other therapy can provide. Its value must not be overlooked.

Hospice can be looked at as pragmatic and utilitarian. It clearly does serve a purpose. However, to ignore its very real spiritual dimension is to miss a significant part of its meaning. This topic is dealt with in detail in Chapter 12, which explores not only the way that hospice deals with the spiritual needs of patients and families, but the whole broad range of nonmaterial aspects of hospice care.

Patient Understanding

Patient and family understanding of diagnosis and prognosis is an important, complicated, and controversial topic. Here we can only touch upon a few practical considerations. The issue of what to tell the terminally ill patient about his or her diagnosis and prognosis has received a great deal of attention (Sheldon 1982). As will be emphasized, "telling" may not be the accurate way to describe this exchange of information. Very often the patient senses the outlook long before being told. What is needed then is confirmation, clarification, and a willingness to answer questions.

No matter requires greater *individualization* than this. Patients vary immensely in the understanding that they bring with them as they enter palliative care, and depending upon a number of factors, they have varying needs for explanation and discussion. Unfortunately, there is no way to be certain that for a particular patient one has selected the best of all possible alternatives.

There is general agreement that in almost all instances the interests of the patient and family are best served when the patient has some understanding of his or her disease and prognosis. For the dying patient, however, one confronts the problem of denial; we must recognize that for some patients at some stages of the pilgrimage, denial is the healthiest possible response. For a few, this may persist until death. To attempt explanations to a patient with a high level of denial is at best frustrating and at worst patently harmful.

If individualization is the first commandment with respect to "telling patients," the importance of *listening* is the second. Listening is in many ways much more important than telling. It is only by first listening that one can determine what can and should be told. Listening, incidently, is used here in its broadest sense, for the patient sends many nonverbal clues. That the patient does not ask questions does not mean there are none. As we listen carefully, we begin to get the feel of what the patient already understands and what further explanation is prudent. In other words, the listener is able to detect the balance between the opposing phenomena of unexpected *awareness* on the one hand and seemingly irrational *denial* on the other. For example, it is very important to distinguish patients who vigorously signal that we must not assault them with information for which they are not ready, from those who already have come to terms with their prognosis but have inaccurate apprehensions about what lies ahead.

A point frequently overlooked is that both listening and telling often need to take place *over a period of time* at multiple visits. Patients' needs and capacities for understanding change and evolve so that an ongoing dialogue is essential. In this connection, it is also important to recognize that understanding is not a consistent progression: a patient may vary immensely from one day to another in what he or she is willing to accept and assimilate.

The stages of understanding do not always seem logical to the professional. Very often, patients perceive the fact that their disease is fatal before they possess much understanding of what the terminal illness is likely to entail. Therefore, even patients who clearly accept the ultimate prognosis may have significant misunderstanding about what is in store for them. So often the expectation is far worse than the reality, particularly when the patient will be receiving hospice care.

Those who first encounter the patient after enrollment in the hospice care program can make certain guesses about a patient's understanding of the disease and prognosis. They are well advised, nonetheless, to listen carefully before they take a particular approach to telling the patient about his or her disease.

Patients vary in their ability and willingness to relate to and share with different individuals. Hinton (1980) has addressed the question "Whom do dying patients tell?" with some surprising findings. One of the virtues of the multidisciplinary team is that it provides a number of options to the patient in this respect. It makes available several sources of information about the patient's understanding and acceptance of the disease. It is very important, therefore, for the members of the team to share information.

This then brings us to the question of *who* should convey to patients information about their disease and prognosis. Again, flexibility and individualization are necessary, but almost without exception the physician should take the lead both in time and in supervision.

As one begins to tell patients about their disease and prognosis, several things should be borne in mind. The first is to recall the importance of nonverbal communication. Just as in listening, what is not said may be as important as what is said. Smiles and frowns tell a great deal and inflection of the voice can make all the difference in the world. Secondly, it is important to remember that there are many options in what to tell the patient; silence, blatant lies, and stark truth are not the only alternatives.

Mount (1976a) and others have gathered data indicating that most patients want to know their diagnosis and prognosis; the same data indicates that usually this is not what happens. In an excellent article on "Telling Patients," Saunders (1965) calls attention to studies demonstrating that hospital staffs usually make an effort to keep the patient in ignorance, although the great majority of dying patients are quite aware of their status. She concludes, "These two facts look very disturbing when put together, for the truth from which the patient is being 'protected' is the truth with which he is being forced to live in isolation."

West and Kirkham (1980) have explored in detail the issue of communication with patients and their families, covering such questions as who should tell, what should be told, and to whom should it be told. Their observations verify what many of us who have dealt frequently with the terminally ill believe: as a general rule, patients are aware of their prognosis even if they have not been "told" it. In most instances they would welcome and profit from the opportunity to discuss with their physicians and loved ones the most important fact of their lives. It has never been clear to the author just who is presumed to be the beneficiary of the cruel deception that tries to deprive the dying patient of a valuable therapeutic weapon.

Although there can be no uniform policy with respect to telling patients about their disease and prognosis, there are some guidelines that can be followed. One must begin by listening and continue to listen carefully. One must individualize on the basis of what is heard. One should be alert, both in listening and in telling, to nonverbal communication. For most patients *the truth presented kindly and at an appropriate time in a suitable setting* can open channels for making dying a little more comfortable and a little gentler.

Antitumor Therapy

A vexing issue in the handling of hospice patients with cancer is the use of antitumor therapy. Such therapy, in the form of surgery, radiation, chemotherapy, endocrine manipulation, and marrow transplantation, is employed only insofar as it contributes to palliation. However, within this framework there are some uncertainties. The likelihood of response of a particular tumor and the severity of the side effects of therapy are often extremely difficult to predict. In addition to the potential side effects of therapy, one must also take into consideration the monitoring that use of a particular form of antitumor therapy may require. The performance of multiple invasive studies in association with such therapy may greatly complicate and even obliterate palliative care. In these matters one can only solicit the best possible advice and then make what seems to be the most reasonable choice.

Beyond this, however, is the question of balancing the quantity and the quality of life; here the uncertainties of antitumor therapy are multiplied by the individual and subjective nature of the assessment of quality of life. It is in dealing with this type of problem that the immense advantage of being able to talk frankly with the patient and family becomes evident. In this connection it is important to remember that all forms of antitumor therapy—especially radiation and chemotherapy—carry different connotations for different people. For the most part patients and their families have far more negative images of these modalities than do physicians, particularly surgeons, radiotherapists, and oncologists. Often it is impossible to overcome these differences in perceptions, but it is important that they be recognized. One never knows whether the right choice has been made in giving or withholding antitumor therapy in a particular instance, but if the decision was based upon the best possible medical opinion combined with a candid assessment by the patient, based on his or her particular values, one has reasonable confidence.

Patient Records

It is important that accurate medical records are kept on each patient. Miller (1984) has provided an excellent source of information on hospice records. The patient's chart serves the same purposes in hospice care as it does elsewhere; these uses need not be reviewed here. Suffice it to say that the use of a multidisciplinary team makes accurate, clear, and succinct record keeping particularly important. Communication is critical to the successful use of a multidisciplinary team; it is the key to avoiding fragmentation. The medical record is one of the avenues of communication; thus it is particularly important to include entries regarding items such as the emotional needs of the patient and family and what the patient and family have been told regarding the disease and prognosis. The system of record keeping and patient charting within a hospice program must be established on the basis of local needs and capacities. In a hospital-based program, the regulations governing record keeping are generally the same as they are for other areas of the hospital, although sometimes a few modifications can be made. Some provision should be made for the coordination of inpatient and outpatient records on each patient. There are a number of ways of accomplishing this.

One of the key functions of the medical record is as an evaluation tool. Hospice care is no exception. Terminal illness does not mean that the quality of a patient's care should not be assessed. In fact, the assessment of some dimensions of care (e.g., meeting emotional needs) is more important than for many other patients. Hospice care should be subjected to the same quality assurance measures as other types of medical care. Such evaluation, incidently, is the key to progressive improvement in the care of the terminally ill. Meaningful research that will enable us to grow and improve must be based on the careful evaluation of what we have done.

Inpatient Care

In a hospital-based hospice program, inpatients are obviously those requiring acute hospital care. There are a number of reasons why the terminally ill patient may require hospitalization. The most common is probably for pain control. As described in Chapter 3, proper adjustment of the patient's pain medication to achieve optimal effect often requires the kind of observation and monitoring that cannot be achieved at home. Intestinal obstruction, respiratory failure, persistent nausea and vomiting, hemorrhage and seizures can sometimes be extremely difficult to control at home; a period of hospitalization may be necessary. Agitation and confusion are also very disruptive in the home environment. In some instances families, either for emotional or physical reasons, are no longer capable of providing care, in which case a period of institutional care may be required. The duration and timing of hospitalization is a highly individual matter in each case. Immediacy of impending death is ordinarily not of itself an indication for admission; a large percentage of patients die at home.

Although the patient is hospitalized because of the need for acute level care, the nature of that care is somewhat different for the hospice patient than for the general medical-surgical patient. Efforts are directed strictly at palliation. Control of symptoms in the broadest definition of that term with the provision of ample attention to the patient's psychosocial needs is the theme of care. Although a great deal of personal attention is provided, little diagnostic or therapeutic technology is employed. No diagnostic studies other than those that will contribute to palliation are carried out; no "routine" admission studies such as complete blood count and urinalysis are done. For most patients entered in the hospice program, it is understood that cardiopulmonary resuscitation will not be undertaken. Although "no code" orders on certain categories of patients have posed administrative and legal problems in hospitals, we have encountered no difficulty in this regard for hospice care patients. Once again, individualization is a critical feature of patient management. One can conceive of an incurable but largely asymptomatic young patient with a relatively long life expectancy for whom the institution of cardiopulmonary resuscitation, if needed, might be warranted.

Standing hospital policies and procedures can and should be relaxed somewhat for hospice patients. Chapter 9 deals with this matter. Our experience has shown that it is possible to do this without detriment to the care of hospice or other patients. Hospice patients may be permitted visitors around the clock, and the visitors may be provided with sleeping facilities. Patient's pets may be permitted to visit. Nursing aides, volunteers, and even family can be asked to assist in giving the patient oral medications. This is helpful because the long time it takes some patients to get down such medication can be very frustrating to a nurse who must dispense medications to a number of patients.

The method of handling an inpatient admission to the program depends upon the circumstances of admission. Patients may already be in the hospital when they enter the program, or they may enter the program concomitantly with admission to the hospital either from home or in transfer from another hospital. In any event, new patients arriving on a nursing unit providing hospice care should be warmly welcomed by the staff. Volunteers are particularly helpful in this. The hospice physician or clinical nurse practitioner should review the available information from the admission materials.

It has been our practice for the clinical nurse-practitioner to meet first with the patient and family and then with the patient alone, obtaining such additional historical information as may seem appropriate; this usually relates to details of symptoms. A complete physical examination is then carried out. Soon after arrival the patient should be seen by the hospice physician. Early in the patient's involvement in the program, usually soon after completion of the physical examination, the clinical nurse-practitioner meets with the family alone to review the goals of the program. The family is introduced to the social worker and such other personnel as appropriate. Concomitantly, attention is promptly directed to relief of pain if this is a problem for the patient. Pain relief must come first before other matters are dealt with.

For patients being *readmitted* to the hospital after a period at home, a similar but abbreviated approach is used. The warm friendly welcome is just as important, as are team conferences to review status and goals.

From the beginning, the clinical nurse-practitioner makes it a point to see each patient daily, usually once alone and once with family members. For most inpatients there are daily physician visits.

A few days after the patient has entered the program or the hospital, it is generally worthwhile to set up a semiformal family conference as described in Chapter 15. This should involve all family members, the clinical nurse-practitioner, the social worker, the home care director and such other members of the team as may seem appropriate. At this time problems are reviewed, plans for future care at home or in the hospital are discussed, and matters such as funeral arrangements can be addressed.

In all respects individualized, high-quality inpatient care should be available to the patient throughout his or her stay. Except for patients for whom death is imminent and for whom death in the hospital is mandated by circumstances, one of the aims of most inpatient stays for hospice patients is discharge as soon as the need for acute general inpatient care has passed. Planning for this should begin as soon as practical and should be properly coordinated with the home care staff. Not only must there be continuity, but the patient must sense that continuity.

Although Chapter 8 is devoted primarily to a description of the organization and operation of *home care*, it also addresses some *general* matters that are equally pertinent to inpatient care. Certain principles of nursing care for the terminally ill are reviewed. Techniques of value in dealing with dying and grief are discussed, as is the handling of the moment of death.

Outpatient Care

For most hospice programs to be feasible and certainly for any hospital-based program to meet its full potential, access to an organized home care service as described in Chapter 8 is essential. Without it, a hospital-based program would be in the position of being able to apply hospice principles only while a patient was hospitalized.

Just as there are a number of options for the organizational structure of hospice care itself, there are a number of options in the provision of home care. Home care services can be obtained under contract with an existing agency such as a visiting nurse association or through public health nurses. On the other hand, a hospice, either free standing or hospital based, can seek the necessary certification for its own home health department. In either event, knowledge of and commitment to hospice principles by the home care staff is imperative; there must be smooth cooperation between the home care and inpatient staffs.

For a hospital-based program that does not have control of or a working relationship with an intermediate care facility, it is important that all patients being considered for admission to the program undergo home care evaluation. Only those patients for whom home care will be feasible (in terms of location and nature of housing, available caregivers, etc.) or those who clearly will require acute general hospital care for the duration of their lives should be accepted. Otherwise the program will repeatedly face the situation of having to abandon a patient's hospice care service or keep him or her in an acute care facility when such is really not required for medical purposes.

The use of a day care center (Wilkes et al. 1978) is an imaginative and promising innovation in hospice care. It may enable the patient to be at home in a family situation where the principal caregiver is employed. It also opens options for respite for weary family members.

Some patients will enter home care at the time of admission to the hospice care program, but many will enter home care after an interval as hospice inpatients. In the latter event, it is important for the home care staff to become familiar with the patient at the stage of discharge planning and to coordinate their activities with those of the inpatient staff. As discussed in Chapters 5 and 8, the home care staff plays a major role in the provision of bereavement service to the family.

There are certain requirements that must be met before home care is possible for a hospice patient:

1. The mechanisms of symptom control must be ones easily employed at home. For example, although some families are capable of giving hypodermic injections, this is often not feasible in the home situation. In actual practice the techniques of symptom control utilized in hospice care (as described in Chapter 3) are such that they lend themselves well to home care.

2. There must be at least one caregiver in the home who is able and willing to provide the care necessary. This is usually a family member, although it may be a close friend. The importance of dealing with the patient and family as the unit of care is evident. It is only after adequate understanding has been achieved that families and friends can provide the type of assistance necessary.

3. A well-trained home care staff that includes nurses, aides, physical therapists, and volunteers must be available. The frequency with which home care visits by these individuals will be necessary depends upon the individual status of the patient.

4. There must be available in the home suitable equipment and supplies. This may include items such as dressings, oxygen, bedside commode, etc. For the patient who is going from hospital to home, it is imperative that these materials be available in the home before the patient is discharged from the hospital.

5. The final requirement for home care is the ready availablity of a higher level of care. The patient and family must know that the patient can be admitted promptly to an inpatient facility if this should be necessary. Simple assurance on this point has made it possible to have many patients begin a successful period of home care when they otherwise would have refused to do so.

Home care policies and personnel must be flexible and adaptable. Treatment modalities change and the home care procedure must be ready to change with them. Advancing technology sometimes makes possible and desirable the use of previously impossible procedures. Intravenous fluids and medications are an example. Although most hospice patients are not given intravenous feedings, much less hyperalimentation through a central line, there are some patients for whom this is useful in palliation, and it is now possible to employ these modalities in the outpatient setting. Bolus intravenous medication such as mithramycin, described earlier, or intravenous morphine drip can make an immense contribution to patient comfort at home.

Special Considerations in a Hospital-Based Hospice Program

A hospital-based hospice program can take a number of forms. For large hospitals there are probably material advantages to having a separate unit, such as the Palliative Care Unit at the Royal Victoria Hospital in Montreal. For smaller hospitals, particularly those with a relatively high occupancy, it may not be suitable to have a separate unit if the inpatient load fluctuates substantially. Having patients spread throughout the hospital in a "scatter bed" arrangement creates a number of problems, not the least of which is the difficulty of successfully educating and training nursing personnel throughout the hospital in hospice care principles in a short period of time. Furthermore, this arrangement dissipates some of the cohesiveness of the hospice care program.

Our experience has been with a "swing bed" arrangement on a single nursing unit; we feel that this model has a number of advantages for the medium size and small hospital. Chapter 10 deals with the details of organization and financing of a hospice program within a hospital. A few remarks here may be helpful.

There seem to be certain advantages that a hospital-based program has over a free-standing program; there are certain additional advantages in the use of a swing bed arrangement on a single nursing unit. As discussed in Chapter 14, hospital-based programs in general tend to ease the problems of the curative-palliative interface. Transition from one approach to the other is usually relatively smooth in such programs. Antitumor therapy for palliative purposes in cancer patients is more convenient in an acute general hospital than it is in a free-standing hospice. Hospitals also can make available to the patient other sophisticated forms of care that can contribute to palliation; these may be somewhat more difficult to procure in a free-standing unit. Naturally, although the hospice patient is not subjected to many tests or treatments, there are times when the easy availability of an x-ray or an intramedullary nail can be most helpful in making a patient comfortable. The other advantage of a hospital-based unit is, in a sense, the other side of the coin. Much of what is generic to hospice care can be of benefit to patients who are not terminally ill. There is the opportunity for hospice principles to influence other types of health care in hospital-based units.

One of the advantages of the free-standing unit has been the presumed inability of hospitals to be sufficiently flexible in implementation of policies to make hospice care workable. Hospitals are seen as cold, impersonal, and rigid. Our experience has been that the same hospital is quite capable of providing both the highest quality curative medicine and topflight care for the terminally ill.

The swing bed arrangement on a single nursing unit serves several purposes. It prevents the segregation of terminally ill patients and the related disadvantages of isolation. For example, there are many patients who, at the time they could begin to profit from hospice care, are unwilling to have anything to do with a place they see as one from which there is no return. Integration of hospice patients minimizes the "death house" stigma. It also provides personnel involved in hospice care with a balance between caring for the terminally ill patient and assisting other patients to reach their maximum health status. This not only facilitates the impact of hospice care on other care, but also minimizes problems of staff stress related to constant exposure to the terminally ill.

It provides far more efficient use of hospital beds by maintaining flexibility according to hospital demand. This may make a swing bed hospice program feasible for a small or medium size hospital when no other arrangement would be workable.

The bed issue is a complex one, subject to a number of misinterpretations. It has sometimes been said that implementation of a hospice care program will fill some of the empty beds in an underutilized hospital. This would obviously be true only if, in the course of undertaking a hospice program, the hospital were bringing in patients who would not otherwise be admitted there. If, on the other hand, a hospital simply provides hospice care to those same terminally ill patients for whom it would otherwise provide conventional care, there will not be any increased bed utilization. Church Hospital, as noted, has had a high occupancy rate and therefore designed its program primarily for patients of members of its medical staff, although it does accept a limited number of other patients.

The use of hospice principles and practices, particularly use of the home care facilities, has resulted in terminally ill patients spending less time in the hospital and more time outside of it. Therefore, a hospital that does not reach out to serve a new population through its hospice care program will in fact, not fill empty beds but will empty full ones. The same line of reasoning, incidentally, can be used to reassure the medical staff in a high-occupancy hospital that is fearful of "filling up all those beds with dying patients." The point is that as a hospital designs a hospice care program, it must look at its own particular circumstances; it can then tailor the program in accordance with its specific situation and needs.

Clinical Research in Palliative Care

For some of the nonphysician hospice staff members — and even for some of the physicians — research may carry unpleasant connotations. It is thought of as experimenting on patients and is presumed to be harmful to all involved. Certainly, no responsible person would recommend using hospice patients for the tesing of untried drugs or other treatments. However, if care for the terminally ill is to continue to improve, we must learn from our experience and subject proposed methods of treatment to scientific scrutiny. It was from such study that much of what we know and use today was derived.

Hospice programs will vary in their commitment to research, but all should make clinical investigation of approaches to palliative care possible. Up to this point the advantages of hospice care over conventional care have been documented in anecdotal fashion. Those of us who are convinced of the superiority of hospice care must be prepared to offer some evidence in the future. Even more important, we must begin to study the relative value of treatments within hospice care. Clinical investigation in palliative care will be arduous and demanding. It will require the development and refinement of measurement tools. Meetings such as the seminar in research methodologies sponsored by the Royal Victoria Hospital in October 1980 have proved encouraging.

Whether or not hospice patients with cancer should be permitted to be subjects of clinical studies of promising antitumor therapy is another somewhat different matter. Obviously, informed consent for involvement is needed from the patient, but even with this, one's initial inclination is to feel that the involvement of hospice patients in such protocols is inappropriate. Generally such protocols require careful patient monitoring, with frequent diagnostic studies of a type quite incompatible with hospice care. However, individualization and flexibility is again the wisest course. One can conceive of a therapy with inconsequential side effects that show striking promise for the complete cure or at least protracted remission of a certain type of tumor. It does not seem right to deny a patient the chance for such a response simply because he or she is in a hospice care program. Although our hospice care committee has been approached on a few occasions about involving our patients in antitumor therapy studies, we have not yet encountered one that we have felt possessed characteristics to warrant recommending participation to our patients.

Administrative and Financial Considerations in Hospice Care

The organizational aspects of hospice care, including its financing, are examined carefully in Chapter 10. However, it would be good at this point to take a brief overview of the administration and economics of hospice care.

Once again, the key to success is individualization on the basis of local needs and abilities. Whatever administrative structure is chosen, however, should be clear, articulate, and understood by all concerned. For an independant hospice suitable bylaws should be established, preferably with the assistance of a qualified parliamentarian. A hospice program that is part of another institution may function under the bylaws of that organization, but the way in which it fits into its parent should be clearly delineated. The lines of authority from governing board through medical director should be established. In setting policy the NHO and JCAH standards can be helpful. Chapters 6 and 7 deal with selection and management of staff. One cannot emphasize too strongly that it is essential that those in charge of the hospice program possess the knowledge and flexibility to deal with changes in the surrounding society and health care delivery system. It is not essential, of course, that the program itself provide all the necessary services; some can be arranged through contract. Decisions do have to be made, however, with respect to the sorts of patients eligible for the program and the services that will be available to them. For example, a hospital-based program with a home care service must decide whether to accept only patients for whom there is an identifiable caregiver or to make arrangements for entry of hospice patients into an intermediate care facility without interruption of hospice services.

It is legitimate to inquire whether hospice care as a principle is sound from a financial standpoint. In other words, what does it cost? For several reasons this is not a simple question. First, the diversity of hospice programs makes it impossible to give a comprehensive answer applicable to all hospice care. Second, hospice care is presently at a stage where very little useful information about costs is available. Furthermore, one must determine the sort of care with which the costs of hospice care are to be compared. At present, all kinds of nonhospice care are provided to terminally ill patients, ranging from virtually no care at all to extremely expensive intensive care. To decide whether or not hospice care offers society an economically attractive option in the management of terminal illness, we must establish which of many alternatives is to serve as the basis of comparison.

Nonetheless, there are certain worthwhile general observations that can be made regarding the costs of hospice care. It involves minimal use of high-level technology, both with respect to diagnostic tests and therapeutic maneuvers. This and the fact that under hospice care satisfactory palliation can often be achieved in the home setting tend to lower the cost of the care of terminal illness. This is true even though there are often substantial costs incurred in providing hospice care at home. On the other hand, hospice care involves a great deal of personal attention, and wherever rendered, this tends to raise cost. However, the fact that much of this personal attention can be provided by volunteers tends to diminish that cost increase. The *net* effect of all of this would appear to be, at this point, a *reduction* in the cost of terminal illness care when hospice care is introduced to replace good conventional care.

The other aspect of hospice care financing is the *reimbursement* of the provider for the costs incurred. The feasibility and survival of most hospice programs rest on this issue. In the United States the situation currently can be described as uncertain and changing; it is also inconsistent from one area to another.

When we speak of reimbursement, we are speaking largely of third-party payors since there are almost no patients who will reimburse the hospice directly for a major share of the care provided. The principal third-party payors are the state and federal government and Blue Cross-Blue Shield. In some areas other commercial insurance companies are important sources of reimbursement.

We will focus on institutional reimbursement. Physician reimbursement, for example through Blue Shield and ordinary Medicare Part B, is much the same as it would be for terminal care rendered outside a hospice care program. However, it is pertinent to note that reimbursement systems do not place a heavy emphasis on a high level of personal attention but tend to be oriented toward disease treatment, episodic care, and procedures.

Institutional reimbursement arrangements, both private and governmental, are evolving. As discussed in Chapter 10, under Medicare an optional hospice benefit is now available to terminally ill patients and hospices, but the restrictions placed on this benefit have limited its use. Under most present reimbursement formulas, institutions receive no payment for some of the important nonmedical services that are a vital ingredient of hospice care. This includes the costs of handling some of the patients' social problems and the provision of bereavement counseling.

Through current conventional insurance arrangements, strictly medical services are reimbursable in part. Hospital-based programs are paid for inpatient care in essentially the same fashion as they would be for inpatients receiving nonhospice terminal care. However, for outpatients reimbursement is very limited. Many patients do not have any home care coverage in their insurance policy. If they do, there are often numerous restrictions on the terms of this reimbursement. For example, the institution may be reimbursed only if there has been a recent prior hospitalization or only if the patient is homebound; these stipulations are often not met by hospice patients. Furthermore, the amounts paid for hospice home care usually do not reflect the longer and more frequent visits that are necessary for hospice patients. Infrequently there is a restriction upon the number of home visits permitted, which may be unrealistic for hospice care patients.

For the free-standing hospice, the reimbursement problem may be even more acute. In some areas such institutions are not recognized as a part of the health care system and therefore are not reimbursed at all.

It easily can be seen that reimbursement for hospice services, or more specifically the lack of adequate reimbursement, poses a threat to the viability of hospice care. The problems in reimbursement are being addressed in a number of different ways in different parts of the country. For example, pilot projects sponsored by the federal government, state governments and insurance carriers have experimented with liberalized reimbursement formulas that recognize hospice care and take into account its special requirements. The hospice benefit under Medicare represents another experiment.

In approaching the matter of reimbursement we must be realistic. If we are to have reimbursement for hospice care, there must be some form of institutional certification in order to protect the public's interests. This raises some very serious problems. Up to this point demonstration and pilot projects have been confined to a relatively small number of hospice programs that can be identified, characterized, and monitored in a way that will not be possible as reimbursement becomes more widespread. Therefore, hospice workers must be ready to accept the application of standards and the implementation of accreditation. It is important that such standards and accreditation permit the maximum flexibility and diversity compatible with safety.

Those of us involved with hospice programs also will need to accept the fact that financial resources everywhere are limited. Consequently, some restrictions will have to be placed upon the services that can be reimbursed. One hopes that an informed consumer public will have some role in determining those services that it wishes to have covered (i.e., for which it wishes to pay) under its various insurance policies.

References

American Hospital Association: Memorandum. *AHA Washington Memo,* no. 513:4, August 10,1984.

Annotated Code of Maryland, supplement, 1981.

Bayer R, Feldman E: Hospice under the medicare wing. *Hastings Cent Rep,* December 1982

Brooks TA: Legal and regulatory issues in hospice care. *Hosp Med Staff,* p 15, June 1980.

Buckingham RW, Lupu D: A comparative study of hospice services in the United States. *Am J Public Health* 72:455, 1982.

Burne SR: Hospice care for children. *Br Med J* 284:1400, 1982.

Burne SR, Dominica F, Baum JD: Helenhouse — A hospice for children: analysis of the first year. *Br Med J* 289:1665, 1984.

Cohen KP: *Hospice: Prescription for Terminal Care.* Aspen Press, Germantown MD, 1979.

Corr CA, Corr DM: *Hospice Approaches to Pediatric Care.* Springer, New York, 1985.

Davidson GW: *The Hospice: Development and Administration.* Hemisphere Publishing, Washington DC, 1978.

Department of Health and Human Services, Health Care Financing Administration, Medicare program: *Hospice Care Proposed Rule,* Federal Register II, vol 48, August 22, 1983.

Didolkar MS, Fanous N, Elias EG, Moore RH: Metastatic carcinomas from occult primary tumors — Study of 254 patients. *Ann Surg* 186:625, 1977.

Eisman D: The second dimension. *Arch Surg* 186:625, 1977.

Gaber AO: Metastatic malignant disease of unknown origin. *Am J Surg* 145:493, 1983.

Garland CA: *Psychosocial Care of the Dying Patient.* McGraw-Hill, New York, 1978.

Gyulay J: *The Dying Child.* McGraw-Hill, New York, 1978.

Hamilton M, Reid H: *A Hospice Handbook.* William B Eerdman Publishing, Grand Rapids MI, 1980.

Hinton J: Whom do dying patients tell? *Br Med J* 281:1328, 1980.

Joint Commission on Accreditation of Hospitals: *Proposed Hospice Standards Manual.* JCAH, Chicago, 1983.

Koff TH: *Hospice: A Caring Community.* Winthrop Publishing, Cambridge MA, 1980.

Krakoff IH: The case for active treatment in patients with advanced cancer: Not everyone needs a hospice. *CA* 29:108, 1979.

Lack SA, Buckingham RW: *First American Hospice.* Hospice Inc, New Haven CT, 1978.

Lamerton R: *Care of the Dying.* Priority Press, London, 1973.

Martinson IM: *Home Care for the Dying Child — Professional and Family Perspectives.* Appleton-Century-Crofts, New York, 1976.

Maryland Hospital Educational Institute: *Hospice: Time for Decision.* Maryland Hospital Educational Institute, Baltimore, 1980.

Miller SC: *A Medical Record Handbook for Hospice Programs.* Foundation for Record

Education of the American Medical Record Association, Chicago, 1984.

Mor V, Hiris J: Determinants of site of death among hospice cancer patients. *J Health Soc Behav* 24:375, 1983.

Mott M: Caring for children with cancer. *In Wilkes E (ed): The Dying Patient — The Medical Management of Incurable and Terminal Illness*, 45. George A Bogden and Sons, Ridgewood NJ, 1982.

Mount BM: The problem of caring for the dying in a general hospital: The palliative care unit as a possible solution. *Can Med Assoc J* 115:119, 1976a.

Mount, BM: *Palliative Care Service: October 1976 Repport*. Royal Victoria Hospital/ McGill University, Montreal, 1976b.

National Hospice Organization Licensure and Reimbursement Committee: *Why State Licensure?* NHO, Arlington VA, 1984.

Parkes CM: Bereavement counseling: Does it work? *Br Med J* 281:3, 1980.

Potter JF: A challenge for the hospice movement. *N Engl J Med* 302:52, 1980.

Pryga EA: Hospice regs pose major hurdles for medical staff. *Hospital Medical Staff*, p 7, November 1983.

Reese WE, Lutkins SC: Mortality of bereavement. *Br Med J* 4:12, 1967.

Rolka HR: Quality assurance for the terminally ill. *Hospital and Health Services Administration*, March/April 1983.

Rossman P: *Hospice: Creating New Models of Care of the Terminally Ill*. Association Press, New York, 1977.

Saunders CM: Telling patients. *District Nursing*, 1965.

Saunders CM: *Management of Terminal Disease*. Yearbook, London, 1978.

Schonberg IB, Carr AC, Peretz D, Kutscher AH: *Psychosocial Aspects of Terminal Care*. Columbia University Press, New York, 1972.

Sheldon M: Truth telling in medicine. *JAMA* 247:651, 1982.

Spencer FC: Competence and compassion. The Gibbon Lecture. *Bulletin American College of Surgeons* p 15, November 1979.

Stedman's Medical Dictionary, ed 24. Williams and Wilkins, Baltimore, 1982.

Stoddard S: *The Hospice Movement*. Stein and Day, Briarcliff Manor NY, 1978.

Taylor G : Helping families cope when a child has cancer. *Resident and Staff Physician*, p 32, July 1981.

Thomas L: *The Lives of a Cell*. Viking Press, New York, 1974.

Walter NT: *Hospice Pilot Project Report*. Kaiser-Permanente, Hayward CA, 1979.

Webster's New World Dictionary, college ed 2. New World Publishing, New York, 1972.

West TS, Kirkham SR: Communication with patients and families. Paper presented at the International Hospice Conference, London, June 1980.

Wilkes E, Crowther AGO, Greaves CWKH: A different kind of day hospital — For patients with preterminal cancer and chronic disease. *Br Med J* 2:1053, 1978.

Relief of Physical Symptoms in Advanced Cancer

Jack M. Zimmerman

General Considerations

Physical symptoms in cancer patients, who comprise the vast majority of hospice patients, can arise from a variety of sources: the tumor, antitumor therapy, intercurrent disease, or sometimes, treatment undertaken to relieve other symptoms. It is in its attitude toward symptom relief that hospice care differs from other medical care. Relief of symptoms becomes the overriding consideration in treatment; symptoms are defined very broadly to include not only physical but also psychological and social problems (Saunders 1982).

This chapter is devoted to the handling of physical symptoms by medical means. The next chapter deals with the psychosocial aspects of care of both the patient and his or her family.

The objective of this chapter is not to provide a thorough discussion of each of the symptoms that may occur in a patient terminally ill with malignancy. More comprehensive and detailed consideration can be found in other sources (e.g., Abeloff 1979; Twycross and Lack 1984), as can information regarding the handling of the symptoms occurring in patients with specific types of tumors (Wilson et al. 1980; Wilkes 1982). Techniques and experiences with symptom relief in other hospice programs have been well presented (Mount 1976; Saunders 1978).

The focus here is upon the treatment of those symptoms that we have seen most frequently in our patients. What follows is designed to provide the guidelines that we have found helpful in managing these symptoms. For some, such as pain, we have been quite gratified by our success. With others, such as weakness, we have been quite frustrated by our results.

One of several approaches may be taken in presenting material about symptoms. The method used here is, for the most part, a listing of symptoms grouped essentially by organ system, without regard to tumor type or underlying condition producing the symptom. Wilkes (1982) has organized his presentation around types of tumors, whereas Abeloff (1979) deals with specific underlying conditions such as hematological problems, renal complications, endocrinological disorders, and the like. Since related pathophysiological abnormalities can create different symptoms, this can be a useful approach. For example, both *hypercoagulation* leading to in situ thrombosis and *hypocoagulation* leading to bleeding can occur in cancer patients (Caprini and Sener 1982).

Although symptom relief takes a higher priority in the dying patient, the methods employed are in most respects similar to those used for other patients. However, experience in hospice programs has taught that certain modifications in approach to symptom control are appropriate for the terminally ill. In other words, relief of symptoms in terminally ill cancer patients often involves simply the application of conventional therapeutic measures; occasionally, however, it includes the use of unconventional techniques.

Of course symptom relief is a continuing obligation of all of the caregivers on the hospice team, but the importance of beginning such relief early must be emphasized. This is particularly true of pain. The physically uncomfortable person cannot come to grips with and resolve complex philosophical issues. At the very outset of hospice care, efforts at symptom relief must begin.

Expectations about what can be achieved in providing physical comfort can create problems. The expectations of the patient, family members, the physician, and other team members may differ considerably, and these differences then disrupt the patient's care. For example, physicians sometimes assume that the patient with advanced malignancy still expects cure of the tumor when in reality the patient is quite ready to accept simply a measure of relief from troublesome sensations.

Three key points in control of physical symptoms deserve emphasis:

1. Adequate communication with the patient regarding his or her symptoms is essential. One cannot treat symptoms effectively unless one takes care to elicit detailed information about their presence, severity, and nature. This requires both time and a proper attitude on the part of those caring for the patient. All members of the hospice care team should be alert to the presence and nature of the patient's symptoms and should relay information about them to the attending physician. Once symptoms are recognized, treatment must be tailored to the symptoms and to the overall situation of the patient. It is important also to determine what drugs or other measures have so far been helpful. It should be remembered in this connection that the act of communication itself may be a valuable component of therapy.

2. Careful follow-up, with adjustment of therapy as needed, is of paramount importance. As therapeutic measures are employed, their effectiveness should be carefully monitored. Ineffective treatments should be discontinued; they add unnecessary costs and, through side effect and interaction, may complicate an already difficult situation. This rule is particularly important in palliative care, in which symptoms are the main focus of attention. It is very easy to allow medications and treatments to accumulate; this should be avoided.

3. Psychological and social problems can aggravate physical symptoms. Support in coping with such problems can greatly simplify the management of physical symptoms. Thoughtful listening, simple explanation, or a helping hand can often minimize the use of drugs or be even more effective than any pharmacological agent.

The provision of symptom control in the terminally ill can demand the highest degree of excellence in clinical judgment. Careful gathering and evaluation of the available information is often required in reaching decisions about relief of symptoms.

Another critical element in the provision of optimal symptom relief is excellence of nursing care. There is really little that is unique about nursing care in a hospice program. If there is anything that distinguishes the hospice nurse from other nurses, it is simply the degree of reliance upon sound nursing practice for success and satisfaction in the work. Hospice care not only draws upon but requires the finest from the traditions of nursing. Constant attention must be directed to the maintenance of patient comfort. To accomplish this effectively the nurse must be active, not passive. One cannot wait for the patient to complain; one must search out problems and anticipate potential difficulties. One must be alert to special dangers such as the development of decubiti. The patient's emotional and psychological needs must be monitored but never to the exclusion of physical needs. It is important to be aware of the sick person's need for independence. One must be not only a team member but also a team leader. All aspects of fine nursing care are essential if symptom relief is to be at its maximum.

Although appropriate use of drugs is central to symptomatic treatment, one must remember that physical measures such as the proper use of positioning, massage, active and passive motion, and heat and cold can contribute greatly to providing comfort. Furthermore, formal physical therapy can be very useful. Cancer rehabilitation has come a long way in recent years, and its techniques often apply as much to the terminally ill patient as to the one who is potentially cured. (Dietz, 1981; Harvey 1982.)

In meeting the patient's needs, sensitivity is essential. The caregiver brings to the situation of terminal illness some perceptions and assumptions that may not conform to those of the patient. It is the patient's needs, however, that must be met. Bingham (1977) has pointed out that needs perceived by the dying patient and needs perceived by those providing his or her care may not always conform. Therefore all members of the hospice team must be alert for and sensitive to what is troubling the patient and the family.

It is not surprising that there is lack of uniform agreement about methods of symptom relief. For many symptoms there are various treatment methods available, with no consensus as to which is best. For some symptoms no therapy has proved consistently effective. Obviously, the clinician must resolve these problems while deciding upon some form of treatment for the patient. One hopes that as time passes we will gather through hospice programs and from other sources the kind of useful data that will permit a more sensible selection of options and through which new and effective forms of therapy can be developed.

Of course, useful information about the quality of the patient's life would be very helpful in making such a selection. At present, measures of this dimension are quite crude. However, as clinical research is beginning to focus on this matter, investigative studies are producing some tools that offer promise of practical usefulness (Spitzer et al. 1981; Sugarbaker et al. 1982).

Some of the most difficult therapeutic choices in the symptomatic treatment of the terminally ill have to do with whether or not to employ antitumor therapy in the form of surgery, radiation, chemotherapy, hormonal manipulation, or bone marrow transplantation. These problems are related to but separate from those at the interface between curative and palliative treatment. In Chapter 2 we discussed the problem of deciding whether the patient has a reasonable chance of *cure*. It is on this determination that the decision to enter the patient in the hospice program is based. However, once it has been agreed that antitumor therapy no longer offers a prospect of cure, whether antitumor therapy will contribute to the patient's *palliation* may still be uncertain.

At this point we really have limited information available regarding the effect of such treatment upon palliative care. As noted, the impact of these measures on quantity of life can be very difficult to predict, but one must also deal with the delicate balance between quantity and quality of life. For example, it would appear that surgical debulking of tumors too large to remove may have a specific but quite limited role in symptom relief (Silberman 1982). The same is probably true of resection of metastatic tumor in the liver and lung (Storm and Morton 1979). Further study of all antitumor modalities, particularly with the use of quality-of-life measures, may help us select antitumor therapy more rationally in the incurable patient.

A similar problem arises with respect to the use of other relatively aggressive forms of palliative treatment. Invasive measures and operative procedures, although initially quite traumatic, may offer better symptomatic relief than do more conservative forms of therapy. The relative benefits and difficulties associated with such forms of treatment must be carefully weighed. Surgical treatment of pathological fractures can be most helpful, as can palliative intubation of an obstructed esophagus (Zimmerman and King 1969). On the other hand, the performance of gastrostomy is of relatively limited value as a palliative maneuver in advanced cancer (King and Zimmerman 1965). Ferrara et al. (1982) have demonstrated that emergency operations for perforated viscus or massive bleeding carry very high morbidity in patients with metastatic cancer. However, technological advances can shift the balance between gain and loss with various forms of treatment. For example, it is now possible to provide, under certain circumstances, intravenous antibiotic therapy at home (Poretz et al. 1982), and with the availability of this, one might be inclined to treat vigorously some infections that previously could not have been treated. In each case, therefore, the decision for or against the use of relatively aggressive forms of treatment must be highly individualized.

This type of decision requires great skill in clinical judgment. Information from a number of sources must be assimilated. The type and extent of the tumor, the nature of symptoms, the likelihood of success, the side effects of therapy, the need for monitoring, and a number of other factors must be weighed in each case. Consultation, combined with frank and thorough discussion, can be invaluable in making decisions about aggressive forms of therapy in the terminally ill. Nonetheless, very often the data about the probability of clinical response may be inadequate.

Another related issue arising in the symptomatic treatment of the terminally ill is the prevention of symptoms. This might be called *prophylactic palliation*. Coping with existing symptoms can confront the hospice staff with some difficult problems and decisions. However, some thought also must be given to the prophylaxis of potential symptoms, which take a variety of forms and may create some very difficult choices. Should antitumor treatment or some other aggressive forms of management be used in an effort to forestall the possible development of symptoms? The use of pulmonary resection as a means of preventing, as well as treating, symptoms in incurable lung cancer has shown some promise (King et al. 1965; Smith 1963). In certain patients with vertebral metastases manifested only by pain, a case can be made for early myelogram and surgical decompression of the spinal cord before symptoms of neurological deficit develop.

Although the matter of prophylactic palliation is controversial, it cannot be ignored by conscientious physicians responsible for the care of terminally ill patients. It is discussed in more detail in Chapter 14. At present there are more questions than answers. However, for each individual patient the hospice physician should stay alert to potential measures that may prevent symptoms. In addition, this is one of those fields in which hospice care programs possess the capacity to provide valuable information through careful study.

Another area in which the hospice physician must often make troublesome choices has to do with the treatment of symptoms themselves as opposed to searching out and treating underlying causes. Certain symptoms, such as nausea and dysphagia, can result from a variety of causes. Sometimes the cause is evident and the choice of whether to treat it or the symptom is easy. Nausea due to digitalis intoxication is best treated by proper adjustment of the digitalis dosage. The dysphagia resulting from recurrent tumor and extensive esophagitis following heavy radiation therapy for esophageal carcinoma does not lend itself to treating the cause of the symptom. However, sometimes the cause of a symptom may be obscure; in such a case, a decision must be made about the vigor and persistence with which the cause will be sought. In other situations the cause will be evident, but a great deal of judgment may be required in deciding whether it is more prudent to attempt to remedy the cause or simply to treat the symptom. The patient with a relatively advanced malignancy and the onset of nausea and vomiting due to intestinal obstruction frequently poses such a dilemma. Once again, it would not be productive to establish comprehensive rules for choosing whether to treat the symptom or its underlying cause in the multiple guises in which this question can arise. Careful assessment of the facts of the individual case, use of good sense, and willingness to make a decision without totally satisfactory evidence are essential.

There are certain underlying problems that occur frequently in patients with advanced malignancy. Some of these are mechanical, such as viscus obstruction or serous effusion. Some are metabolic, such as hypercalcemia or hyponatremia. Others are hematological such as hyperviscosity syndromes and alterations in coagulability. For the most part, once the decision has been made to treat one of these underlying disorders, the therapeutic approach is generally the same for hospice patients as it is in other clinical settings.

Finally, questions regarding symptom control may arise in regard to intercurrent problems not immediately related to the advanced malignancy. Renal failure, congestive heart failure, pulmonary insufficiency, and pneumonia are examples. Obviously, decisions must be made on the basis of particular circumstances in individual cases. Early in the course of terminal illness, appropriate treatment of intercurrent disorders can provide additional quantity and quality to life. On the other hand, to apply aggressive treatment to these problems late in the course of terminal illness not only may subject the patient and family to unnecessary discomfort, but may actually deprive the patient of what would have been his or her most comfortable mode of demise.

The aim of reviewing each of these problems areas has not been to provide ready-made solutions, but rather to alert the hospice worker to the kinds of choices that have to be made. An awareness that others have faced these problems and that there are no definitive answers will, we hope, be of some help. Chapter 14 deals in greater detail with some of these issues.

Specific Symptoms

In the treatment of individual symptoms described, the dosages noted for medications are those that we employ in the medium-sized, middle-aged terminally ill patient with only moderate debility and wasting. Appropriate adjustments of dosages for other types of patients are required.

Pain

Pain, although not uniformly present in the terminally ill, is an extremely common symptom. For a number of reasons, it has received the largest share of attention among symptoms in patients dying of cancer. This is partly due to its frequency as a symptom but also to the fact that deeply interwoven in the fear of cancer in our society today is fear of pain. Oster et al. (1978) provide some quantitative information about pain in advanced malignancy. Through the studies of Twycross (1974) and others, hospice workers have made basic contributions to better pain control in the terminally ill. Outside of formal hospice programs, relief of pain in such patients has continued to receive careful attention (Shimm et al. 1979). The literature on pain relief in the terminally ill is voluminous; there are several excellent reports that provide more scope and depth than is possible in this chapter and that give some varying views (Black 1979; McGivney and Crooks 1984; Reuler et al. 1980; Twycross and Lack 1983; Wall 1985). Kenton (1983) has done a complete search of the recent literature on chronic pain in terminal illness.

For those dying patients who have pain, it must be controlled before other symptoms can be handled effectively. Almost all patients with advanced malignancy fear both uncontrollable pain and the possibility of being so mentally obtunded from pain relief that they are rendered subhuman. They must be assured from the beginning, and shown thereafter, that it is possible to be kept pain free and alert throughout much of their terminal illness.

The first step in pain control is to determine the cause of the pain. Symptoms originating from sources other than the tumor (e.g., dental caries, constipation, hemorrhoids, etc.) must be dealt with appropriately. If pain is due to the tumor, first consideration should be given to the possiblity that antitumor therapy in the form of excision, radiation, or chemotherapy might be helpful. If these do not offer a reasonable promise of pain relief, other measures must be undertaken. For this, many modalities are available: nerve block, neurosurgical procedures, electrical stimulation, hypnosis, acupuncture, and analgesics, including intrathecal agents. It has been our experience that although there are circumstances in which other measures are preferable, for most patients pain can be well controlled with the proper use of analgesics. Because analgesics offer certain advantages over other measures, we have usually selected this approach.

As in all pain relief by pharmacological measures, the mildest agent capable of producing relief should be employed. For some patients aspirin and acetaminophen prove quite satisfactory; for many, codeine-like drugs are needed, while for others morphine derivatives are essential.

There are two important points to remember in alleviation of pain from advanced malignancy: it is easier to prevent than to relieve intense pain, and fear of additional pain is an important symptom in the terminally ill. For these reasons the use of analgesics on an as-needed basis plays little role in the management of chronic pain. Analgesic medication must be given on a regular basis.

Relief from chronic pain can be seen as a *spectrum*, with uncontrolled pain at one extreme and unconsciousness at the other; in the center there is, with most potent analgesics, an area within which chronic pain is relieved and the patient is alert. The aim of pain treatment is to titrate the dosage regimen so that the patient is in this portion of the spectrum.

The way in which the patient is entered into this spectrum of pain relief depends upon the severity and duration of the pain and the patient's attitude toward it. For the patient who has relatively mild pain and who is extremely fearful that efforts to relieve the pain will result in impairment of mental function, it may be desirable to begin with low doses of mild analgesic, gradually increasing these until the patient is comfortable. For the patient for whom pain has been a serious problem over a period of time, it is usually best to begin with the assurance that the pain can be relieved and to provide ample narcotic initially. The first aim should be a good night's sleep.

Oral medication is preferred. Liquid preparations are easier to manage than pills and capsules. Occasionally, severe pain is better relieved by parenteral than by oral analgesics, but for most patients the oral route is effective and much more satisfactory.

Aqueous morphine, which is relatively soluble, serves as an excellent potent analgesic for the patient with severe chronic pain from advanced malignancy. It can be mixed with many vehicles for palatable administration. Treatment with aqueous morphine is initiated at regular 4-hour intervals, selecting a dosage that appears appropriate for the particular patient. The morphine dosage and timing then can be adjusted to bring the patient into that central portion of the pain relief spectrum in which he is pain free and mentally alert.

The dosage of analgesic required to place the patient in the central portion of the pain relief spectrum is a highly individual matter. As a guideline to *initiation* of therapy, we have used an equianalgesic dosage schedule. The following are regarded as essentially equivalent to morphine, 30 mg by mouth: oxycodone (Percocet, Percodan), two to three tablets; hydromorphone (Dilaudid), 6 mg rectally, 4 mg by mouth, and 2 mg parenterally; morphine, 5–10 mg subcutaneously. Thus the patient who had been receiving two to three tablets of Percodan without relief would be started on 30 mg of aqueous morphine by mouth.

Surprisingly large doses of morphine may be necessary to produce pain relief, but as long as they do not produce excessive drowsiness, there is no harm in these large doses. The principle of a central portion of the spectrum where the patient is pain-free but alert holds through a very wide dosage range, depending upon the severity of the underlying pain. In other words, as increasing pain requires an increased dosage of morphine, there is a concomitant increase in tolerance to the drug, so that the new high doses do not reduce the patient's level of alertness. It has been our experience, and that of others, that side effects such as drowsiness and depression are largely related to the patient's overall condition and nutritional status. In other words, a generally robust patient with severe pain will require substantial doses of morphine to relieve the pain but at these doses will remain quite alert. However, the severely debilitated patient is likely to have a much narrower pain-free and alert zone in the central portion of the spectrum.

During this period of titration, very careful observation and questioning of the patient is essential. One needs to be certain that pain is indeed relieved. It is also important to avoid repetitive overdosage and to establish the minimal dose that will keep the patient pain free. As Potter (1980) has observed, the aim is to have "a patient who is free from pain but who is alert enough to enjoy the benefits of pain free survival." Once the proper dosage and timing of morphine are established, they are likely to remain stable over a protracted period of time until there is some major change in the patient's condition.

An interesting legal consideration related to patients receiving high doses of potent narcotics is the matter of mental competence. It has been customary, in most hospitals, not to accept as valid a consent form signed by the patient within several hours of receiving a narcotic. This poses some problems for the hospice patient who has been nicely titrated into the central portion of the pain relief spectrum. To all intents and purposes the patient seems to meet any reasonable test of mental competence but technically is unable to provide informed consent. This can be a practical consideration if some type of invasive procedure is planned. The author has encountered the situation in which the alert patient and his lawyer were revising the patient's will, which began "Being of sound mind and body . . . ," but this same patient was ineligible to sign a consent form for a minor surgical procedure. We have dealt with this problem by creating a form on which two physicians, one usually the hospice physician, certify to the patient's competence to make the decision in question.

However, caution should be exercised in permitting patients to take their own narcotics. Should for any reason a patient's mental acuity be diminished, no care giver will be aware of exactly how much narcotic has been taken.

Narcotics tend to produce nausea; anxiety potentiates pain. Therefore, the patient initially may be given prochlorperazine (Compazine) syrup (5 mg every 4 hours) for its antiemetic and tranquilizing effects. Its dosage and timing also can be adjusted as necessary. Once stability of dosage and timing of morphine and Compazine is achieved, the two medications can be combined.

It should be remembered that constipation is a problem with most potent analgesics. Accordingly, the patient should be given ample stool softener while receiving these drugs. We often routinely give patients on narcotics a senna pod laxative.

Bone pain due to osseous metastases can be intense and resistant to therapy. The addition of a nonsteroidal anti-inflammatory agent, such as aspirin, ibuprofen (Motrin), phenylbutazone, or indomethacin, is sometimes helpful. Some have found that dexamethasone or prednisone, combined with antacid, is safer and more effective than the nonsteroidal anti-inflammatory agents. Corticosteroids are particularly useful when pain is due to nerve compression or a tumor in a confined space, such as the head or pelvis.

In patients with intractable vomiting or dysphagia so severe as to prevent swallowing even small quantities of liquid, 3mg hydromorphone (Dilaudid) suppositories are often effective. Morphine sulfate suppositories can be used, but if the patient is being shifted to these from other routes of morphine administration, needed changes in dosage are somewhat variable. If rectal medication is not effective, parenteral therapy, usually with morphine plus Compazine, may be used. At this point we give consideration to other measures of pain relief, such as intrathecal morphine, transcutaneous electrical stimulation, nerve block, and neurosurgical procedures.

There are two matters with respect to pain relief in the terminally ill that deserve comment because they have been the source of some misunderstanding and controversy.

The first is Brompton's mixture. This combination of heroin with cocaine, alcohol, chloroform water, and flavoring agent was the analgesic agent that many of the first English hospices used for pain relief. Although the substance took its name from Brompton's Chest Hospital in London and was presumably used for treatment of patients with chest diseases, its name became, in the minds of many, intertwined with the term hospice. The rationale of the mixture was that cocaine and alcohol provided some euphoric effect to potentiate the action of heroin. It is not totally clear what the chloroform water was to contribute; unless the English sense of taste is vastly different from that of Americans, it is hard to imagine that it was to contribute to the palatability of the solution. In any event, various hospice programs made modifications in the composition of Brompton's solution. American hospices had to substitute morphine for heroin. Like others, we made our own modifications at Church Hospital. It is not surprising that as experience has grown, Bromptom's mixture largely has been replaced by aqueous morphine or heroin. Single-agent drugs are usually more satisfactory than multiple-agent ones. The euphoric effect of cocaine proved somewhat unpredictable and its side effects were disturbing, particularly in older patients. Alcohol, in the volume used, contributed little of therapeutic value. It can be administered better as the liquor of the patient's choice. Like most other hospice programs, we have abandoned the use of Brompton's mixture and find it today of little but historic and sentimental interest.

The other matter is the issue of heroin. It is, of course, available for medical purposes in the United Kingdom but not in the United States. There are those who feel strongly that Americans should be allowed to use it for therapeutic purposes, most particularly for the management of terminal illness. Heroin (diacetylmorphine) is, milligram for milligram, about 1.5 times as potent as morphine; it is somewhat more soluble and has a questionably greater euphoric effect than morphine. It appears that for oral use heroin probably has few advantages over morphine. Aqueous morphine is reasonably soluble, and the volume of oral solution for each dose is small with either agent. There are other means of achieving whatever euphoric advantage heroin may have over morphine. Therefore, the effect of a given oral dose of heroin can be achieved by giving one and one-half times as many milligrams of morphine.

It is the author's opinion that two arguments can be made for legalizing the medical use of heroin in the United States. The first is that because of its greater solubility, it is more satisfactory for parenteral administration. However, in hospice care parenteral analgesics are employed infrequently. The second has to do with the individual variation of the patient in response to medications. Patients do indeed differ in their reactions to particular medications; what is helpful and innocuous for one patient may be useless or harmful for another. On these grounds an argument can be made for having available as many medications as possible. Obviously, these arguments for the availability of heroin must be balanced against whatever increased difficulties in narcotics control would result from such availability. Evidence of a recent substantial rise in heroin abuse, particularly among the middle and upper classes, must be taken into consideration.

An interesting observation that we have made, as has been noted by other hospice programs, relates to the matter of drug dependency in the terminally ill patient with pain. From time to time pain in such patients abates for one reason or another, either spontaneously or as a consequence of antitumor therapy such as radiation. In contrast to the individual who has become addicted by virtue of drug abuse, the terminal patient on running doses of morphine can often be dropped back to lower doses or completely withdrawn from the drug without serious side effects. We have had a number of patients for whom radiation therapy was selected as the primary means of controlling pain but who had been placed on substantial doses of oral morphine pending the effect of radiation. Once their pain was relieved, their analgesic was reduced or discontinued with ease. The relatively short duration of narcotic administration might explain this phenomenon in these patients; it does not do so for those who have experienced spontaneous relief of pain after a long-standing lesion has, for some reason, burned out its capacity to produce pain.

Systemic and Constitutional Problems

Weakness   This is a common symptom in patients with advanced malignancy. It can be due to any one of a number of causes: some evident, some not; some treatable, some not (Theologides 1982). It is not surprising, then, that the results of treatment of this distressing symptom are variable.

The first step is to look for a specific treatable cause. Common sources of weakness are surgical convalescence, chemotherapy, radiation, anemia, infection, dehydration, malnutrition, hypokalemia, depression, and prolonged bed rest. As much as possible these should be dealt with appropriately. Encouragement of activity and formal physical therapy can be helpful in combating weakness. A proper balance is necessary between encouraging the patient to move around and "nagging."

When such measures fail and weakness is a predominant symptom, the use of corticosteroids (prednisone or dexamethasone) or a testosterone preparation may be helpful. Dexamethasone is usually begun at a dosage of 0.75 mg three times per day; if no effect is achieved, this is increased gradually up to 1.5 mg three times per day. Prednisone is usually started at 5 mg three times per day; if no effect is achieved, this is increased to 10 mg three times per day. For an anabolic steroid, we have used either nandrolone decanoate (Deca-Durabolin) at 200 mg intramuscularly each week, or fluoxymesterone (Halotestin) at 5 mg three times per day. Undesirable side effects of corticosteroid and testosterone preparations must be watched for. As a practical matter muscular wasting clearly attributable to corticosteroid usage has not been observed, presumably because the time span has been relatively short. On a few occasions we have used a central nervous system stimulant with good effect for the patient in whom weakness was a predominant symptom. Methylphenidate (Ritalin) at a dosage of 10 mg three times per day has been our choice.

Thirst The combination of narcotics, dehydration, and mouth breathing often results in a combination of troublesome thirst and dry mouth. For this, careful attention to mouth care, the provision of frequent small sips of fluid, and sucking on ice chips can provide remarkable relief. An artificial saliva containing methylcellulose and glycerin is prepared in our pharmacy and has been helpful in dealing with thirst and dry mouth.

Hypercalcemia Although it is a metabolic disorder rather than a symptom, the management of hypercalcemia deserves some special comment. It is not uncommon in patients with advanced malignancy, and it is easy to overlook, particularly in patients who are not subject to frequent laboratory tests. It can produce a wide panorama of symptoms in many different organ systems. Also, successful treatment can be quite elusive.

When hypercalcemia occurs late in the course of terminal illness, within a few days of death from an overwhelming tumor, it is best treated by acceptance as a part of the final constellation of problems. However, when it occurs earlier and there is reason to believe that treatment of it will produce symptomatic relief, it should be dealt with. The usual measures (intravenous fluids including saline, loop diuretics, corticosteroids, and phosphates) can be employed. Mithramycin is particularly useful in treating hypercalcemia associated with advanced neoplastic disease. As little as 1 – 2 mg two times per week given intravenously can produce dramatic symptomatic response without serious toxic side effect. It can be given safely for as long as 6 months; no monitoring is necessary. It is usually given as an intravenous bolus with about 250 ml of saline. It is important to be certain that there is no extravasation of solution, because mithramycin is irritating to the tissue.

Hemorrhage Bleeding can originate from a number of sources in the terminally ill patient and can range from trivial to exsanguinating. Hemorrhage can occur from the primary tumor, whether it is located on the surface of the body or in viscera such as the intestine, urinary tract, or bronchus. On the other hand, severe bleeding can occur from nontumor sources such as peptic ulcer or erosive gastritis. It must be remembered that through a number of mechanisms, malignant tumors and various forms of antitumor therapy can produce alterations in coagulability.

Bleeding of a minor nature usually requires no treatment by members of the hospice care team. Team members must remember, however, that even slight bleeding can be an unexpected and frightening experience for the patient and family. In such circumstances prompt and effective reassurance can be of inestimable value. It is when bleeding is more substantial that some critical choices must be made regarding the patient's treatment. Management of severe hemorrhage involves two basic elements: control of hemorrhage and maintenance of adequate blood volume. A number of factors must be taken into account: the patient's general condition, the extent and distribution of the tumor, intercurrent conditions, the cause and site of bleeding, and so forth. For patients in good general condition with relatively limited tumor and an evident site of bleeding that can be controlled simply, the decision is obviously an easy one. For already moribund patients with widespread tumor and hemorrhage from an obscure source, the choice is also easy. However, between these extremes the hospice staff may be called upon to decide how vigorously to search for a site of bleeding, how aggressively to look for a coagulation abnormality, whether or not to undertake complex treatments including operations, and how much blood should be expended in transfusion. To treat too strenuously may not only be costly but may be counterproductive to true palliation. However, failure to treat adequately may unnecessarily shorten a patient's life.

There are really no useful guidelines that can be articulated to cover the handling of all possible combinations that can occur in difficult cases of hemorrhage. This is a situation in which ample consultation can be most helpful. It is also one of those points at which the wishes of the patient and the family must be given special consideration.

Fever   In patients with advanced malignancy, fever can arise from a number of causes including the tumor itself and lysis of the tumor by radiation or chemotherapy. It can also result from intercurrent infection either directly related to the tumor (e.g., pneumonia behind an obstructing bronchogenic carcinoma) or from an incidental infection perhaps due to compromised host defense mechanisms. The first step in dealing with fever is to attempt to locate and treat the cause, if possible. If there is no extraneous cause and fever appears to be due to the neoplasm itself, aspirin and acetaminophen are often ineffective. In this circumstance indomethacin (Indocin; 25 – 50 mg three times a day) may be helpful (Warshaw et al. 1981).

Jaundice   In and of itself jaundice is not a particularly troublesome symptom, but its appearance can be alarming at times to the patient and his or her family. Of course, jaundice can arise from a number of causes but its occurrence is usually an ominous sign with respect to the prognosis for quantity, if not quality, of life. When jaundice is due to extrahepatic biliary obstruction, it may be associated with severe pruritus, which is indeed a very difficult symptom to relieve. Until recently there was often little that could be done to relieve obstructive jaundice due to tumor located close to the hepatic hilum. Recently, however, more aggressive approaches to this problem have been associated with some success. For their effect on increasing the quantity of life and in ameliorating the troublesome symptom of pruritus from obstructive jaundice, these aggressive measures often deserve consideration (Blumgart et al. 1984; Cameron et al. 1982; Jones et al. 1983). In prolonged biliary obstruction lack of vitamin K absorption may lead to coagulopathy and consequent hemorrhage. For this, vitamin K at 10 mg intramuscularly per week can be used.

When jaundice is the result of multiple hepatic metastases, there is usually little that can be done. Hepatic artery perfusion with chemotherapeutic agents seldom improves the quality of life at this stage.

One must remember that certain drugs, particularly chlorpromazine, can produce jaundice. Cessation of the drug will generally improve the patient's status.

Gastrointestinal Symptoms

Anorexia Loss of appetite and an unwillingness to eat are common occurrences in the terminally ill. There are number of possible sources of anorexia in patients with advanced malignancy. A detailed examination of this interesting topic is beyond the scope of this book. What does deserve attention here is the fact that anorexia has varying significance in terminally ill patients. It may be a symptom of hypercalcemia occurring in a patient with a life expectancy of several months, in which case the metabolic disturbance should be dealt with as described earlier. Similarly, anorexia due to other correctable causes should be treated appropriately.

If loss of appetite occurs early in patient's course as a relatively isolated symptom, the consequent acceleration of malnutrition may seriously compromise both the quantity and quality of the patient's remaining life. In such circumstances it is worthwhile not only to direct efforts at the correction of any underlying problems, but to try to encourage by any means possible the intake of adequate nutrition. Dietary supplements may be very helpful. Except in the most unusual circumstances, however, elemental diet and intravenous hyperalimentation are best avoided in the terminally ill. Consideration can be given to these measures if, for some reason, the appetite impairment is clearly going to be temporary or results from some correctable underlying problem.

For patients with more advanced tumors and in the later stages of their disease, nutritional replenishment becomes of little importance. Anorexia in this situation is often more distressing to the family than to the patient. As a consequence they exhort the patient to eat and present the individual with large quantities of nutritious food, often aggravating the anorexia. This is an area in which understanding by the family can be most helpful. They must learn that emphasis should now shift from maintenance of nutritional status to enhancing the patient's comfort through the provision of small appetizing meals. Success in making this transition usually results in considerable relief to the patient and the family. Careful discussion of meal planning with the dietitian can be very helpful. Chapter 6 reviews some of the contributions the dietitian can make. Alcoholic beverages usually stimulate appetite.

A corticosteroid (in the dosage as described for weakness) will for some patients produce improvement in appetite. Tricyclic antidepressants such as doxepin (Sinequan 50 mg at bedtime), also increases appetite in some patients. These measures may be tried, but their success varies unpredictably between spectacular and nil.

Dry Mouth   Dry mouth can result from a number of causes including mouth breathing, damaged buccal mucosa, or decreased secretion of saliva. For patients with this symptom, meticulous mouth care including mouth washes and use of lemon-glycerine swabs is important. Frequent sips of water and the liberal use of candy such as Lifesavers can give relief, as can an artificial saliva.

Dysgeusia   An altered sense of taste is a symptom that occasionally occurs in patients with advanced malignancy. At times one sees a patient whose only symptom is a bad taste in his mouth, which he finds extremely annoying. Naturally, poor oral hygiene, dental caries, and obvious contributing factors should be dealt with. If none of these exist, zinc sulfate in 220-mg capsules three times per day can be tried. Its use has been recommended for dysgeusia, but controlled trial has not supported its value. Our results with it have been variable. Some have suggested that reducing the urea content of the diet by increasing white meat, eggs, and dairy products may be helpful. Others have tried the use of strong seasonings in food, increased fluid intake, and the use of food that leaves its own taste, such as fresh fruit and hard candy. This is one of a number of symptoms that warrants further investigation of its palliative care, as it can be most distressing to the few patients who experience it.

Dysphagia   For the patient who complains of trouble swallowing, it is important to establish the cause. This may be quite apparent but sometimes is difficult to detect. Most frequently it is due to obstruction in the hypopharynx or esophagus; other causes are not uncommon.

Dysphagia due to pain from radiation-induced esophagitis may respond to oral viscous lidocaine (Xylocaine Viscous). When *Candida* esophagitis is at fault, nystatin suspension (Mycostatin 600,000 U four times per day) often provides relief. We have encountered a number of patients who have not responded to nystatin, and for these we have employed ketoconazole (Nizoral), 200 mg per day by mouth.

Aguilar et al. (1979) have reviewed the complex and somewhat specialized deglutition problems occurring in patients with head and neck cancer. Although the emphasis in that report is on rehabilitation to establish nutritional adequacy, some of the relatively sophisticated techniques that they employ are worth study by those who deal with terminally ill head and neck cancer patients.

For most patients with severe dysphagia and very advanced tumors, adequate hydration and nutrition can be maintained by patiently giving small, frequent feeding of liquids. For those with a less advanced tumor, more aggressive measures such as the passage of a feeding tube or the insertion of an intraluminal esophageal tube (e.g., Celestin) may be warranted. The use of gastrostomy or intravenous fluids is seldom called for in patients with advanced malignancy, although these measures may be helpful in a few circumstances. In handling dysphagia, there is need for individualization of treatment based upon a careful assessment of the particular situation.

Nausea and Vomiting   These symptoms can result from the patient's tumor, various medications including morphine, or factors unrelated to the patient's advanced malignancy. The underlying cause should be sought and dealt with appropriately. The liberal use of antiemetics such as prochlorperazine (Compazine) is usually the most effective measure when the underlying cause cannot be corrected. Compazine syrup is begun in a dosage of 5 mg every 4 hours and is increased up to a level of 25 mg four times per day until nausea and vomiting are satisfactorily relieved. Alternatively, 25-mg Compazine suppositories may be given two or three times per day. However, nausea and vomiting can be stubborn symptoms, and a trial of various combinations of medications may be necessary (Frytak and Moertel 1981).

Recently, some reports have been published about the use of delta-9-tetrahydrocannabinol (THC), a derivative of marijuana, for treatment of nausea and vomiting in cancer patients undergoing chemotherapy. This agent, which is presently available only for investigational purposes, has shown promise. Nausea and vomiting in the terminally ill are not only common symptoms, but are also extremely troublesome ones; they sometimes can be quite refractory to all presently available forms of treatment. Therefore, the trial of THC, or synthetic analogs, in patients not receiving chemotherapy seems warranted.

Constipation   The combination of inactivity, decreased dietary bulk, and the use of narcotics sets the stage for constipation in many terminally ill patients. The use dioctyl sodium sulfosuccinate (Colace) in dosages of 200 – 600 mg per day plus two to six tablets per day of a senna pod preparation (Senokot) generally keeps the patient free of this distressing symptom. Of course, it is important that the patient be kept as well hydrated and as active as possible. There should be prompt response to the patient's request to defecate, and it is best to avoid using bed pans. Appropriate nursing measures such as bracing the abdominal muscles and supporting the feet on a footstool are useful. When the above measures are unsuccessful, stronger laxatives such as milk of magnesia and cascara can be tried. The judicious use of suppositories and enemas can be helpful. Fecal impaction must be watched for; if it occurs, it must be dealt with in the conventional fashion.

Diarrhea   When diarrhea occurs, an underlying cause such as medication or fecal impaction should be looked for and treated appropriately. Diphenoxylate with atropine (Lomotil; two tablets four times per day) or loperamide (Imodium; 2 mg four times per day) has proved effective in patients with severe diarrhea.

Intestinal Obstruction   Planning suitable treatment for intestinal obstruction in the terminally ill requires individualization. The level and cause of obstruction, the extent of the tumor, and the general condition of the patient are all factors to be considered in the selection of appropriate therapy.

For example, when complete distal colonic obstruction occurs in a patient with relatively limited, although incurable, tumor, the performance of colostomy can provide excellent palliation. On the other hand, the patient with partial small bowel obstruction from a widely disseminated intraperitoneal tumor can often be kept quite comfortable by nonoperative means without the use of a nasogastric tube.

For some patients, pain can be controlled with adequate analgesics, as described earlier. Nausea is generally a much more bothersome symptom to the patient than is vomiting. Therefore, without the use of a nasogastric tube and intravenous fluids, the patient can be given large doses of antiemetics and stool softeners and be allowed to eat and drink. Under these circumstances, the patient will be largely free of pain and nausea but will vomit periodically while remaining surprisingly comfortable. One of our patients has described the sensation of vomiting under these circumstances as similar to that of voiding or defecating; it relieves an uncomfortable fullness. Although not an ideal situation, this method allows the patient a more comfortable demise than that which results from the performance of a futile laparotomy at which the peritoneal cavity is found seeded with extensive tumor producing multiple points of obstruction (Brown et al. 1977; Osteen et al. 1980).

Ascites   Symptomatic ascites sometimes occurs as a dominant problem relatively early in the terminal illness. In such cases aggressive conventional therapy including diuretics and paracentesis can produce considerable palliative effect. For patients with a reasonably long prognosis, peritoneovenous shunts have been reported to be valuable. Somewhat surprisingly, neither enhanced tumor spread nor disseminated intravenous coagulation have been a problem although the technique is not useful when the ascitic fluid is of high viscoscity (Souter et al. 1983). Lacey et al. (1984) have reviewed some of the other measures that can be utilized in the management of malignant ascites. Asymptomatic ascites and ascites occurring in the moribund patient do not require therapy.

Respiratory Symptoms

Foul Breath Halitosis can arise from a number of causes, ranging from oropharyngeal sepsis to intestinal obstruction. It is sometimes an early manifestation of candida infection in the upper airway. Underlying causes should be dealt with to the extent possible. Beyond that, hydrogen peroxide gargle or a mouthwash solution should be used liberally.

Cough Treatable causes of troublesome cough should be handled in conventional fashion. For example, postnasal drip should be managed in the usual way, and except for the patient with very advanced tumor, pneumonia should be treated with appropriate antibiotics.

Beyond this, several measures directed at treatment of the cough itself are useful. Adequate humidification of the air by using a vaporizer is important. Expectorants such as potassium iodide (SSKI) and guaifenesin (Robitussin) are sometimes helpful if the patient has thick, tenacious sputum. For these patients the use of mucolytic agents and bronchodilators may also be helpful, and if the patient is otherwise in reasonably good condition, physical therapy including postural drainage may be tried. Codeine alone and codeine-containing preparations such as terpin hydrate with codeine can be used as cough suppressants; so can the more potent narcotics.

As a consequence of dehydration and mouth breathing, many patients complain of dry scratchy throat as the trigger mechanism for their cough. For them adequate humidification of the air, the use of viscous lidocaine and a cough-suppressant medication can provide some relief. Hard candy and Lifesavers are also useful.

Dyspnea The causes of dyspnea that can be treated by specific therapeutic measures should be dealt with appropriately. Pleural and pericardial fluid accumulations should be drained. If pleural effusion recurs, an intracavitary sclerosing agent may be employed; we have preferred the use of tetracycline for this purpose as it has been effective in most instances and has produced less side effect than cytotoxic agents such as nitrogen mustard. If pericardial effusion recurs, creation of a pericardial window or even pericardiectomy may be considered. *The Medical Letter* ("Treatment of Malignant Pleural and Pericardial Effusion" 1981) has briefly reviewed the topic of malignant pleural and pericardial effusions. Bronchospasm should be relieved with the use of bronchodilators, and congestive heart failure should be treated in the conventional fashion. If such measures do not produce relief, provision of ample reassurance, careful positioning of the patient, use of oxygen, and administration of sedatives and narcotics can offer quite satisfactory palliation in many instances. Dexamethasone (in the dosage pattern described for weakness) has sometimes proved useful, particularly when dyspnea is associated with substantial wheezing.

Congestion   A symptom perhaps slightly different from cough and dyspnea is a deep, moist, noisy respiration associated with a rather ineffectual, nonproductive cough. It usually occurs relatively late in the patient's course and has given rise to the term "death rattle." Although usually not a source of distress to the patient, it can be quite bothersome to his or her family. We have found that 0.4 mg of scopolamine intramuscularly or one Transderm Scop topically every 72 hours usually makes the patient sound better. Placing the patient in semi-Fowler's position may help. Only when troublesome congestion occurs at an earlier stage is postural drainage suitable for treating this symptom. Rarely, oropharyngeal suction may be employed in the deeply unconscious patient for the relief of a greatly distressed family.

Hiccups   Hiccups occur occasionally in the patient with advanced malignancy. Although they are frequently due to extensive intraperitoneal or hepatic metastases, other causes that are treatable, such as gastric dilitation, should be sought and dealt with appropriately if present. In the absence of such treatable causes, hiccups can be a very refractory symptom. The simple mechanical measures such as rebreathing, carotid pressure, and pressure over the eyeballs are seldom beneficial. Amphetamine (10 mg three times per day) is occasionally successful, as is chlorpromazine (Thorazine; 25 mg three times per day), but neither of these has proved consistently effective. Even phrenic nerve block does not uniformly produce relief.

Cardiovascular Symptoms

Edema   Various factors combine to make edema a relatively common symptom among the terminally ill: inactivity, hypoproteinemia, venous obstruction, renal insufficiency, cardiac causes, and the like. The vigor of the investigation for underlying cause and the aggressiveness of treatment depend upon the severity of edema and the stage of disease. Mild swelling requires no specific treatment. When more severe edema occurs, diuretics such as furosamide (Lasix) may be employed. However, the advantages to be gained must be weighed against the disadvantages: the possiblity of aggravating disorders of fluid-electrolyte metabolism and the need for monitoring of serum potassium. Physical measures such as elevation and elastic support may be helpful.

Thrombosis   As noted, patients with advanced malignancy are prone to the development of a number of different coagulation disorders. The hypercoagulable state may be manifested by thrombosis in veins or arteries or by disseminated intravascular coagulopathy (DIC). Thrombophlebitis may be either superficial, manifested by an inflamed superficial vein, or may be deep, manifested by diffuse swelling of a limb. The manifestations of arterial thrombosis will depend, of course, upon the anatomical site. DIC is manifested by diffuse bleeding; the diagnosis can be difficult to establish.

Superficial phlebitis may be treated with appropriate analgesic plus local compresses; anticoagulants are not required. For the patient with deep vein thrombosis, a variety of factors must be considered in selecting treatment. Moore and co-workers (1981) have questioned whether conventional anticoagulant therapy is safe or effective in cancer patients. However, except for the individual with a relatively long life expectancy, venous interruption techniques are seldom suitable. The choice must be made on an individual basis.

Optimal handling of acute arterial occlusion depends upon the circumstances and location of the occlusive process and the stage of malignant disease. Mesenteric arterial occlusion, for example, usually produces extensive bowel infarction and is diagnosed late and thus is not amenable to treatment. In the limbs, proximally located thrombosis in a patient who is in generally good condition can be handled by thrombectomy, with gratifying results. However, sometimes the occlusive process is distal, in situ thrombosis in diffusely sclerotic vessels, occurring late in the course of the disease and related to low-flow states. Under such circumstances anticoagulant therapy, amputation, or simply supportive care may be the wisest approach, depending upon the patient's general condition.

Unfortunately, DIC usually responds definitively only to irradication of the causative focus, an option not open to the patient with advanced metastatic malignancy. The use of fresh frozen plasma and heparin, which in other circumstances might be employed as a temporizing measure, is seldom of value. Thus, when DIC occurs, it almost always is a terminal event.

Urinary Tract Symptoms

Symptomatic Urinary Tract Infection   Patients with symptoms of frequency, dysuria, and the like from urinary tract infection should be dealt with in the conventional fashion: urine culture and the prompt institution of appropriate antibiotic therapy. Urinary tract analgesic agents such as phenazopyridine hydrochloride (Pyridium; 200 mg, three times per day by mouth) can be employed to relieve symptoms of pain, burning, urgency, and frequency associated with irritation of the lower urinary tract.

Incontinence   For the patient with urinary incontinence, Foley catheter or "Texas catheter" can be employed in the usual way.

Urinary Retention   In the late stages of terminal illness from malignant disease, urinary retention due to either obstruction or neurogenic factors can be handled quite satisfactorily by bladder drainage utilizing either the urethral or suprapubic route. Earlier in the patient's course, when obstructive uropathy or hemorrhage may be of long duration, a variety of urinary diversion procedures can contribute significantly to palliation (Perinetti 1982).

Bladder Spasms   The intense pain caused by spasm of the detrusor muscle can be caused by tumor, radiation, indwelling catheter, or cystitis. Anxiety often is an exacerbating factor. A treatable underlying cause should be dealt with and adequate analgesics should be provided. In addition, drugs that reduce detrusor sensitivity, such as phenazopyridine, nonsteroidal anti-inflammatory agents, and anticholinergic drugs, may be helpful.

Neurological Symptoms

Depression   In handling the depression that is so common in dying patients, the provision of simple psychological support by members of the hospice care team can often be extremely effective. This, combined with relief of pain and the easing of some of the social and financial burdens, can improve the patient's mood and should be the first step in the treatment of depression.

The use of tricyclic antidepressants is frequently beneficial; 50 mg of doxepin (Sinequan) at bedtime has been our choice because amitriptyline (Elavil) sometimes causes hallucinations and agitation. Cocaine (10 mg by mouth three times per day) may be employed for its euphoric effect, but side effects, particularly in elderly patients, can be troublesome. Methylphenidate (Ritalin), in the dosage pattern described for anorexia, has been utilized for short-term depressive reactions with some success. Psychiatric consultation has rarely been necessary for our hospice patients; it usually has been required for a psychiatric condition that antedated the terminal illness.

Insomnia   Sleeplessness is a common problem in the chronically ill. It can range from a mildly bothersome complaint to a devastating problem. In its severe form it can contribute to the patient's overall debility; its effect on the family can be the factor that tips the scale to make home care impossible, necessitating hospitalization. In addition, daytime sleeping interferes with psychosocial support and disintegrates family interactions.

For mild insomnia it is helpful for the patient and his or her family to understand that loss of sleep is not unexpected and that in its mild form it is not harmful. The availability of nighttime activities such as reading, television, and painting can be helpful. For more severe insomnia, drugs can be employed. The tricyclic agents given at bedtime (as described for depression) can be helpful. Diphenhydramine (Benadryl), hydroxyzine (Vistaril), triazolam (Halcion), or flurazepam (Dalmane) may be useful. It should be remembered, however, that barbituates and benzodiazapines such as Dalmane and Halcion may contribute to depression.

In attempting to relieve insomnia, communication is very important. There are a variety of conditions that may contribute to sleeplessness: pain, incontinence, caffeine, for example. Elimination of a causative factor may obviate the use of potent hypnotics.

Dementia Dementia in the terminally ill patient with advanced malignancy can be due to a number of factors. Treatable causes such as medications or correctable metabolic disturbances should be sought and dealt with. If hypoxia is felt to play a role, the use of oxygen can be tried; if this does not produce improvement relatively quickly, it should be discontinued.

When there is no treatable cause of dementia, attention should be directed primarily to combating restlessness and agitation and at support of the close family members for whom this is a particularly trying symptom. Haloperidol (Haldol; 0.5 mg three times per day) has been useful on occasion when there is little agitation. When agitation is the predominant problem, chlorpromazine (Thorazine; 25 mg three times per day) can be tried.

Paralysis Palliative care for local paralysis, paraplegia, and quadriplegia must be individualized. The extent of tumor spread and life expectancy are the major determinants for the institution of rehabilitative measures. If there is reason to believe that aggressive physiotherapy will restore function for a time, it should be pursued. However, for most terminally ill patients with paralysis, rehabilitation is not a consideration. In such circumstances attention should be directed to the provision of comfort and the avoidance of skin breakdown.

An area requiring special attention is metastatic disease of the vertebral column with or without spinal cord and nerve root compression. Pain and potential, developing, and established neurological deficits are all sources of concern in providing palliation. Onofrio (1980) has addressed the interesting and challenging topic of metastatic disease to the spine. The considerations in managing such patients can be rather complex.

Usually, the first evidence of spinal metastasis is bone pain, although occasionally asymptomatic metastases are detected on x-ray. In addition to direct symptomatic treatment of the pain, consideration must be given to the matter of antitumor therapy to the metastasis. This can be in the form of radiation, chemotherapy, or hormonal manipulation. Furthermore, at this point some thought must be given to the potential for spinal cord or nerve root involvement. A decision must be made as to whether or not a myelogram should be done in the absence of neurological findings. In other words, the difficult issue of prophylactic palliation must be faced.

In this connection, in addition to other factors such as extent of tumor, general condition of the patient, and life expectancy, the source of the primary tumor must be taken into account. Certain tumors, such as prostatic and breast cancers and multiple meyloma, usually have a longer interval between the onset of back pain and the development of cord compression than do lymphomas or tumors of lung, colonic, or renal origin.

Ordinarily, we employ radiation therapy in the treatment of vertebral metastases occurring relatively early in the patient's terminal illness. We have not routinely performed a myelogram nor even obtained neurosurgical consultation. The latter is usually sought at the first signs of neurological deficit. A decision regarding further management is then made jointly between the neurosurgeon and the hospice physician. In those cases in which the potential for spinal cord involvement is high, neurosurgical consultation is sought in the absence of neurological findings.

Although we mostly have been satisfied with our approach to the problems of metastatic disease to the spine, we recognize that it is an area deserving further study.

Skin Problems

Decubitus Ulcers In the course of the patient's routine daily care, it should be remembered that the terminally ill are particularly susceptible to developing troublesome decubitus ulcers. Prevention is more effective than cure; the earlier a decubitus ulcer is detected the more satisfactorily it can be handled. Because no totally satisfactory means of handling an established decubitus has been agreed upon, and because our thinking with respect to its management is in the same evolutionary stage as that of others, we will make no specific recommendations here regarding decubitus care. We have a routine that has proved relatively successful, but we have no reason to believe that we have found the ultimate answer to this vexing problem. Constant alertness to the potential for development of decubitus ulcers, provision of good nursing care for their prevention, early recognition, and prompt institution of the locally favored method of treatment are really all we have to offer. Sometimes an enterostomal therapist can be helpful in managing decubitus ulcers.

Pruritus For some patients with advanced malignancy, particularly those with unrelieved obstructive jaundice, pruritus can be a maddening symptom. Insofar as possible, underlying causes of itching such as dehydration, skin rashes, and contact dermatitis should be eliminated.

Good general skin care is imperative. Emollient creams and methylated lotions often provide relief. Pharmacological agents with presumed antipruritic action, such as trimeprazine (Temaril; 2.5 mg four times per day), can be tried; they may be helpful in a few instances. Sometimes a corticosteroid (as described for weakness) produces some relief.

Alopecia Although alopecia rarely occurs as a manifestation of advanced malignancy alone, it is not an uncommon concomitant of chemotherapy. Though generally a temporary phenomenon, it can be a most distressing one to the patient and his or her family. There is nothing that can be done to prevent it after the administration of the numerous chemotherapeutic agents that produce it. Therefore, it is important for the patient and family to recognize this problem as choices are made about the use of antitumor therapy. Some of our patients have pointed out that it is as much the "ratty" appearance of the hair as the baldness itself that is distressing. For many patients the services of an excellent wigmaker are a worthwhile investment. However, this doesn't solve all of the problems: one of our male patients was unable to overcome his instinct to remove his "hat" during the playing of the national anthem.

Fungating Growths, Draining Fistulas, and Similar Lesions Appropriate care is critical to the proper management of the terminally ill patient with a seminecrotic, fungating growth on the body surface, a fistula, or a malignant ulceration. An enterostomal therapist may be of assistance.

As with decubitus ulcers, there is no standardized method that is uniformly effective for an ulcerated or fungating mass on the skin. The objectives, of course, are to keep the exposed growth clean, dry, and odor free while avoiding the development of frank infection and hemorrhage. In accomplishing this we have found hydrogen peroxide solutions and mild oxidizing agents such as dilute Dakin's solution quite helpful. In a good review of this topic, Wood (1980) has suggested the use of acetic acid and some of the agents used for burn therapy, such as mafenide acetate. We have found substances such as silver nitrate and potassium permanganate messy and of little use. If bloody oozing does occur, the topical application of a vasoconstrictor such as Adrenalin or a hemostatic agent such as Gelfoam may be helpful.

Consideration must always be given to the role of local or systemic antitumor therapy. Electrocoagulation, cryotherapy, excision, radiotherapy, chemotherapy, and hormonal therapy are all approaches that should be considered; a decision should be made on the basis of the individual circumstances in the particular case. On the extremities excisional therapy may require amputation, which in some situations can be a most rewarding maneuver.

Intestinal, urinary tract, and bronchial fistulas can be the source of considerable discomfort and may require imaginative local care. Particularly troublesome are fistulas in the perineal area, which may originate from either the urinary or intestinal tract. In such instances a choice must be made between local care, which is often quite unsatisfactory, and performance of a urinary or fecal diversion procedure. In this connection we have found Turnbull's (1978) technique of diverting loop colostomy very useful. It permits adequate diversion by a procedure that is of less magnitude than the ordinary diverting colostomy.

References

Abeloff, MD (ed): *Complications of Cancer: Diagnosis and Management*. Johns Hopkins University Press, Baltimore, 1979.

Aguilar NV, Olson MD, Shedd DP: Rehabilitation of deglutition problems in patients with head and neck cancer. *Am J Surg* 138:501, 1979.

Bingham CA; A study of the relationship between perceived needs of dying patients and the needs perceived by nurses providing care to these patients. Masters thesis dissertation, Catholic University, Washington DC, 1977.

Black P: Management of pain. *In Abeloff MD (ed): Complications of Cancer: Diagnosis and Management*. Hopkins University Press, Baltimore, 1979.

Blumgart LH, et al.: Surgical approaches to cholangiocarcinoma at the confluence of the hepatic ducts. *Lancet* 1:66, 1984.

Brown PW, Terz JJ, Lawrence W, Blievernicht, SW: Survival after palliative surgery for advanced intraabdominal cancer. *Am J Surg* 1:66, 1984.

Cameron JL, Broe P, Zuidema GD: Proximal bile duct tumors — Surgical management with silastic transhepatic biliary stents. *Ann Surg* 196:412, 1982.

Caprini JA, Sener SF: Altered coagulability in cancer patients. *CA* May/June, 32:162, 1982.

Dietz JH: *Rehabilitation Oncology*. John Wiley & Sons, Inc. 1981

Ferrara JJ, Martin EW, Carey LC: Morbidity of emergency operation in patients with metastatic cancer receiving chemotherapy. *Surgery* 92:605, 1982.

Frytak S, Moertel CG: Management of nausea and vomiting in the cancer patient. *JAMA* 245:393, 1981.

Harvey RF, Jellinek HM, Habeck RV: Cancer Rehabilitation *JAMA* 247:2127, 1982.

Jones RS, et al.: The combined use of percutaneous transhepatic drainage and irradiation for carcinoma of the extrahepatic bile ducts. *Contemporary Surgery* 22:59, 1983.

Kenton C: *The Care of Patients with Severe Chronic Pain in Terminal Illness*. Literature Search, National Library of Medicine, Bethesda MD, 1983.

King TC, Zimmerman, JM: Gastrostomies in patients with incurable cancer. *Am Surg* 31:251, 1965.

King TC, Ramos AG, Zimmerman JM: Surgical palliation for lung cancer. *Am J Surg* 109:432, 1965.

Lacy JH, Wieman TJ, Shively EH: Management of malignant ascites. *Surg Gynecol Obstet* 159:397, 1984.

McGivney WT, Crooks GM: The care of patients with severe chronic pain in terminal illness. *JAMA* 251:1182,1984.

Moore FD, et al.: Anticoagulants, venous thromboembolism and the cancer patient. *Arch Surg* 116:405, 1981.

Mount BM: *Palliative Care Service: October 1976 Report*. Royal Victoria Hospital/ McGill University, Montreal, 1976.

Onofrio BM: Metastatic disease to the spine. Mayo Clin Proc 55:460, 1980.

Osteen RT, Guyton S, Steele G, Wilson RE: Malignant intestinal obstruction. *Surgery* 87:611, 1980.

Oster MW, Vizel M, Turgeon LR: Pain of terminal cancer patients. *Arch Intern Med* 138:1801, 1978.

Perinetti ET: Palliative urinary diversion. *Surg Clin North Am* 62:1025, 1982.

Poretz DM, et al.: Intravenous antibiotic therapy in an outpatient setting. *JAMA* 248:336, 1982.

Potter JF: A challenge for the hospice movement. *N Engl J Med* 302:53, 1980.

Reuler JB, Girard DE, Nardone DA: The chronic pain syndrome: Misconceptions in management. *Ann Intern Med* 93:588, 1980.

Saunders CM: *Management of Terminal Disease*. Yearbook, London, 1978.

Saunders CM: Principles of symptom control in terminal care. *Med Clin North Am* 66:1169, 1982.

Shimm DS, Logue GL, Maltbie AA, Dugan S: Medical management of chronic cancer pain. *JAMA* 241:2408, 1979.

Silberman AW: Surgical debulking of tumors *Surg Gynecol Obstet* 155:577, 1982.

Smith RA: Surgery in treatment of locally advanced lung carcinoma. *Thorax* 18:21, 1963.

Souter RG, Tarin D, Kettlewell MGW: Peritoneo-venous shunts in the management of malignant ascites *Br J Surg* 70:478, 1983.

Spitzer WO, et al.: Measuring the quality of life of cancer patients. *J Chronic Dis* 34:585, 1981.

Storm FK, Morton DL: Treatment of metastatic disease. *Adv Surg* 13:33, 1979.

Sugarbaker PH, et al.: Quality of life assessment of patients in extremity sarcoma clinical trials. *Surgery* 91:17, 1982.

Theologides A: Asthenia in cancer. *Am J Med* 73:1, 1982.

Treatment of malignant pleural and pericardial effusion. *The Medical Letter* 23:59, 1981.

Turnbull RA:*Diverting Loop Transverse Colostomy*. Current Surgical Techniques, Schering, Kenilworth NJ, 1979.

Twycross RG: Clinical experience with diamorphine in advanced malignant disease. *Int J Clin Pharmacol Ther Toxicol* 9:184, 1974.

Twycross RG, Lack SA: *Symptom Control in Far Advanced Cancer: Pain Relief*. Pitman Publishing, London, 1984.

Twycross RG, Lack SA: *Therapeutics in Terminal Cancer*. Pitman Publishing, London, 1984.

Wall R: Cancer pain management. *Infections in Surgery*, p 195, March 1985.

Warshaw AL, Carey RW, Robinson DR: Control of fever associated with visceral cancers by indomethocin. *Surgery* 89:414, 1981.

Wilkes E: *The Dying Patient — Medical Management of Incurable and Terminal Illness*. George A Bogden and Sons, Ridgewood NJ, 1982.

Wilson CB, Fulton DS, Seager ML: Suppportive management of the patient with malignant brain tumor. *JAMA* 244:1249, 1980.

Wood DK: The draining malignant ulceration. *JAMA* 244:820, 1980.

Zimmerman JM, King RC: Use of the Souttar tube in the management of advanced esophageal cancer. *Ann Surg* 169:867, 1969.

Chapter 4

Psychosocial Issues in the Care of the Terminally Ill

Milton Buschman

A number of psychosocial issues emerge as the patient and the family deal with impending death. These issues include an appreciation of the basic human condition as it relates to mortality, denial and stages of realization, the problems faced by the dying patient in the stages of fatal illness, the problems faced by the family of the terminal patients, the physician's experience, and bereavement.

Death and the Human Condition

Weisman (1972a) explores the concept of the primary paradox, hope, and the condition for appropriate death in the face of terminal illness. On the one hand, man intellectually acknowledges the universality of death, but "he cannot imagine his own death." Other people may die, but our own death, perhaps, can be somewhat avoided. Consequently, the occasion of our terminality finds us surprised, poorly prepared, even numbed. How can the world continue without us? Yet hope is not seen as based simply on avoiding death, but rather on our belief in "the desirability of survival." While originating from a positive self-image, with the notion that we have at least some modicum of influence on the external world, hope ultimately is determined more by the acceptance of self. Ironically, psychiatric patients with a markedly depleted self-esteem appear more hopeless than dying patients, experiencing their suffering as if from the midst of an endless black hole. It is not simply survival but "significant survival" that is pertinent, as it is only the latter that contains the human personal aspect beyond the mere continued functioning of organs.

Weisman (1972a) cites three factors that he feels constitute significant survival: biological survival, competent behavior, and responsible conduct:

> Biological survival in the course of serious illness means physical continuity, pain relief, reduction of suffering, and adaptation to diminished strength and capacity. Competent behavior means that, to some extent a sick person can choose the way in which he solves daily problems and carries out his customary tasks. Responsible conduct is determined by how closely a patient's competence permits him to fulfill the directives and avoid the prohibitions dictated by his ego ideal.

Ego ideal is the part of the personality that contains the goals and the aims for the self. It usually refers to the conscious or unconscious identification of significant figures. It emphasizes what we feel we should do or be.

Physicians, historically, have been imbued with magical powers. In turn, they participate in mankind's universal fear of death and especially in our cultural tendency to view death as somehow bad. Thus, their preconceptions can be generationally passed along.

Weisman (1972a) lists seven popular *fallacies* about the dying used by doctors to defend themselves from involvement with death:

1. Only suicidal and psychotic people are willing to die. Even when death is inevitable, no one wants to die.
2. Fear of death is the most natural and basic fear of man. The closer he comes to death, the more intense the fear becomes.
3. Reconciliation with death and preparation for death are impossible. Therefore, say as little as possible to dying people, turn their questions aside, and use any means to deny, dissimulate, and avoid open confrontation.
4. Dying people do not really want to know what the future holds. Otherwise, they would ask more questions. To force a discussion or to insist upon unwelcome information is risky. The patient might lose all hope. He might commit suicide, become very depressed, or even die more quickly.
5. After speaking with family members, the doctor should treat the patient as long as possible. Then, when further benefit seems unlikely, the patient should be left alone, except for relieving pain. He will then withdraw, die in peace, without further disturbance and anguish.
6. It is reckless, if not downright cruel, to inflict unnecessary suffering upon the patient or his family. The patient is doomed; nothing can really make any difference. Survivors should accept the futility, but realize that they will get over the loss.
7. Physicians can deal with all phases of the dying process because of their scientific training and clinical experience. The emotional and psychological sides of dying are vastly overemphasized. Consultation with psychiatrists and social workers is unnecessary. The clergy might be called upon, but only because death is near. The doctor has no further obligation after the patient's death.

For most of us sickness is of the temporary variety, even though painful or ill timed. If an illness continues unabated, however, independent functioning in everyday activities is jeopardized, if not sacrificed entirely; then the issues of mere survival can become the central focus. Thus one must deal not only with the life threatening illness, but also maintenance of a viable sense of self in light of progressive deterioration, with most of the activities lost that previously had given pleasure and definition to one's life.

Denial

In the technical, strictly psychoanalytical sense, denial refers to "the defensive distortions of one's perception of some aspect of one's environment, of what is usually called external reality" (Brenner, 1982). A more colloquial sense of the meaning includes a defensive distortion or disavowal of one's own wishes, affects, memories, and the like. Since every defense denies something, denial in the latter sense has no special or technical meaning and simply becomes a synonym for defense.

Patients with terminal illness may exhibit any one of three types of denial. The first type includes denial of the "facts of the illness." For example, the patient will deny the diagnosis. The second type is a denial by the patient of the "implication and extensions of the illness." Here the patient acknowledges having a tumor but sees the accompanying symptoms as unrelated to that fact. The third type represents a denial of mortality itself. The diagnosis and progress of the illness are accepted, but the patient speaks as if somehow he or she will recover. Most terminal patients, regardless of how recently diagnosed, show only the second and third types of denial. Very infrequently is there a patient that appears completely free of denial. Patients seem to oscillate in the degree of denial versus acceptance, but generally denial gives way to acceptance. A persistent, marked degree of denial is often fostered by fear of alienation and endangerment. Also, if others reinforce denial, then alienation may increase, with more and more withdrawal by the patient (Weisman 1972b).

Elizabeth Kubler-Ross (1969) is well known for her enumeration of the five stages that a terminally ill patient tends to experience sequentially: denial, anger, bargaining, depression, acceptance. While these may be common experiences, Kastenbaum (1975) feels that "clinical research concerning the dying process by other investigators does not clearly support the existence of the five stages or of any universal form of staging."

Stages of Fatal Illness

Weisman (1972b) outlines three stages of fatal illness. Stage I consists of the time from the onset of symptoms until the diagnosis is made. It is here that the majority of the psychosocial problems focus around delay and denial. Most people are not under medical treatment at this time, and friends and family may need to forcefully insist on medical consultation. Stage II is the period between diagnosis and the beginning of terminal decline. Most of the medical treatment is performed during this period. The psychological problems are often understood in the context of shifts in the spectrum between denial and acceptance. In Stage III we see the period in which active treatment appears to have less and less usefulness and purpose. The treatment then tends to shift from cure to symptomatic relief and care. Physicians are apt to withdraw at this point. Simultaneously, patients are faced with the dual prospect of having to relinquish much control to others and of no longer being. "Stage III is the sickness until death." Weisman (1972b) reminds us that

Salient psychosocial problems occur at any stage of fatal illness, and we must realize that such problems not only differ from stage to stage but also from person to person, depending on the diagnosis, age, social and cultural resources, interpersonal affiliations, and disengagements, economic independence, and ethnic customs, as well as upon physical and personal incapacity. We cannot oversimplify, nor should we overgeneralize even though three stages of fatal illness can be outlined.

He continues,

At each stage, the psychosocial problems of the patient's potential survivors should be anticipated. These are not only general problems of bereavement, but also highly practical issues, such as contending with the disruption of households, financial problems, critical communication, or what to tell children. Planning is both long-and short-range. Bereavement does not start at the moment of death, but at any stage when a significant person realizes the loss is inevitable and that drastic change cannot be avoided.

The person with a terminal illness faces a number of problems that force catastrophic changes in his or her living pattern (Garfield 1978). The first change often involves having to give up one's work. Hence one moves from an independent role to a sick person role in the midst of a society that places heavy emphasis on the state of independence. Second, physical changes lead to need for more and more assistance from others. This can range from being driven to the doctor's office to complete personal care. Obviously, one's self-esteem is at high risk when one is forced to assume the infant's position once again. Third, increasing physical discomfort and symptoms may occur that make difficult even the most ordinary activity, such as breathing, walking, eating, and talking. A fourth problem stems from reactivation of numerous and varied unresolved conflicts. The earliest universal calamities of childhood include feared and/or perceived object loss, loss of love, castration, and superego demands and prohibitions (Brenner 1982). Although these appear sequentially, each persists once it has appeared and continues to play an important role in psychic life thereafter. As a result of psychological regression during this terminal period, the resolution of these early calamities can become undone, leading to rather primitive and inappropriate emotional responses. In addition, ongoing unresolved conflicts and tensions between the patient and those around him in his adult world can become exacerbated.

The patient's anger is one of the more difficult responses with which the hospital staff of the caregivers in general must deal. This anger may represent the patient's searching for some explanation, any explanation, for the terrible thing that is happening. The explanations considered may include "a random and meaningless universe or worse, a tyrannical and capricious god, operating without plan or with malevolent intent" (Garfield 1978). Then, too, patients may vent their anger against a "whimsical death sentence." However, it is important to observe whether the anger also is directed to the hospital staff, who may be perceived as ignoring the patient's needs, or to the doctor and his or her diagnosis and treatment, or to relatives who may be withdrawing. Not infrequently, the anger represents a defense from the various fears, if not terror, that the patient may be experiencing. It is usually helpful to assist the patient in articulating this anger and in clarifying, with as much specificity as possible, the issues that have aroused it. Anger is a natural, potentially adaptive affective response and should not be summarily categorized as inappropriate or pathological (Garfield 1978).

Depression represents another common response of patients to a terminal illness. Most probably the patient has a depleted self-esteem, often due to repeated hospitalizations, real or perceived emotional withdrawal by friends and relatives, impersonal care by hospital staff, and frequently severe financial distress. Generally, when one sits with the patient a sufficient length of time to obtain the details, one or more of these complaints will be voiced. Some of the circumstances, then can be corrected or improved. Preparatory depression is seen as basically an anticipation of the threatened "loss of oneself." Rather frequent reactions include loss of appetite, general irritability, nightmares, and apathy. This is actually viewed as a mourning period. Much can be achieved by simply being with the patient. Sometimes it is helpful to assist the patient in coming to a "sense of closure (i.e., a sense of completing life's unfinished business — personal, interpersonal, spiritual, and financial)" (Garfield 1978).

The patient's degree of acceptance of impending death varies and, indeed, can often fluctuate, depending on the amount of pain, state of consciousness, and mood, as well as other emotional factors. Many people, particularly the elderly, may have a sense of the timeliness of their own death. They may well feel a completion of their life's work, be it economic, emotional, religious, or interpersonal. Perhaps it is more possible while dying than at any other time in one's life cycle for personal change and maturation to occur (Garfield 1978).

Terminal Patients — Psychosocial Management and Appropriate Intervention

The purpose of psychosocial management of terminally ill patients is to prevent or at least control "secondary suffering." Weisman (1972b) lists the following symptoms exhibited by dying patients: impairment of self-esteem, endangerment, annihilation anxiety, and alienation anxiety. Self-esteem impairment is expressed as heightened feelings of worthlessness, avoidance of usual interests, and an excessive propensity to play back the perceived staff's expectations. Endangerment represents excessive regression. This regression may take the form of hallucinations,

projection (an unconscious defensive maneuver in which the emotionally unaccept-
able in the self is unconsciously rejected and attributed or projected to others), and
marked denial. Even though few terminal patients actually attempt suicide, implications of such may appear in the guise of a cavalier attitude towards one's
symptoms or an excessive concern with tangential, if not totally irrelevant issues.
Annihilation anxiety is defined as a fear of dying and disintegration. Frequently
there is an impairment of reality testing as well. Usually the patients don't voice the
fear directly but rather express complaints and ideas that in turn clearly reveal the
annihilation anxiety. Weisman (1972b) cites some instructive examples of annihilation anxiety:

This food doesn't taste right. Don't they care what they feed me anymore?" "I'm
just a number to these people here. Why do they want to get rid of me? Do they
think I'm dying or something?" "People don't make sense. They say I'm sick and
I've got to believe them." I'm an old woman; I wish they would leave me alone
to die in peace. But they seem to want to drive me crazy, first!"

He continues

The emphasis upon impersonality is almost diagnostic. The staff and family
become "they" or "those people," just as the patient fears becoming only a
number or a thing. Fear of losing sanity means fear of losing whatever makes
sense and becoming nothing at all. "Doctor, I look in the mirror every morning
and see my face hanging on the bones. Everything I do goes wrong, nothing
works right anymore. What is becoming of me anyway?" Most dying patients
wish to talk about their situation, but our own annihilation-anxiety may cause us
to withdraw.

Interestingly, Annas (1974) cites seven studies that point out that approximately
90% of all patients interviewed preferred to know their diagnosis, even if it were terminal. Correspondingly 60% to 90% of their physicians opposed telling them.

With respect to the alienation anxiety, Weisman (1972b) states the following:

Alienation-anxiety stems from fear of separation, especially separation from
key supports and regarding activities. It is important to appreciate that much of
one's personality is attached to things in the world and that we die not only *from*
illness but also *to* many other activities that generate our sense of being alive.
Alienation refers to both major and minor losses, partial worries about his or her
home, job, or children; and as life ebbs away, "the future is an illusion."

We should keep in mind that no rules are carved in stone and that dying is an individual matter. Nevertheless, Weisman (1972b) lists a number of helpful reminders
for the therapist:

Accept the terminal patient according to what he would be like *without* the illness and disease. Otherwise we may fall victim to a tendency to confuse the
person or the patient with the disease, lesion, or symptoms.

Make allowances for the deterioration and disability caused by illnesses. But
this should not mean supporting regressive defenses.

Permit, encourage the patient to talk about how illness has changed him. But
emphasize the patient that is sick, not disease in the abstract.

Be sure you understand the difference between disease, fatal sickness, and the sickness unto death (terminality itself).

Ask the patient about possessions and pursuits that meant the most during the patient's healthy life. This includes both factors that supported his ego ideals and self-esteem and factors that made him feel discouraged, demoralized, or defeated.

Preservation of the highest practical communication and behavior also preserves self-esteem. This is even more important than the fact of illness itself.

Monitor your own feelings: You are not immune to denial, dissimulation, and antipathy, and fears of personal annihilation. Do not be ashamed to admit that caring for the dying is, itself, exposure to endangerment. Therefore, do not hesitate to enlist the assistance of significant key persons, and other kinds of support.

Safe conduct requires acceptance, clarity, candor, compassion, and mutual accessibility.

Time your confrontations to meet what is relevant to the moment. Do not rush to talk about death or to underscore the gloomiest side of the illness, nor should you persist with empty optimism when facts no longer justify it.

Unless a patient's physical condition and state of consciousness have compromised his judgment, do not exclude him from decisions and information about illness.

While we do not allow the family to make decisions for the patient, we encourage decisions with the patient, since he will yield control to others as the illness progresses.

Do not hesitate to assess the specific changes the death will bring the family. The optimal attitude toward the terminal situation is one of compassionate objectivity. A therapist who is stringently clinical is scarcely a therapist, but a technician. If he becomes a surrogate mourner he is not very helpful, since he displays his helplessness. The therapist remains sufficiently detached to be the intermediary between family and the other professional staff, without usurping the perogatives of either.

Help survivors to accept the inevitable death, but do not force a theory of bereavement and mourning upon anyone. In addition to bereavement, families may need help with the practical problems of readjustment to the altered life.

Recognize signs of iatrogenic distortions and psychosocial complications that the terminal situation creates. False hopes, displacement of interest to illusory or to the trivial, withdrawal of personal concern, and premature burial are but a few signs of iatrogenic problems.

The qualified therapist for the terminally ill is not defined as much by professional degrees or areas of specialization as by an ability to truly be with the patient. Those therapists who assume primary responsibility for the safe conduct and management of the terminally ill patient need to be aware of their own biases and distortions. If we are experiencing too much despair, it may suggest our own unrealistic expectations. On the other hand, if we feel that we are working in vain, more than likely we are contending with our own narcissistic conflicts. To be a significant figure does not require either omnipotence (all powerful) or omniscience (all knowing). Therapists will be most effective when they see themselves functioning as an important part of the psychosocial picture and consider the main task to be assisting patients to "die their own deaths. An appropriate death, if such exists, is, after all, not an ideal death. Rather an appropriate death is one that a person might choose, had he a choice" (Weisman 1972b).

Garfield (1978) reminds us that to be effective supports for the dying patient we must:

1. Realize that role models appropriate to laboratory science are largely inappropriate to the effective emotional support of patients and families facing life-threatening illness. That is, we are emotionally involved with our patients and we need to be able to discuss this involvement both with our patients and our colleagues in order to maximize the supportive nature of these basically interdependent relationships.
2. Recognize that the psychosocial aspects of patient care require a great deal more than "hand holding." Almost without exception, physicians who take the psychological and social issues surrounding life-threatening illness seriously can develop a real mastery of this increasingly important aspect of patient care.
3. Examine carefully physician attitudes concerning death and the dying patient and realize that when it comes to a subjective understanding of the nature of the dying process most patients know a great deal more than those who care for them.

Garfield (1978) feels we use a set of faulty operational assumptions in our attempt to understand the emotional realities of terminal patients:

1. We rely on summary information about the patient's emotional world, that is, notes in the chart or brief word-of-mouth explanations, and on modal or normative data.
2. Our values as health professionals are most firmly footed in middle-class thinking that makes it difficult to comprehend cross-cultural variation and value systems.
3. We are unable to effectively incorporate or interpret experiential and behavioral extremes in a meaningful fashion.
4. We have great difficulty dealing with emotional expression, for example, extreme anger, long-term depression, and so on; the somewhat presumptuous yet frequently invoked assessment of the patient's chosen form of expression as *inappropriate affect* is often a signal of our inability to cope.
5. We attempt to deal reasonably with what is most often an unreasonable life situation.

Garfield (1978) suggests the following outline as useful in determining the psychosocial needs of terminal patients:

1. With the assistance of the patient, define the major areas of emotional distress.
2. Respond to the patient's request for information with an honest, complete, and accurate presentation of the major aspects of illness and treatment.

3. Inform the patient's family of the status of his health so the family members can assume their rightful status as members of the treatment team.
4. Make it possible for the patient to be aware of staff expectations concerning treatment, patient-staff relationships, etc., and conversely be aware of patient expectations.
5. Always compare your perceptions of the patient and his situation with those of your colleagues. It is hazardous to make unilateral judgments about a person's emotional reality.
6. Remember that psychosocial evaluation, like medical appraisal, is a continuous process. Two innovations that have proven successful in maintaining ongoing evaluations are (a) the institution of interdisciplinary psychosocial rounds, the specific purpose of which is to evaluate staff success in meeting the emotional needs of all patients (the option of inviting patients to talk to staff about how to best care for them has been a successful aspect of these rounds); and (b) the use of a psychosocial log in which all health providers may record their feelings and thoughts on various aspects of working with the seriously ill patients. This log can serve as a catalyst for discussion during psychosocial rounds.

When therapists are able to listen carefully and respond to patients in their terminal setting, it sometimes provides a unique opportunity. Patients' usual defenses may be put aside at this time, allowing them to deal in a most authentic manner with their here and now (Schmale 1974). Garfield suggests the use of a patient advocate or companion to be available for each patient. He sees this as offsetting a perhaps unconscious attitude the therapist may have that in some way equates *professional* with being correct and *patient* with being incorrect. Garfield also discusses certain unique aspects of thanatological work. First, the goals are different. It is a time-limited effort and the goals are considered more finite. The overriding goal is to provide psychological comfort. There is no specific measure of personal insight or self-knowledge that a patient must have. Surely everyone's life is incomplete. Also the rules are seen as different. For example, the degree of professional distance may vary: the depth of the relationship may well become more intense between therapist and patient than the usual guidelines for psychotherapy might recommend. While it should be psychotherapeutic, it may in fact not be psychotherapy in the familiar sense of the word. Doing psychotherapy with the terminally ill person may have aspects of the usual psychotherapy but may well include other more general aspects of human interaction. Then, too, therapy continues until interrupted by death. There is no plan for termination of therapy. It is also suggested that the main focus be on "benign intervention." The dying patient is the one that sets the pace. Here the emphasis is on the therapist's continued presence. It should also be kept in mind that denial will be present, not simply as a stage of dying, but rather as a universal aspect of the dying process. One should not be surprised to find it surfacing throughout the dying period. Finally, the importance of the therapist having a good support system for him- or herself cannot be underestimated. The work is intense;

the therapist too is vulnerable and bereaved as the patient dies. The support systems should include outside pleasant activities and interests, vacations, friends, relatives, and understanding peers.

Other techniques or approaches also have been suggested for the therapist (Peretz 1972):

1. To help the patient come to value the quality of companionship and close relationship, not for the length of its duration but for the quality of inner experiences.

2. To attend dressing changes by the surgeon as he cares for the patients who are being "eaten away" by their disease, thus smelling and accepting the patients' odors as a reality and not repugnant experiences to be avoided.

3. To concentrate with the patient on the positive in addition to the approaches described above. This means that living, the 'doing,' and includes allowing that there are still possibilities for life and helping the patient discover them, such as extra flowers, a book, someone to talk to, extra company, knowing who is coming to visit.

4. To set up a therapeutic atmosphere in the ward or room (patients seem to do better when they eat in a common room, when one patient brings in a tray to the bedside of another, when reasonable human demands are made upon a patient by the staff rather than allowing him to retreat.)

The Dying Patient's Family

Maddison and Raphael (1972) suggest understanding the problem by considering the family under three categories: individual family members, the family group, and the family in its relationship to society.

The reactions of the individual family members suggest certain pairings. They include marital partners, the parent and dying child, the child and dying parent, and finally the sibling-to-sibling relationship. These reactions can range from quite healthy to markedly pathological. Regarding marital partners, numerous studies have shown that there is an increase in morbidity and mortality in the survivor, widow or widower. Conflict may be mobilized in the family member for a number of reasons. The dependency needs of the family member are quite possibly threatened; this is particularly true of a child. Reactions may be numerous, including a variety of overt psychiatric symptoms, as well as depression and somatic complaints. Aggression may be expressed as dependency needs cease to be gratified. However, there also may be numerous types of aggressive fantasies toward the dying person. In addition, a significant amount of hostility may have accumulated as a result of caring for the terminal person over a period of time, especially if the nature of the care were particularly disagreeble. Then, too, a number of sexual conflicts may occur. For example, if one has experienced prior feelings of sexual inadequacy, these feelings may become conscious by identification with the dying patient. If there is a potential loss of the parent of the same sex, there may be a reactivation of oedipal issues, including prior hostile fantasies toward the parent, with concomitant guilt. Of course, for children this issue is potentially more damaging because they are actually in the midst of experiencing the universal calamities of childhood. Hence the potential parental loss threatens to interfere with sufficient resolution of these preoedipal and oedipal issues. Then, too, dealing with the patient's pain may arouse sadomasochistic feelings. Finally, the surviving spouse may well have to contend with his or her own unsatisfied sexual expression (Maddison and Raphael 1972).

The Physician's Conflicts

Important problems include imposing emotional isolation on the terminally ill, making routine the treatment, treating the patient as an incapable child, inadequately communicating with the patient, and insufficiently recognizing and assuming the responsibility for the dying patient. Like patients, physicians react to loss with denial, anger, depression. "The prospect of losing one's own life or the loss of a patient, the end of a relationship with the dying person or the sad conclusion to a battle with an illness all may generate similar psychological repercussion" (Kastenbaum and Aisenberg 1972). Anger may be used as a defense against anxiety. Then too, denial may be as blatant in physicians as in the terminally ill themselves. Finally, continued contact with their terminally ill patients can certainly lead to depression, particularly for physicians with excessive work loads and unbalanced life-style that does not include sufficient emotional support and revitalizing play.

Bereavement

Bereavement may be viewed as "the state of thought, feeling, and activity which is a consequence of the loss of a loved or valued object" (Peretz 1970). The loss may be gradual or sudden. Bereavement can be seen as an illness since it does tend to represent, at times, a dramatic departure from the person's usual state of behavior, thought, and feelings, and is associated with both physical and emotional symptoms. Recovery is seen when the symptoms have receded; it may be complete or partial. Comparing bereavement to a wound or infection is sometimes helpful in that the outcome may be quite varied. For some there is little or no scarring, "while for others healing leaves serious scars which later interfere with function or produce weakness in a system which is then predisposed to later failures in function" (Peretz 1970). Very often bereavement states are self-limited and require no specific treatment (grief). Other bereavement states are seen as maladaptive, last indefinitely, and cause extended dysfunctions and problems for relatives and friends as well as the bereaved . Peretz (1970) lists ten bereavement states: 1) "normal" grief; 2) anticipatory grief; 3) inhibited, delayed, and absent grief; 4) chronic grief (perpetual mourning); 5) depression; 6) hypochondriasis and exacerbation of preexistent somatic conditions; 7) development of medical symptoms and illness; 8) psychophysiological reactions; 9) acting out (psychopathic behavior, drugs, promiscuity); and 10) specific neurotic and psychotic states.

Normal grief is characterized as

intense suffering and distress, deep sorrow and painful regret. Initially, the bereaved experiences shock and numbness and denies that the loss has really happened. His incomprehenson soon gives way to, or alternates with, bewilderment and weeping, despairing acknowledgment of the loss with constantly returning thoughts and memories of the deceased (Peretz 1970).

In addition, physical reactions such as shortness of breath, sighing, sensations in the throat, insomnia, anorexia, and feelings of emptiness may be present. Tension, anxiety, agitation, and handwringing may be seen soon after the loss occurs. This emotional reaction may appear intermittently and last up to an hour, gradually decreasing in frequency. There may be painful yearning or loneliness, feelings of unreality, guilt feelings, irrational anger, depression, and feelings of numbness and helplessness. This period may last up to a year although the first several months may represent the more acute phase. Recovery is seen when there is an interest in new relationships and a return of capacity to enjoy without undue shame or guilt. Bereaved persons may not understand the intensity of their feelings and may be frightened by them. At this time communicating to them that their loss is understood and appreciated, as well as general support for their grief, is quite important. In addition, it can be useful to explain to bereaved persons that their reactions are normal and that expression of their feelings will help facilitate their own recovery (Peretz 1970).

Anticipatory grief is an attempt to prepare ourselves in advance for an impending loss (Reed 1974). In anticipation of imminent loss, those persons involved experience the beginnings of grief. These may cover considerable range; they may be "quiet periods of sadness and tears and those symptoms usually associated with grief over actual loss. However, anticipatory grief may deprive both the dying patient and the bereaved-to-be of the possibilities still remaining in the relationship" (Peretz 1970).

The immediate absence of emotion may simply represent initial shock or denial. Also there are persons who only grieve away from the public. Others simply may not show very deeply a state of grieving, perhaps due to strongly ambivalent feelings toward the lost object. Persons with delayed grief are more apt to experience "anniversary reactions," such as their wedding date, birthday of the deceased, and the like. Chronic grief, another type of bereavement, really represents persistent mourning. In this setting it is as if the home and life-style became fixed in time, almost awaiting the return of the deceased. Obviously, such a condition represents denial of the loss of the object, largely to protect against the pain and suffering that would be experienced if it were acknowledged (Peretz 1970).

Acute grief may have signs and symptoms seen in depression. Nevertheless, the two conditions substantially differ. Depression may be present as the main feature of the state of bereavement. It may have an immediate, gradual, or delayed onset. Clearly, it is important to distinguish a major depressive state from the normal grief reaction, so that antidepressant medication and psychiatric follow-up may be initiated. With depression, feelings of sadness, tension, and depletion predominate. There is anorexia, constipation, loss of sexual interest, and decreased verbalizing. When the person does communicate, there may well be self criticism. The grieving person will likely show a quicker mood shift from sadness to a more normal state during the period of a day and will usually respond to general support. The depressed person remains pessimistic, although there may be some daily relief toward evening. There is a consistent inability to experience pleasure. The depressed person will actually seem more preoccupied with self rather than the lost object. While the grieving person may experience the world as empty, the depressed person will feel this more persistently. Also, the depressed person will show a marked lassitude, difficulty concentrating, and even thinking, and may suffer from early arousal and intermittent awakenings. There is a tendency to feel more empathic towards the bereaved than toward the depressed, almost as if the preoccupation with self is experienced as a hostile act by onlookers.

Hypochondriasis also may be one of the reactions toward loss. It may be transient, become an important symptom of depression, or remain as an independent illness. Sometimes it may be manifested as a complaint similar to the one that caused the death of the lost object. Such people are expressing a great deal of hostility, guilt, and anxiety in the fabric of the symptoms. While they do obtain attention, it is at great cost. They need reassurance as well as symptomatic treatment of their symptoms. Gradually, with patient care, the bereaved may become more open and discuss the varieties of feelings and conflicts that actually lay behind the hypochondriacal symptoms.

Another result of loss may be psychophysiological reactions. These include such conditions as ulcerative colitis, duodenal ulcer, hypertension, and rheumatiod arthritis.

Another type of bereavement is acting out. The bereaved may become excessively active in an attempt to avoid the painfulness of the bereaved state. Also, they may impulsively remarry or find a series of substitutes for the lost object. They may throw themselves into a flurry of unusual activity, be it work, travel, or avocations.

Drug dependence may become a problem for some bereaved individuals. Addiction may occur to both alcohol and prescribed psychoactive medications. In addition, other specific neurotic or even psychotic states may appear or worsen following object loss (Peretz 1970).

Chapter 5 describes some measures that have been useful at Church Hospital in providing bereavement support to family members.

References

Annas G: Rights of the terminally ill patient *J Nurs Adm* 4:40 – 43 (1974)

Brenner C: *The Mind in Conflict*. International Universities Press, New York, 1982.

Garfield CA: *Psychosocial Care of the Dying Patient*. McGraw-Hill, New York, 1978.

Kastenbaum R: "Is death a life crisis? On the confrontation with death in theory and practice *In Datan N, Ginsberg LH (eds): Life-Span Developmental Psychology: Normative Life Crisis,* 19 – 50. Academic Press, New York, 1975.

Kastenbaum R, Aisenberg R: *Psychology of Death*. Springer, New York, 1972.

Kübler-Ross E: *On Death and Dying*. Macmillan, New York, 1969.

Maddison, Raphael: The family of the dying patient. *In* Schoenberg B, Carr AC, Peretz D, Kutscher AH (eds): *Psychosocial Aspects of Terminal Care,* 185 – 200. Columbia University Press, New York, 1972.

Peretz D: Reaction to loss. *In* Schoenberg B, Carr AC, Peretz D, Kutscher AH (eds) *Loss and Grief: Psychological Management in Medical Practice,* 20 – 35. Columbia University Press, New York, 1970.

Peretz D: Psychotherapy workshop *In* Schoenberg B, Carr AC, Peretz D, Kutscher AH (eds) *Psychosocial Aspects of Terminal Care,* 185 – 200. New York, 1972.

Reed AW: Anticipatory grief work. *In* Schoenberg B, Carr AC, Peretz D, Kutscher AH, et al. (eds): *Anticipatory Grief*. Columbia University Press, New York, 1974.

Schmale A: Principles of psychosocial oncology. *In* Rubin P (ed) *Clinical Oncology for Medical Students and Physicians*. American Cancer Society, Rochester NY, 1974.

Weisman AD: *A Psychiatric Study of Terminality*. Behavioral Publishing, Pasadena CA, 1972a.

Weisman AD: Psychosocial considerations in terminal care. *In* Schoenberg B, Carr AC, Peretz D, Kutscher AH (eds): *Psychosocial Aspects of Terminal Care,* 162 – . Columbia University Press, New York, 1972b.

Bereavement Care

Yvonne M. Leacock

In the preceding chapter it was pointed out that bereavement is a highly stressful event, frequently evoking powerful emotional, physical, and/or intellectual reactions. It creates the need for changes and social adjustments that cannot be made quickly or easily. Grief, a response to bereavement, presents a syndrome similar to depression, but it should be viewed as "distress" rather than illness or disease (Osterweis et al. 1984).

Since we are primarily concerned with the implementation of complete hospice care, a review of the growing body of literature related to bereavement is not included. The report of the Committee for the Study of Health Consequences of Bereavement (Osterweis et al. 1984) should be a part of every hospice library and is an excellent resource for the staff member who coordinates bereavement care. The committee was appointed by the Institute of Medicine at the request of the Office of Prevention of the National Institute of Mental Health. The committee's report is a comprehensive, analytical review of the current status of grief and bereavement research, theory, and intervention.

A brief note of caution is in order on this point. A few years ago many of us with an interest in the delivery of bereavement care lamented the paucity of readily available information and resources. Recently, there has been a groundswell of interest in the handling of bereavement and grief responses. Workshops and conferences are promoted at the local, regional, and national levels. Bookstores devote sections to the subject; information and advice appear regularly in the popular press. Thus the layman and the professional need to be informed consumers when seeking information and services.

Background of Present Programs

Any description of hospice principles includes a provision for follow-up services to the patient's family. Even without this philosophical guideline, the Church Hospital team feels a strong sense of responsibility to the bereaved, born of a common humanity and a commitment as professional health care providers.

Not unlike the experiences of many hospice programs, our bereavement care evolved with the growth and development of the program as a whole. Services were provided by nurses, volunteers, and chaplains. Ultimately, the need arose to balance limited resources against the commitment to provide the most effective and comprehensive follow-up services possible. The necessity for an identified team member to plan, coordinate, and supervise services was recognized. Since members of the existing staff carried full work loads in their combined hospice and nonhospice duties, staffing became a practical problem. There was and continues to be an essential lack of funding for this important service. The Church Hospital solution to the problem was to create a part-time staff position for a bereavement coordinator on the home care hospice staff.

In planning to expand and formalize bereavement services at Church Hospital, some existing models of care were examined. The most helpful resources were a site visit to Hospice of Northern Virginia with the bereavement coordinator; the *Bereavement Care Manual* (Lattanzi and Coffelt 1979) of Boulder County Hospice, Inc; and the work of Silverman and colleagues (1972, 1974) on the widow-to-widow format. Additionally, an interest survey was conducted of all hospice caregivers who were between 5 and 25 months post bereavement. The purposes of the survey were to learn what, if any, type of group format our bereaved population would like; to identify the interest population by age and relationship; and to determine scheduling preferences. The results directly influenced the plan to offer several modalities of care.

Our services currently include one-to-one follow-up; periodic two-hour workshops with a specific theme; a structured seven-session growth group spanning ten weeks; a caregivers group; and an annual memorial service and reception.

Purpose and Goals

The purpose of our bereavement care program is to provide comfort, understanding, support, and information to surviving relatives and friends in an effort to alleviate the distress of bereavement and promote the most favorable outcome possible. Grief is recognized as a process and has been characterized as "a succession of clinical pictures which blend into and replace one another" (Parkes 1972). The general goal is to provide appropriate care as the grief response changes. Specific program goals are to

1. assess the coping ability of the survivors
2. encourage and facilitate the expression of feelings regarding the loss
3. reassure survivors that this process, though painful, is normal
4. reinforce new patterns of behavior that are adaptive
5. identify maladaptive behavior and encourage exploration of alternative behaviors or make appropriate referral
6. provide opportunity for the bereaved to appreciate their increased growth and maturity resulting from the loss experience
7. provide an opportunity for feedback about program effectiveness (Leacock 1984).

The temporary nature of hospice support is kept in mind as goals are implemented. The grieving person is encouraged to develop inner strengths and to utilize family and community resources.

Description of Team

The work of the bereavement team is an integral part of the process of hospice care. The bereavement coordinator works under the supervision of the Director of Home Care and reports to the hospice care committee. This individual is responsible for planning, coordinating, and supervising the services provided by the bereavement team. The coordinator works in close collaboration with the Director of Volunteers and consults with social work, nursing, and chaplaincy staff as needed. The qualifications for this position include

1. a master's degree in psychology, counseling, or social work.
2. one year of clinical work experience
3. knowledge of the dynamics of grief
4. skills in program planning and development, teaching, and supervision
5. ability to function effectively as a member of an interdisciplinary team.

Volunteers are recruited by the Director of Volunteers specifically for bereavement work. The one-to-one outreach is designed as peer support. Therefore, a concentrated effort is made to recruit volunteers from the most heavily represented communities in the catchment area. After completing the application, they are interviewed and selected for training jointly by the Volunteer Director and Bereavement Coordinator. The qualities described in Chapter 7 are used in screening bereavement volunteers. Additional qualifications looked for during training are

1. the resolution of a close personal loss (In our experience those who have adjusted to such a loss are the most effective volunteers.)
2. the serenity and strength to be still, to listen, and to bear the pain and anxiety of others
3. the ability to work independently, often without immediate feedback or gratification.

Volunteer Training

The 6-session, 12-hour orientation is experiential and didactic. In the first two sessions, the volunteers discuss their goals, motivations, and personal loss experiences. The sharing fosters the development of team spirit and helps in the process of knowing and evaluating the prospective volunteer. The discussion is used to emphasize that there are universal and unique experiences in the response to bereavement and other losses. Throughout training the content of these sessions is used for illustration. Topics covered in subsequent sessions include

1. process and symptomatology of grief
2. the tasks of mourning (Worden 1982)
3. family systems perspective on loss and grief
4. effective use of the telephone
5. responsibilities and risks of being a helper.

This orientation is sufficient to begin the process of helping; education is ongoing. The monthly team meetings are mandatory and well attended. They provide team support, case management, and continuing education.

One-to-One Follow-Up

The basic procedure for one-to-one follow-up is formalized

1. When the patient has been on the home care service, the primary nurse assures that the initial bereavement contact is made.
2. Depending upon the individual caregiver, a letter signed personally by the Home Care Director is mailed ten days to three weeks postbereavement.The letter expresses sympathy and the hope that the team and services have been helpful. It reminds the caregiver of the follow-up program and gives the coordinator's name and phone number to be used if needed before contact is made.
3. In most instances the initial bereavement team contact is a home visit made by the coordinator. The purpose is to complete a comprehensive assessment. A semistructured interview is conducted, being the best technique for also facilitating expressions of grief, normalizing experiences, and demonstrating the continued caring and concerns of the hospice team. These visits require one to three hours.
4. A written assignment is prepared for the volunteer who will follow the bereaved person. The assignment sheet includes important dates, a description of the lost relationship, identified needs of the client, and any known information relevant to the loss.
5. Subsequent contacts may be either home visits or telephone calls or a combination of both.
6. Frequency and duration of contacts depend upon individual and family needs.
7. Follow-up services may continue up to 13 months; this allows the bereaved to experience each significant occasion of the calendar year with support available. Final contact is made at 13 months in an effort to make an accurate assessment of adjustment by eliminating the possible effects of the one-year anniversary of the death.

8. Assessment is continuous, and referral for professional services is made whenever the individual or family needs are beyond the scope of the program.

9. Each bereavement contact is documented in the patient's chart, which is maintained in the files of the Home Care Department for 13 months before being sent to medical records. All notes are submitted by the date of the monthly meeting following the contact.

Groups

Three support groups are offered through the Home Care/Hospice office. At the periodic Sunday afternoon groups, a single topic is presented and discussed. A brief social gathering follows. The meetings are open to everyone who has had a loss in the last 2 to 18 months. The members of the bereavement team host the meetings, encourage interested but reticent individuals, and provide transportation to those who need it.

The seven-session, structured group addresses the personal loss experience of the participants. It is limited to between 5 and 12 participants, who are screened for appropriateness. Some issues for examination when making selections are

1. time since loss; minimum 2 months preferred
2. history of substance abuse
3. multiple crises
4. history of disordered behavior.

The content of the weekly meetings are designed to

1. allow expression of grief
2. promote understanding of the process of grief
3. provide guidance and support with emotional, social, and practical adjustments
4. develop coping skills and strategies
5. create a network of support.

Two Hospice/Home Care staff members co-lead the sessions. Several groups are offered throughout the year.

The caregivers group has an open, mutual-help format. It is scheduled bimonthly and is facilitated by two of the Home Care/Hospice staff. The purpose of this group is to provide a safe environment where the caregivers can talk openly. Themes of grief, frustration, fatigue, fear, isolation, and anger arise. Understanding, caring, and coping strategies are shared within the group.

Memorial Service

The follow-up program includes an annual nondenominational memorial service. Chaplains, lay staff, and family members officiate. It is attended by staff and relatives and friends of patients who died in the previous two years. Families vary in their readiness for this event. The second invitation is appreciated by those who couldn't face it the first year. The reception following the service has the nostalgic quality of a reunion. The afternoon is meaningful to both staff and families.

Bereaved Children

Church Hospital services relatively few young families. Middle-aged daughters make up our second largest group of caregivers; wives over 50 comprise the largest group. The young children and adolescents needing bereavement care are primarily the grandchildren of patients. Our approach in either instance is to provide information, guidance, and support to the adults. Honest communication of both information and feelings is encouraged within the family during the dying, death, and bereavement. Important information for parents and grandparents to have is

1. what reactions to expect in children, according to their developmental needs and understanding of death
2. how to help the child with his or her questions and fears
3. what adult actions and statements are harmful
4. indicators that a child is troubled beyond the expected sadness and distress.

When a parent with young or adolescent children dies, more assistance may be required than hospice can offer. Timely referral for family counseling is indicated when a family has a history of disturbed interaction or when there are complicated or difficult adjustments to be made.

Refusal of Services

Occasionally, follow-up services are refused. Some families may have needed assistance only through the terminal illness. As in terminal care, the goal is to encourage and nurture functioning within the familial and social network. Where there is no need, none should be created. If there is cause for concern when care is refused, that single contact is used to review some common reactions to loss and to reinforce our availability. With permission, the grieving person will remain on the mailing list for announcements about group programs. Every family is invited to the memorial service.

Networking

The mobility and resulting dispersement of families can have a profound effect on the adult child who lives in another area of the country. When the grieving individual returns to a distant residence following a parental death, there are no supportive relatives and friends who know the family and understand the meaning of the lost relationship. Whenever possible, a contact is made with a hospice or other resource for bereavement services. With permission, the contact person is asked to initiate follow-up with the bereaved client.

References

Lattanzi M, Coffelt D. *Bereavement Care Manual*. Boulder County Hospice Inc, Boulder CO, 1979.

Leacock YM: Bereavement follow-up. *The Hospice-Care Program Manual*, ed 3, p 7-1. Baltimore, 1984.

Osterweis M, Solomon F, Green M (eds): *Bereavement : Reactions, Consequences and Care*. National Academy Press, Washington DC, 1984.

Parkes CM: *Bereavement: Studies of Grief in Adult Life*. International Universities Press, New York, 1972.

Silverman PR: Widowhood and preventive intervention. *The Family Coordinator,* pp 31 – 38, January 1972.

Silverman PR, MacKenzie D, Pettipas M, Wilson E: *Helping Each Other in Widowhood*. Health Services Publishing, 1974.

Worden, JW: *Grief Counseling and Grief Therapy*. Springer, New York, 1982.

Chapter 6

The Hospice Care Team

Jack M. Zimmerman and Kathleen A. Roche

A comprehensive approach that deals with the patient's medical, social, psychological and spiritual problems over a period of time and in a variety of settings is among the important objectives of a program for the care of the terminally ill. Hospice care addresses these objectives through the use of a multidisciplinary team. In this chapter we will examine the individual components of that team and the way in which they are selected, trained, and evaluated. Administrative considerations of staff strength, work load, and similar matters are covered in Chapter 10.

Life-threatening disease creates a variety of problems. In addition, the patient and family bring to the terminal illness all of the baggage of life, including preexisting personality, marital, and financial problems. In coping with all of these complexities, a team approach is of immense help; it is sometimes necessary to draw upon professional expertise from a variety of fields in order to resolve difficulties. Furthermore, patients are highly individual in their ability to relate to other people; therefore, the availability of many team members provides the opportunity for support from a number of sources. It is not uncommon for the most important emotional support to come from a nonphysician member of the team.

This feature of hospice care serves as the enabling link between the kind of personal attention that the revered family physician could provide and the sophisticated techniques of modern health care. There are few circumstances left in which it is possible for one kindly and well-trained physician or nurse to provide the breadth and depth of care that a well-organized hospice care team can offer.

The benefits of a multidisciplinary approach derive from the diversity of talent it brings to the task, but it is most vulnerable in its need for coordination among team members. Coordination requires both communication and leadership. There must be an opportunity for the various members of the hospice care team to communicate freely regarding each individual patient and about the program in general. Each team member must be able to offer his or her knowledge and experience and to hear the contributions of others. Various mechanisms can be developed to permit this kind of interchange. The responsibility for coordinating the activities of team members rests primarily with the physician. In our program, the clinical nurse-practitioner has been of immense help in assisting the physician with this chore.

An important feature of multidisciplinary care in a hospice program is the lack of sharp distinction between the functions of the various team members. Although each has an area of expertise and primary responsibility, each must be alert to the problems and needs of the patient in other areas. All should share in providing psychological and emotional support to the patient and family. This role is important because team members are in the strongest position to offer this service. It is far better that they do this than that there routinely be a separate "psychological counselor." There is no dearth of people who are willing to volunteer to provide advice to terminally ill patients and their families, but our experience has been that the impact of such counselors is negligible compared to that of the team members who are meeting the patient's physical needs day by day.

Team Members and Their Roles

The details of composition of a hospice care team will vary from program to program. Described here are the roles of the most common team members. The precise makeup of the team in each program will depend upon local circumstances, including program objectives and available personnel. What follows, then, are general guidelines based upon what we have found to be helpful.

For obvious reasons, our emphasis here will be upon those roles that are somewhat different for hospice patients than they are for other patients. Thus, we are looking specifically at the role of each team member in hospice.

Study and reading are very useful beginning points for individual team members to learn about hospice care, particularly if they are to avoid repeating the mistakes of others; however, the bulk of such learning comes from experience. It is only by active involvement in a program that a hospice worker truly begins to see hospice principles and to understand his or her own particular role.

Physicians

Physician attitudes and involvement are critical to the success of any program for the care of the terminally ill. In hospice care, physician leadership is necessary for the program as a whole and for coordination of the team efforts with each individual patient. In addition, it is imperative that physicians not involved directly in the hospice program accept it as a legitimate and worthwhile contribution to the care of the dying.

As will be seen, the participation of individual physicians in hospice care extends over a spectrum, from total abstinence to full-time patient care and administration. Physicians with limited exposure to hospice often fear loss of control of their patients. One of the interesting aspects of this field is that as a physician's experience with a good hospice program increases, this fear diminishes because the need for the contributions of the physician becomes increasingly evident. It is a fact that many physicians are not equipped to provide services that other team members do. This is not a unique situation. There is no need for the ship's captain to be as expert in every field as each of the specialized members of the crew. It is important, however, that the program not take away from the physician those things that he or she *is* able and anxious to do.

Hospice Physician   We use this term to designate a physician who devotes a significant share of time to the care of patients in the program. Many hospice physicians will also be immediately concerned with the organization and operation of the program. Such physicians are often called hospice medical directors.

Physicians may come to hospice work from a wide variety of backgrounds. A hospice physician must be familiar with the principles and practice of hospice care and must have an understanding of malignancy and other diseases that affect hospice patients. Much of what he or she needs in these fields, and in pharmacology and other areas that will be important to his or her work, can be learned through experience in hospice work. What is needed to begin with is competence as a physician, the ability to learn and the personal characteristics that lend themselves to success in hospice work. These are difficult to define but obviously include compassion, patience, maturity and confidence. The hospice physician should be able to use the healing power of his or her words, hands, and unique humanity (Benjamin 1984).

Once involved in the hospice program, the hospice physician will often serve as the personal physician for terminally ill patients in the program, directing attention to palliation and employing the techniques described in Chapter 3. As he also must serve as a consultant for other patients he should understand and be comfortable with that role. For new patients and for those considering whether or not to enter the program, it will often be the hospice physician who will provide explanations of the hospice concept. The physician member of the hospice team is obviously responsible for the planning and ordering of the patient's medical care. It is the hospice physician who sees the patient in the context of his or her prior medical history and who possesses the knowledge of the natural history of the disease process, which is so important to planning medical care. It is this physician who must make some of the difficult decisions described in Chapters 2, 3, and 14. To make hospice care work properly, the hospice physician must be prepared to work with team members from other disciplines, drawing upon their knowledge of other fields and of the patient. He or she must be prepared to properly deploy and direct the various members for maximum benefit to the patient and must communicate comfortably with other physicians. The hospice physician should be able to play a useful role in the events surrounding the patient's death (Tolle and Girard 1983).

Attending Physicians for Hospice Patients   In the Church Hospital hospice program, a member of the Church Hospital medical staff referring a patient for hospice care has the option of continuing as the patient's attending physician, using the hospice physician as consultant; alternatively, he may simply turn the patient over to the hospice physician. In both options the attending physician is a critical member of the hospice care team. In some other programs, the hospice team serves as a support service in a consultant capacity; the patient, in all instances, remains under the care of the attending physician. His or her performance profoundly affects the success of hospice care. It is important that the attending physician be philosophically in tune with the objectives of the program and be familiar with the principles of hospice care. He or she must be fully and consistently commited to having the patient in the program and must be able to work with and utilize the hospice care team. It would be nice if every attending physician with patients in a hospice program possessed the personal characteristics and understanding of hospice principles that make a good hospice physician, but it would be unrealistic to expect this. Individualization is necessary, but the hospice care team, including the hospice physician, will sometimes have to provide some to the elements of support and comfort that are not forthcoming from the patient's attending physician. Through constant and continuing education of attending physicians as a group and as individuals, they should increasingly gain knowledge of, and sympathy with, the principles of hospice care. It is in this way that hospice programs grow.

Referring Physicians Physicians who turn patients over to the hospice physicians and care team are still, in a sense, team members. These physicians need not have a detailed knowledge of techniques in hospice care, but it is imperative that they thoroughly understand hospice philosophy and have a general acceptance of the approach. Although detailed, ongoing reports are not necessary, referring physicians should be informed of major developments with respect to their patients. The avenues of communication should be kept open.

In a hospice care program for the patients of staff members of a single hospital, particularly if it is the first program in the area, the demand for hospice care will be immense. Some physicians who are not members of the hospital's medical staff will refer patients to medical staff members for the sole purpose of making them eligible for the hospice care program. This can create problems if such patients fail to meet the criteria for admission to the program or if the program is overloaded. Medical staff members should be urged either to direct these referrals to the hospice physician or to check with the hospice care staff before accepting such patients.

House Officers The way in which interns and residents relate to a particular hospice program will depend upon local circumstances, but it is a matter that should be addressed very carefully by program leaders. There are obvious advantages to encouraging house officer participation in hospice programs, but there are some problems that come with this approach.

The advantages are those of disseminating understanding of hospice care to young physicians during their period of specialty training (Mathew et al. 1983). In addition, the participation of capable, interested house officers enlarges the team's capacities. However, the routine rotation, particularly for short intervals, of interns and residents through a hospice program can result in misunderstandings and misadventures from lack of knowledge about, and sympathy with, hospice care.

It is important that to the extent that house officers are to be involved, they should be carefully oriented to the elements of hospice care and to their responsibilities. The lack of proper orientation can lead to troublesome frustrations for other members of the hospice team, particularly the nursing staff. Periodic reeducation is necessary. For example, the organizational structure of a hospital may be such that the house officer will be the one who is charged with the responsibility for pronouncing patients dead and completing the death certificate. In such instances, the house officer needs to know how to do this expeditiously and unobtrusively. Many families of hospice patients wish to remain with the patient for awhile after death; the cooperation of house officers in not dismissing families from the room while the act of "pronouncing" goes on is a small but often important point. Young house officers also frequently have problems with the larges doses of narcotics employed for pain control unless they have been provided with adequate instruction. As in other areas of graduate training, physicians should not be expected to provide service without concomitant education.

Nurses

Much of hospice care rests in the hands of nursing personnel. Hospice care draws heavily on the high tradition of nursing; fundamental principles of sound nursing practice are foundations upon which hospice programs are built. The nurse brings to the hospice care team a familiarity with the physical and psychological function of the patient that is critical to making decisions about the patient. Observations regarding pain, appetite, bowel habits, and other symptoms, as well as the assessment of the patient's mood and attitudes, are essential to good palliation. The provision of sound nursing care in the form of positioning and mouth and skin care is critical to patient comfort. Nursing personnel in the home care setting may make it possible for the patient to spend much of the terminal illness in the familiar surroundings of his or her own home.

Nursing care in a hospice program is basically no different from good nursing care elsewhere, except that it reflects the change in orientation from cure to palliation. However, certain attributes are particularly valuable for the hospice nurse. One must be astute in determining what the patient and family perceive as needs and problems. One must be able to assess the nature and severity of symptoms, paying close attention to nonverbal signals. Very often patients are reluctant to ask for medication, and as noted in Chapter 3, satisfactory pain control depends upon titration of appropriate analgesic, which in turn depends upon an accurate perception of the patient's pain.

The hospice nurse must possess a sound understanding of hospice philosophy, principles, and practice. Often the team member to whom patients and relatives will turn for counsel, the hospice nurse should be comfortable in dealing with problems of impending death. One should be able and willing to leave oneself open to questions from the patient and family, responding to them as well as possible and not being unduly discomfited when unable to provide specific answers. Fortunately, there is evidence that hospice nurses have greater personal comfort in working with death and dying than do comparable nonhospice nurses.[1]

The hospice nurse is well advised to be prepared for certain things that occur rather frequently in the care of the terminally ill. Discharge planning often requires a great deal of time. The potential for emotional involvement with patients is enormous. Although hospice care has its satisfactions, the frustrations are substantial and often very graphic.

Since the patient's family is a part of the unit of care in a hospice program, there must be more exacting attention to observation of the family members in order to recognize stress and conflicts. There must be a greater willingness to intervene for the purpose of providing support and assistance to loved ones than there is with nonhospice patients.

The hospice nurse, in additon to providing direct nursing care, serves as a supervisor and consultant for nonprofessional workers. One must be alert to lack of understanding or acceptance of hospice principles on the part of other personnel.

As will be discussssed, volunteers are used more extensively and in an expanded role in hospice care. The nurse must accept volunteers and be able to work with them, and must provide the appropriate balance of supervision and independence for each volunteer.

The special features of home care nursing, as well as some general principles of hospice nursing, are dealt with in detail in Chapter 8. It must be understood that the home care nurses are an integral part of the hospital team. It is only through excellent cooperation between those responsible for nursing care in the hospital and those who handle it at home that true continuity in terminal care can be provided. The home care staff in our program visits hospitalized patients as necessary and maintains constant liaison with the unit nurses and the clinical nurse-practitioner.

Clinical Nurse-Practitioners and Physician's Assistants

In our program, as in many others, the clinical nurse-practitioner (CNP) or physician's assistant (PA) has played a major part in the management of hospice patients, particularly those in the institution. Precisely how such individuals function will depend, of course, a great deal upon local circumstances. CNP-PAs can participate in the initial screening of patients being considered for admission to the program and assist in determining whether specific patients should be accepted on the basis of established criteria. They are particularly helpful to the hospice physician in this respect because they are familiar with the work load on the inpatient nursing unit.

---

1. Bateman et al., 1984, A study of comfort with death and dying: oncology versus hospice nurse (unpublished data).

They may carry out the admission history and physical examination, write routine orders, and play a vital part in titrating analgesics for pain control. Of course, CNPs can begin the nursing care plan. Soon after completing the initial history and physical, a CNP-PA can set up meetings with the patient and family to review the goals of the hospice program and elicit special problems that may exist in each individual case. The CNP-PA can assure that the patient and his or her family are introduced to the members of the hospice team with whom they will have contact. If possible, it is advisable that the CNP-PA daily see each patient alone and with family members.

CNP-PAs maintain communication with the referring physician, the patient's attending physician, other nursing personnel, and the various members of the hospice care team. In many respects they can serve as coordinators of the patient's care. They monitor the patient's status and make recommendations for adjustments in the treatment program. They can initiate discharge planning. We have found that they can provide some of the services performed by house officers in hospitals with residency training programs. In addition to all this, CNP-PAs are important contributors to the clinical conferences and continuing education programs.

By virtue of their special training and experience, CNPs form an important link between nursing care and physician care. PAs also can obviously be valuable members of a hospice care team (Kuhrts 1977). As noted, the way in which CNPs and PAs function will depend upon the particular institution and individuals involved.

Nursing Assistants

Nursing assistants or aides are a vital part of the hospice team. They are intimately involved in the day-to-day care of the patient. In developing a hospice program, careful attention should be paid to the proper selection and training of nursing assistants. For the program to function effectively, these individuals must have a knowledge, understanding, and acceptance of hospice principles and must possess those personal traits that enable them to work effectively with the dying patient and the family. The unique role which those providing the physical elements of patient care have in meeting the emotional and spiritual needs of the terminally ill has already been emphasized. Patients and families vary immensely in their capacity to relate to various members of the hospice team. Periods of "opening up" may be transient and brief, but they are extremely important. The confident reassurance or the gentle touch at the right moment by an understanding aide can sometimes be an irreplaceable therapeutic measure.

Social Workers

The goal of the social work service is to help the patient and family deal with the personal and social problems of illness, disability, and impending death. In hospice care this is particularly important. The social worker assesses the problems, needs, and capacities of patients and their families and brings to the hospice team a special knowledge of community resources that can be of help. All hospitalized hospice patients and their families are seen by the social worker so that the social, emotional environmental, and financial impact of the terminal illness may be evaluated.

A social worker involved in hospice care obviously needs to be familiar with hospice philosophy and principles. He or she should have a special interest in working with the terminally ill and have those special talents that make it possible to work cooperatively with a multidisciplinary team. The social worker is involved in supportive and therapeutic counseling, discharge planning, direct assistance to the patient and family, and bereavement counseling. The social worker is often one of the team members who is involved with both inpatients and outpatients.

Our social workers have found themselves doing a number of interesting (and some not very interesting) chores. They often serve as a sort of travel agent for out-of-town family members, arranging for food, lodging, and transportation. When family members are fearful of losing their jobs because of time away from work, the social worker speaks directly with employers. Social workers have been to court on behalf of hospice patients when there had to be guardianship arrangements, and they have been involved with juvenile authorities concerning the custody of children after their mother's death.

Dietitians

The approach to nutritional management of the terminally ill patient must be individualized. For example, the patient with a substantial life expectancy may be materially helped by improvement in nutritional status, whereas for the patient with a very limited expectancy, this consideration becomes irrelevant.

A profound state of malnutrition and wasting frequently accompanies malignancy and is often the most significant and disabling feature of the patient's disease. Anorexia is often compounded by a perverted sense of taste and smell. Patients frequently say that food just doesn't taste right.

To overcome or minimize these problems, the patient's cooperation, to the extent possible, is required. The individual should be allowed a free choice of types and quantities of food. Special attention must be paid to the appearance, aroma, and temperature of food. Portions should be small, with frequent snacks. Families can often provide special ethnic foods that may stimulate a lagging appetite. The patient should never be forced to eat. Although augmentation of basic diet with supplemental feedings may be helpful in some circumstances, it must be remembered that a diet is only beneficial to the patient when it is individualized to meet that patient's particular needs.

For some patients considerable dietary manipulation may be advisable in order to improve nutritional status relatively early in the course of their terminal illness. Diet supplements may be useful. However, later in the course of illness, emphasis should shift away from maintenance or improvement of nutritional status and should be directed entirely at patient comfort. Therefore the dietitian must maintain communication with the physician and nurses so as to be familiar with the therapeutic objectives of dietary management at any given time.

The social aspects of food should be kept in mind. Appetite is often poor when patients are eating alone, so arrangements should be made for guest tray service if at all possible. Light food and liquid refreshments should be available on a complimentary basis for the patient's family. Birthdays, anniversaries, and special events can serve as an occasion for a celebration, with patient, family, and staff sharing together.

The dietitian must remember that for many patients, and particularly for family members, eating is of symbolic importance. It is a sign that life is still going on normally. This can have a profound impact on the care of the patient and must be dealt with. Except for the tumor itself, in a cancer patient there is probably nothing that destroys appetite as effectively as a feeling that one *must* eat. The dietitian, along with other members of the hospice team should be alert to such pressure from family members and caregivers, helping them to draw back and deal with the patient as he really is, not as they would like him to be. The complex relationship between nutrition, palliation, and eating is also discussed in Chapter 3 and 14.

Thus, although special diets for therapeutic purposes are seldom necessary, the dietitian must be constantly alert to the often changing dietary preferences of the patient and be ready to suggest alternatives when foods become unappealing. An individualized dietary care plan should be based on the dietitian's assessment of the appetite, food preferences, tolerances, and the physical capabilities (chewing, swallowing, ability to feed self) of the individual patient. This requires periodic discussion with the patient and the family; there is no substitute for observing the patient at meal time. Conferences with other members of the hospice staff regarding the patient's nutritional care and possible need for changes in diet can be invaluable.

Pharmacists

In hospice care, drugs are used both in conventional and unconventional fashions and dosages, particularly in pain relief; it is important that the hospital pharmacy staff be conversant with principles of hospice care. Certain agents such as high-dose morphine solution, Dilaudid suppositories, and artificial saliva are seldom used in non-hospice patients.

Because of the complex nature of the problems presented by the terminally ill and the multiplicity of the medications with periodic dosage changes, the services of a clinical pharmacologist can be very helpful for hospice patients. A hospice program is very fortunate if it has access to such a professional.

For work with outpatients it is often helpful for a hospice care program to involve at least one private pharmacy outside the hospital. The pharmacist there should be thoroughly oriented to hospice care and be considered part of the hospice operation. It may be advisable, incidentally, that the identity of such a pharmacy be kept secret or at least not publicized because of the problems that arise when a pharmacy is known to stock substantial amounts of narcotics. The selected pharmacy should provide emergency and delivery services. The pharmacist needs to be imaginative in the preparation and packaging of materials for hospice patients.

Physical Therapists

Physical therapists can be of significant help to many kinds of hospice patients. Their value should not be overlooked in establishing a hospice team.

The aim of physical therapy in hospice care is, in actuality, somewhat different from its aim in other patients. For nonhospice patients, the objective of treatment is usually improved function, but usually for hospice patients the objective is relief of discomfort.

Again, individualization is necessary; it depends upon the particular patient and the type and stage of the disease. The goals of the physical therapist are usually to help the terminally ill patient adapt to physical limitations and to permit the individual to function at the highest possible physical level. An effort is made to maintain function as long as possible. While doing this, it is important for the physical therapist to provide emotional and psychological support, for as the patient's condition deteriorates, he or she often becomes increasingly concerned about lessening ability to perform the activities of daily living. Generally speaking, the physical therapist will find it helpful to allow the hospice patient to talk more than other patients and perhaps to use recreational therapy more frequently. In addition to working directly with the patient, the physical therapist must be prepared to offer professional assessment of the patient's functional status and physical capabilities.

Because of the somewhat different orientation of physical therapy for hospice patients, not all physical therapists are suited to this type of work. It is generally best that one member of the physical therapy department be selected for this role. The prime requirements are a special interest in working with the terminally ill, the ability to work cooperatively with the multidisciplinary team, adaptability, and some knowledge of the issues of death, dying, and grief. Naturally, the physical therapist must have an understanding of, and agreement with, hospice care principles.

The physical therapist must be prepared for a level of emotional involvement with hospice patients that is seldom achieved with nonhospice patients. There must be a willingness to accept the fact that the overall course of hospice patients is one of deterioration, rather than of rehabilitation and improvement. The physical therapist must be ready to discontinue physical therapy when, in his or her judgment, it clearly is no longer helpful or in the patient's best interests.

Within this framework, techniques employed are much the same as they are for nonhospice patients. Certain measures such as chest physical therapy and breathing exercise can be particularly helpful.

Psychiatrists and Psychiatric Nurses

Hospice programs have varied in the extent and manner in which they have utilized psychiatric services. In our program, staff psychiatrists and the psychiatric liaison nurse have been available to hospice patients, as they are to other patients in the hospital. They have been used in the evaluation and management of problems of a truly psychiatric nature occurring in terminally ill patients and their families. The special expertise of psychiatrists with respect to the psychosocial dimension of patient care has been very useful to *hospice team members* through formal and informal education (See Chapter 4).

In these roles psychiatrists have been invaluable. However, we do not regard dying itself as a psychiatric disorder. As indicated in Chapter 3, we have generally felt that except in unusual circumstances, straightforward psychological support to patients and family members in handling serious illness and impending death is best provided by members of the hospice care team who are immediately involved in meeting the patient's physical needs.

Other hospice programs have, of course, used psychiatric support services much more liberally in planning, policy making, patient care and staff support. Psychiatrists have played a critical role in the development and implementation of some hospice programs. It can be argued that by virtue of their training and experience psychiatrists provide special skills of value to terminally ill patients, their families and the staff caring for them, and that therefore the psychiatrist should be a member of the hospice care team, rather than a detached consultant as described above. It must be recognized, though, that psychiatrists with requisite skills may not be available to all hospice groups.

Obviously, each developing hospice program must make its own decision with respect to the role of psychiatrists. That decision will be based largely upon local circumstances.

Chaplains

By the nature of their function in the hospital, chaplains often play a critical role in hospital-based care. Chaplains have been deeply engaged in most hospice programs. Their ministry is available to all involved in hospice care. In addition to providing spiritual support to the patient and family in an unusually demanding situation, the chaplain must be alert to their physical and psychological needs.

Primary attention is to the spiritual needs of patients and family. "Spiritual" is used in its broadest sense and must be distinguished from specific religious concerns. The distinction is important in order to respect the wishes of those persons who do not profess or care to align themselves with a religious affiliation. Those who do wish to receive religious ministrations such as the sacraments are accommodated appropriately.

The chaplains routinely visit hospice inpatients and see hospice outpatients as appropriate, often through referral from the home care staff. Contact is established with the patient's own clergyman where indicated. As can be readily appreciated, other members of the hospice staff often play a role in the spiritual aspects of hospice care, so that the chaplains make themselves available as a resource to the staff. In this capacity they help the staff to deal with difficult questions that patients and families may raise. They also help the staff to deal with pressures and stress and, as a consequence, enable them to expand and deepen their own capacity to provide excellent hospice care.

When the chaplain functions as sole pastor for the patient and family, he or she should be available for extended pastoral counseling when needed. Also, the chaplain may be asked to officiate at the funeral upon the death of the patient and participate in bereavement follow-up. Patients and their families should be encouraged to attend and be made welcome at regularly scheduled services in the hospital chapel. Special hospice memorial services are often very meaningful to all concerned with hospice.

Because of their interest in and knowledge of the hospice program, our chaplains have played a variety of other roles. They have participated in staff training and continuing education and are available for educational activities in the community. They also assist the director of volunteers in interviewing and evaluating recruits for positions as hospice volunteers.

For hospitals that do not have a chaplain, the appointment of a volunteer or part-time salaried chaplain-coordinator from the community should be considered for the hospice program. There are several possibilities for locating such a key person.

Most communities have a ministerium, which is usually ecumenical and fairly representive of the clergy in the area. Some are more effective or representative than others. Appeal can be made to such a ministerium for help in identifying a suitable candidate for hospice chaplain-coordinator. It can also be helpful to identify the clergymen in the community most distinguished for strong pastoral ministry; these may not be the most popular or celebrated clergy. This person or persons could be invited to participate, along with key representatives from the hospice program or committee, in locating a suitable chaplain-coordinator.

Prerequisites for a position as chaplain-coordinator include strong commitment to the program, highly developed pastoral skills (marked by a caring and loving nature), flexibility so far as ecumenical considerations are concerned (this would require a good understanding of traditions other than his or her own), leadership ability (which would include the respect of other clergy in the area), strong counseling experience, and some background in health care (particularly regarding the needs of the dying and their families). Such a candidate must be a person with whom the staff is comfortable and in whom staff members have confidence. Interviews with the medical director, administrative coordinator, social worker, and at least one member of the nursing team should be required.

The chaplain-coordinator would recruit suitable clergy from the community to assist in hospice chaplaincy on a regular, shared, scheduled basis. These clergymen would be on call at specified times and be responsible during that time for regular visits to the hospice patients and families. These chaplains should be considered members of the hospice staff and should be utilized as such for consultation, referral, education, and voluntary attendance at staff meetings.

The chaplain-coordinator or chaplain is expected to participate regularly in staff sessions and preferably should be included in the hospice committee or governing agency for the hospice program. He or she is held accountable for the chaplaincy service and like other members of the team, is regularly observed and reviewed.

Volunteers

Volunteers have played a vital role in virtually every hospice program. Because their role in hospice care represents a greater departure for volunteers than it does for other team members, Chapter 7 is devoted to a consideration of volunteers in hospice. Proper selection, training, and supervision is imperative; with this, volunteers are in a position to make tremendous contributions. For example, those who are interested can provide many of the same comfort measures that would be assigned to lay caregivers in the home. They are also sometimes in a position to provide emotional support in ways that other staff members are not. This effectiveness may be due in part to the fact that they don't *have to* be there. Volunteers are a heterogeneous group. Some are most comfortable in the hospital setting, whereas others prefer home care. We encounter some who wish to contribute to the care of dying patients but don't wish to have direct patient contact. There is a place for them. We have found volunteers an essential component of hospice care.

Other Needs, Other Answers

Terminally ill patients and their families can present problems that require the specialized techniques and knowledge of professionals from areas other than those described. One of the advantages of a hospital-based program is the relatively ready availability of such individuals, even though they may not be, in the strictest sense, members of the hospice care team. The enterostomal therapist, for example, can often be of immense assistance, not only to the patient with a poorly functioning colostomy but also in the treatment of decubitus ulcers and intestinal fistulas. For some head and neck cancer patients, the speech therapist can offer useful assistance. We have been pleased by our experience with art therapy, and the music therapist can also be helpful. There are other members of the hospital staff, such as housekeeping and maintenance personnel, whose contact with hospice patients is, for the most part, casual. For all such individuals a brief basic orientation to hospice philosophy and practice can be most worthwhile.

As discussed in Chapter 5, someone should be in charge of bereavement care. We elected to have a part-time professional in this position.

To be truly comprehensive in its care of the terminally ill, the hospice care team must be prepared to draw upon all available resources to meet the needs of patients and their families.

Staff Selection, Education, and Evaluation

Selection

No matter what other attributes a hospice program possesses, in the final analysis it is only as good as its staff. It is surprising therefore that very little has been written about the criteria for and process of staff selection. Five qualities seem to be of utmost importance for staff members: competence, sensitivity, flexibility , maturity, and spirituality.

Competence Professional competence is of tremendous importance. This is particularly true for home care staff members, who work with minimal supervision and opportunity for immediate collaboration in their day-to-day patient contact. For all hospice workers assessment skills must be highly developed. Naturally, as an individual gains experience, capacity for accurate diagnosis and effective intervention will increase. Nonetheless, there is no substitute for a high level of professional competence even as a staff member begins his or her work as part of the hospice care team.

Sensitivity   Hospice care was born out of a holistic need for low technology and high caring. Sensitivity is the very foundation and fabric out of which hospices are made. The person who chooses to work in hospice must have done so out of a personal desire to serve, experience, and grow. While it is recognized that staff members will to some extent meet some of their own needs as they attempt to fulfill those of others, those responsible for selecting hospice staff must be on the alert for manifest or hidden agendas such as proselytization, resolution of previous guilt or grief, and acquisition of personal gain.

Sensitivity is a key requirement affecting all levels of the program. If a hospice team is to be durably constructed, its members must integrate hospice principles into their own attitudes, caring not only for their patients, but also for each other and for themselves. The concept cannot survive unless the team is alert and its members are available to each other in times of need.

Sensitivity is somewhat intangible and abstract; it is difficult to define. Yet it conveys a sense of activity rather than stagnation. One is reminded of the story of the "warm fuzzies," in which the recipient learns he can replenish his supply only by giving it away. As hospice staff members learn to trust their intuition and to act upon it, they gain confidence in themselves and in their ability to meet those very subtle needs that can so greatly enhance the quality of living and dying. This positive feedback encourages the development of even greater sensitivity. In other words, not only must staff members be selected in part because they possess sensitivity, but also that sensitivity must be nurtured throughout their hospice experience.

This process requires mutual trust, understanding, and patience. Advanced development of skills and attributes are acquired over time, but their potential for development can be readily detected by a sensitive administrator. In a hospital-based hospice, the hospital administration must not only approve of the hospice philosophy, but also must actively encourage the development of new skills and techniques that enhance humanistic care in general. Sensitivity training, popular in the 1960's, may be a valuable tool to assist in coping with the intimacy experiences in hospice care.

No one will deny that sensitivity and caring together with a high level of competence are vital to humanistic health care. Each potential staff member must be evaluated for these talents, but alone they are not really enough.

Flexibility   Hospice care requires the courage to deviate from the safe and conventional. It demands a willingness to improvise and an ability to adapt.

In a sense, fear of change is related to fear of death, the ultimate change. Acceptance of change involves the ability to surrender the old, comfortable, and familiar for new involvements. It presumes a strong sense of self and a trust of one's own intuition and the support of colleagues.

The journey with each patient and family is unique. No single staff member can ever expect to be able to accomplish total problem solving and fulfillment of needs. This is the purpose of a team approach. Some situations are a challenge to the resources of the whole team. Intuition may be the best means available to plan care creatively. What was useful yesterday may be irrelevant today. Thus flexibility is essential to the team's ability to function. If a staff member only feels secure by following the letter of the law, by ritual or by a repetitious care plan, he or she may feel extremely anxious in a setting that strives to individualize patient care. A secure, imaginative individual, on the other hand, will feel fulfilled in an environment that not only permits, but also encourages flexibility and creativity. The point is that an effective hospice staff member should not only be capable of being adaptable but also should enjoy it.

Maturity   Maturity may be difficult to define, but it can usually be sensed; it is an important attribute for the hospice team member. It is related to age and experience, but it is not limited to these components. One's philosophy of life, death, and afterlife is important in maintaining balance through difficult situations, such as the death of a favorite patient or many patients in a short time. It is also critical to maintaining a sense of priority during times of stress or fatigue. Staff members should be able to admit mistakes in order to learn from them and each other without fear of hard reprisal. They should accept responsibility for their actions and behavior. They should be able to accept their own feelings and be willing to forgive themselves as well as others. Those who cannot do these things have no place in a high-caring milieu; they will contaminate it.

Spirituality   Modern society convinces us that if we only work hard enough, learn enough, and become strong and self-sufficient enough, we can control our destiny. In this way we can impose peace and fulfillment on ourselves and everyone else. Yet the voice of sanity tells us that there must be more to life than the struggle of the will to be its own master (May 1982). The hospice worker, daily confronted by intense physical, emotional, and spiritual anguish, must be able to find meaning in his or her role, which provides numerous opportunities to make a difference by being present and possibly easing human suffering. Viktor Frankel (1946) speaks eloquently of the striving of human nature to find meaning in life.

Close association with those facing death leaves staff with an increased awareness not only of the real priorities and truth of life, but also with the emptiness of a philosophy of life that tricks society into the belief that individuals are completely in charge. Acknowledgment of a Supreme Power much higher than man will be observed in experienced hospice staff. An enhanced personal relationship with God results from contact with the dying. "Burnout" in this sense may be the refusal of the human will to relinquish its claim to absolute power. Conversely prevention can be accomplished through our willingness or ability to say "yes" to the process of living and all that entails rather than struggling, saying "no" or more commonly, "yes, but . . ." Willingness or surrender of will unites with God and gives strength while willfullness isolates and increases human loneliness. It is this strong faith and spirituality on which the hospice team depends for its continued replenishment (May 1982).

In addition to the five attributes just discussed, there are a number of other features of staff selection that should be commented upon. In selecting hospice staff it is important to look for individuals with varied personal and professional experience. In other words, one should aim for a team with some heterogeneity. The process not only ensures expert care for a larger variety of patients, but also expands the perceptions and attitudes of the staff. For example, a nurse with strong psychiatric experience can have her dormant medical-surgical skills refreshed by a nurse who is strong in these areas, while teaching and sharing her psychosocial skills. The whole staff will become more holistically oriented.

The ability of staff members to function dependently as well as independently is important. Some hospice functions require the capacity for acting on one's own spontaneously, whereas others demand integration in team activities.

Some attention should be given to the history of the hospice applicant's life experience. Frequently, an individual who has experienced a loss in his or her own life and has coped well is not only sensitive but also less anxious (Kübler-Ross 1975). In a sense the individual has been there and survived and thus is an excellent role model for the family. On the other hand, a newly bereaved individual who has not had the time necessary to develop coping and distancing would seem to be a high risk for serious stress problems.

No one is entirely exempt from occasional guilt feelings when his or her patients die. This is especially true when several patients die in a short period of time, suddenly or unexpectedly. Staff members with a low self-image may be plagued with serious doubts in such circumstances, much to their own as well as the program's detriment.

Because there has been some misunderstanding about it, one attribute that does not seem to be of any importance in selecting hospice staff nurses deserves mention. This is the type of educational background. There is no place for educational prejudice or for blanket rules regarding possession of a specific type of degree in the initial appointment of staff nurses. The important focus must be on what an individual can bring to his or her patients. Theoretical background that may be lacking can easily be made up by a motivated individual.

It is probably wise to make all appointments to the hospice staff on a trial or probationary basis. Transfer into other types of work environment should be easy and graceful if things do not work out for an appointee.

Similarly, seasoned hospice personnel may at times wish a temporary transfer for a change of pace, as well as environment, and to permit some reeducation in other areas. It is worth pointing out that this may be extremely difficult to accomplish for the home care staff, since experienced temporary replacements are almost impossible to find. For home care staff some type of contractual arrangement outside of the home care department may allow for the provision of back-up service during such temporary reassignments or during vacation and sick leave. An occasional change of duties may prevent an immense amount of wear and tear. In the home care department, a period of "respite" care is given to staff. This is a period in which no new hospice patients are assigned to a particular staff member and the patients already assigned are temporarily given to others. Staff has found this helpful and patients and their families do not object. Usually there is a natural break in the caseload when the sickest patients have died and those remaining on the caseload are stable enough to permit this type of change in assignment. Thus a staff member on respite may assist with teaching new personnel, students, and visitors or may take on some administrative functions. For qualified workers who enjoy public speaking, there are usually numerous lecture requests that can be assigned. Imaginative innovation in staff deployment is very helpful in keeping the staff fresh, happy, relaxed, and effective.

Education

Orientation Orientation of new staff members needs to be as flexible and individual as the care plans of the hospice patients. It should consider whether the employee is new to the organization, hospice care, or particular aspects of hospice care. The orientation will aim to supplement the individual's knowledge and clinical experience. Most staff members will require fairly basic education and training in the fundamentals of hospice care. Although this must include some theoretical background, much of the training must be practical and experiential. It is only when intellectual knowledge meets emotions and feelings and becomes integrated and congruent that hospice education is complete; this is a never-ending process. There really is no substitute for an experienced mentor working one-to-one with a new hospice staff member. This not only results in highly individualized instruction with immediate feedback, but also provides some anxiety-reducing support.

The Church Hospital orientation to hospice care includes contact with key members of the hospice team (both inpatient and home care) who introduce the orientee to the services they provide within their roles and how they interface with each other. This not only establishes a resource system, but equally important, effectively establishes rapport.

Orientation should include education on matters relating to death and dying, palliative care, hospice concepts, pharmacology, concepts of pain and symptom control, local policy, nursing procedures, and other matters particular to the area that the staff member is entering. For example, an experienced general medical-surgical nurse entering the home care program will be provided with instruction and techniques of home visitation, as well as an introduction to thanatology, grief and bereavement, and stress reduction. Pedestrian topics such as automobile first aid and street safety may prove very useful for a home care nurse. Staff input into the orientation process of new employees is extremely valuable.

Because there is a practical limit to the amount of individualization that can be provided in the initial orientation, it will be necessary in most hospice programs to set up a basic instruction course that includes some classroom time, which then can be supplemented by individual instruction on the nursing unit or in the home care situation.

Continuing Education   Hospice care is not a "once trained, always trained" proposition. There is need for continuing education. This can be accomplished in a number of ways. Regular conferences utilizing cases available in the program are an extremely valuable teaching tool. This often needs to be supplemented by periodic topic-oriented instruction covering such matters as the control of specific symptoms, techniques of dealing with grief reaction, and new methods in symptom control. There is great value in sending staff members off from time to time to other hospice programs and to hospice meetings. Maintaining an up-to-date indexed list of recommended readings can be very helpful.

Within the structure of a hospice program, someone responsible for planning, organizing, and executing initial orientation programs and continuing education programs can be very helpful. However, such an individual must draw upon all members of the hospice team for input into the educational process.

Evaluation

No hospice program meets its full potential unless there is careful evaluation of what is being done. This should be done for individual hospice patients and for individual hospice staff. The precise method of evaluation is a local and individual matter depending upon the particular program. The method chosen should strike a balance. To some extent it should be formal and systematic to ensure completeness and fairness; however, it also should be individualized, subjective, and supportive, to ensure the maximum benefit from the evaluation process.

Each program must devise audit criteria to demonstrate its degree of compliance with regulations and standards such as those developed by the Joint Commision on Accreditation of Hospitals (JCAH) or federal and state agencies. Church Hospital, a JCAH-accredited hospital, has chosen not to participate in the Medicare hospice benefit program or in separate JCAH hospice accreditation. Nevertheless, many of these standards serve as guidelines for our policies and in delivering excellent quality patient care.

Screening criteria developed for inpatient and home care can be designed to discover or follow up problem areas. These results lead to change in program policy.

For example, in the first year of operation of the Church Hospital hospice program, a trend in frequent readmissions to the hospital was noted. Since this was the first program in the area, there were numerous requests for "emergency" initial admission. Most frequently the requests were made for patients experiencing severe pain. It was learned that the request for pain control could not be equated with the readiness or ability of family members to accept a hospice program or commit themselves to the 24-hour home care of their relative. The admission criteria guidelines were revised, and the family meetings were initiated to better orient and prepare its members. Both have succeeded in limiting readmissions to those of clinical necessity.

Occasionally, when a patient or family has been extraordinarily difficult, a post-mortem discussion and review of the care is an important means of learning how to deal with similar situations in the future. It is also helpful for the team members to recognize that they as individuals were not alone in their dilemmas and difficulties and to learn from the experience. Staff must understand that there is no such thing as a perfect or even "classic" hospice patient-family unit; each has its strengths and weaknesses with which the team will struggle. Some patients whose ability to meet the criteria is questionable may be admitted to the program. Such patients are frequently those in most need or whose families need the chance, under the guidance of team, to test their ability to provide care. When someone of questionable status is admitted, those team members providing primary care must be aware of the problems that may jeopardize hospice so that they can be dealt with immediately. On the other hand, someone labeled as an "inappropriate candidate" should not be given up on so quickly that a fair trial is not given. An informed staff will not feel they have failed a patient if after an honest attempt they cannot sufficiently meet the needs.

The support of an extended care facility that is interested in learning hospice care and working in harmony with the hospice program can be a back-up support for the team. Such facilities can provide greater opportunity for patients who fall into the questionable area to have hospice care, even if home care is not appropriate.

Hospice care is not for everyone. Those responsible for admissions must be able to identify patients who do not meet admission criteria and be prepared not only to back the decision to a distraught family, but also to provide assistance in offering alternatives for care. Audits can be useful in exposing inappropriate admissions whose needs were not met.

The design of forms and checklists is an important and easy mechanism to ensure that quality care, hospice priorities, and regulatory compliance is achieved on an ongoing basis. The forms may be the focus of periodic audits, staff self-audit, or hospice team meetings. Staff members can be most helpful in providing input for the design of these tools: they know what they are most apt to forget to document and where they have fallen short of goals. These forms are a useful reminder to ensure adequate patient care documentation.

Evaluation for hospice staff can be a time for honest feedback, as well as creative sharing and setting of goals and expectations for the future. Each staff member brings unique gifts into the hospice experience. The evaluation process presents an opportunity to acknowledge these attributes and to inform the staff member how these relate to the hospice program in general. Naturally, praise breeds a positive atmosphere for continued good work; it needs to be administered in regular doses rather than saved for a yearly overdose.

The evaluation process often can be a useful two-way street. Staff members need to be actively involved in program development and policy making. Their practical day-to-day experience and awareness of trouble spots can be extremely helpful in obtaining the maximum from the program. Furthermore, when staff is involved in the development of guidelines and policy, they are more likely to understand their rationale and to comply effectively. Evaluation should be careful and honest, but to the extent possible it should be carried out in a nonthreatening fashion.

Staff Stress — "Burnout"

Stress is a normal part of life. Without stress life is devoid of an important dimension. Stress can be a positive factor leading to growth and progress. It can also be paralyzing and can contribute to illness (Selye 1956, 1976; Pelletier 1977, 1978).

Thoughout the medical care system, there are many sources of stress and many stressful situations. The care of the terminally ill in general and hospice care in particular can be the source of both beneficial and harmful stress for personnel.

We will be looking here at the harmful aspects of stress among members of the hospice care team. In hospice care, as in some other areas, this goes by the term "burnout." Although some feel that problems of staff stress and burnout in hospice care have received more attention than they deserve, it would be unrealistic to overlook it as a potential source of difficulty for the hospice care team.

It is important to recognize that everyone is prone to the harmful effects of stress; many people are reluctant to admit this propensity or to recognize the unfavorable effects of stress when they occur. Conversely, for some the *fear* of stress may in and of itself be anxiety producing and enervating (Shealy 1976). Once staff stress occurs, it tends to be invasive and contagious. This is not the place for a detailed consideration of the cause, prevention, recognition, and treatment of psychological stress syndromes, but it is worthwhile to make certain observations with respect to staff stress among the hospice care team.

Causative Factors

There are a number of factors in hospice care that foster development of unfavorable stress reactions. The day-in, day-out close contact with dying patients brings the hospice worker into frequent confrontation with his or her own mortality. In such a setting it is difficult to avoid contemplation of one's own death. A hospice team member's unresolved concerns in this regard provide a fertile ground for stress reactions. Furthermore, for individuals with a background in the health professions, death indeed conveys an element of defeat that, even in the absence of unresolved fears, can be a source of frustration.

Many hospice care workers tend to be idealistic. Some adopt an unrealistic view of what it is possible to accomplish for the terminally ill. The discrepancy between their expectations and reality can be the source of severe disappointment, frustration, and distress.

The nature of hospice care deprives team members of some very effective and comfortable defense mechanisms in dealing with terminal illness and death. Depersonalization, detachment, clear definition of responsibility, and stereotyped response can be most helpful defenses when one is threatened by the death of a patient. However, hospice care is characterized by a high degree of personal attention and involvement, lack of strict role definitions for team members, and an emphasis upon flexible and innovative responses to situations (Pelletier 1977). These and a number of other factors, added to the usual stress-provoking aspects of medical care, make the hospice team member particularly vulnerable to staff stress.

Effects of Stress

Excessive stress leads to a number of undesirable effects. For the individual team member, unpleasant symptoms of anxiety, depression, sleeplessness, and change of appetite can be most troublesome (Flynn 1980). The net result is greatly depleted energy and concentration. These in turn lead to impairment of the team member's capacity to provide excellent patient care. In addition, intrastaff friction and scapegoating may develop among team members, which again is both unpleasant for the individuals involved and harmful for patient care. Finally, unhealthy stress responses lead to a high turnover rate among hospice personnel; this not only results in considerable dissatisfaction for individual team members, but also impacts unfavorably on the quality of care provided to patients.

Prevention of Stress Reactions

Prevention of staff stress is more satisfactory than is its treatment. Prophylaxis is not always possible, however, and every mature hospice care program has experienced some adverse stress reactions. It is important, however, to take certain steps to manage stress and minimize its serious risks.

The selection process for team members is important and deserves the careful attention of program leaders. Mismatching a person to a job can create an environment favoring the occurrence of severe, stressful reactions. It is best to avoid appointing to hospice teams individuals with clearly unhealthy attitudes toward death and dying. People vary immensely in their capacity for physical work and psychological stress; work assignments should take these variables into account.

The interview process in selecting new staff members is the beginning of their stress management program. Careful assessment of the previously mentioned qualities (flexibility, competence, maturity, sensitivity, and spirituality) is of utmost importance. Additionally, since few candidates have hospice experience, particularly in the home care setting, a detailed description of the job and the expectations of both candidate and supervisor must be discussed. Examples from anonymous case histories that depict frequently encountered situations and problems help the candidate to understand more clearly the differences between hospice care and previous work settings. It is important not to shock or frighten away a good candidate by sharing the most difficult or sad case histories, as this may be overwhelming. During the interview, when a potential team member is feeling a bit more relaxed, it is most important to discuss what the individual understands about the program in which he or she is applying for a position. What has the applicant heard about the hospice program? The interviewer needs to know something of the person's motivation for choosing to work with the terminally ill. If recent bereavement is a factor in his or her history, these risks need to be considered in the decision to hire. Ascertaining the candidate's stress-related behavior and self-awareness is an early step in staff support. Answers to the question of how the person reacts when feeling emotional discomfort, anger, or repulsion can be very enlightening. When actual behavior matches described behavior, this reveals a high degree of self-awareness. A supervisor can then often provide a great deal of support by gentle, insightful nudges. On the other hand, an employee who reacts much differently than described during anxiety-provoking situations will need more supervision and coaching to recognize his or her symptoms early and make effort to change negative behavior.

Once staff members have been selected, proper orientation can be a valuable tool in preventing staff stress. Each team member should understand hospice principles and practices, accept the hospice approach, and comprehend the way in which he or she fits into the team and its spirit. Most important, however, the team member should be given a realistic picture of what it is reasonable to expect to accomplish in the care of the patient terminally ill from malignancy.

Hospice program leaders should create an environment in which team members are able to help each other. Mutual sharing and assistance among the members of the hospice care team have proved to be the most effective weapons in the prevention of harmful staff stress reactions. There must be ongoing efforts at communication between team members. Regular meetings of the hospice team play an important part in this respect. Topflight educational programs encourage personal growth, which in turn enhances personal satisfaction. Patient care conferences not only provide an improved sense of understanding about individual patients, but if properly conducted, also permit the venting of some concerns, fears, and feelings by team members.

Certain team members are particularly suited to the provision of support to other team members. The chaplain and the psychiatric staff come immediately to mind, as does the hospice physician. However, the important point is that *all* team members must accept responsibility for preserving their own mental and physical health. This means that they take the possibility of stress overload seriously and devise realistic plans of prevention for themselves (Shealy 1976).

In a sense hospice can borrow Dorothea Orem's theory of self-care nursing process and apply it to itself. She theorized that persons who take actions to meet their own self-care requirements (or those of teammates) have a unique set of action capabilities. She defines self-care as "the practice of activities that individuals initiate and perform on their own behalf in maintaining life, health and well-being" (Orem 1980; Fawcett 1984).

The team can rightfully look to the leaders of the hospice program to create a milieu conducive to good working conditions and to encourage several methods of supportive team interaction. On the other hand, it is unrealistic and ineffective for the employees to expect the program to attempt to meet all their needs. The question that first must be asked is what is the team doing for itself individually and collectively? Stress is produced through both internal and external means. Each individual must have the maturity to recognize and meet his or her own needs for adequate rest, recreation, exercise, reflection, and the like. No one can do this for the individual. Naturally team members who share interests and mutual support can draw from each other's resources as needed so long as no one is in the role of giving or taking continuously. The giver can become depleted and the taker, dependent.

Some effective conventional modes of coping with stress are regular exercise or other diversionary activity, good eating habits, and adequate sleep. While such measures obviously promote health and well-being, they are particularly important for caregivers who may habitually think of the needs of others and rarely of their own.

Stress management can also include such innovative self-regulation techniques as yoga or eliciting the relaxation response, including biofeedback (Brown 1974, 1977). Progressive relaxation of bodily parts, rhythmical breathing exercises, or meditation by means of focus of attention and concentration may allow the stress response to decrease, and each is said to be an effective coping tool when taught and used properly (LeShan 1974; Benson 1975; Carrington 1977; Braillier 1982).

Although stress management for staff is vitally important, it is often crucial for family caregivers. Once mastered by staff, these self-regulatory mechanisms then can be taught to patients to enhance symptom control and to families for their general well-being.

At Church Hospital a four-part series is presented to staff (limited to 10 to 16 participants) once or twice a year. Sessions are held one week apart to allow practice time for techniques learned in each session and to more fully integrate the content, which includes general stress theory, the relaxation response, progressive relaxation, visualization and guided imagery, autosuggestion, experience guiding another through process as well as being guided, the use of touch, therapeutic massage indications, and contraindications for various techniques and precautions. Staff members do not attempt to use these techniques with patients or attempt to teach them until they have completed the series and feel comfortable with them. If an individual is not comfortable with the techniques and attempts to use them with another anxious person, his anxiety will transfer. These sessions can serve as a microscope for participants to discover insights into their own attitudes and behavior that they may pass on consciously or unconsciously (Korn and Johnson 1983).

Because working with the terminally ill invoves a high degree of introspection and self-awareness, all staff, particularly in home care where intimacy is even more intense, are encouraged to keep a personal journal (Brown 1983). Frequent brief entries are encouraged on one half of a page. Later *retrospective* notes can be added as clearer insights come into focus. Such journals are naturally the private concerns of the writer and would never be subject to supervisory scrutiny, but supervisory staff can be effective mentors for those who choose to share sections of importance. The journal is particularly useful for enabling staff members to appreciate their growth, changes of attitude, and meaningful actions. It also can enhance their awareness of a negative shift, indicating a need for rest or respite.

Another useful tool is self-scoring on the Templer Death Anxiety Scale. Awareness of the degree of death anxiety, based on a 15-point scale, can enable a staff member to more carefully plot exposure to such anxiety-provoking stress or perhaps assess motives for becoming involved.

Sometimes a staff member is not particularly anxious regarding death issues for him- or herself but will unconsciously or consciously try to protect younger, more inexperienced staff from exposure to complicated hospice patient-family situations. This is particularly evident in middle-aged staff members relating to younger staff approximating the ages of their own children. In our experience this overprotection is not only unnecessary but also unhelpful to staff for whom the concern is directed. All staff members, no matter what their ages and professional experiences, can rightly feel pride in their accomplishments in working with people facing death. To deprive qualified and sensitive staff members by protecting them from the accompanying pain does not do them justice.

Journal Keeping to Combat Stress   Journal keeping is a particularly useful self-help method of assisting staff members to grow in hospice care and maintain a healthy perspective. During orientation each staff member is encouraged to obtain a notebook for this purpose. The suggested format is as follows: Divide pages in half and make a short, dated entry daily on the left-hand column of the page, leaving the right side empty for later comments. This entry is often technical or factual in the beginning. Later entries tend to show more insight and staff feelings.

Periodic Entries

11/1 Admitted Mrs. J to hospice today. She doesn't seem like someone who is dying.

11/7 Mrs. J's pain was severe today and she is beginning to talk about dying. I wanted to reassure her that everything would be OK. It was hard not to offer false hope and instead encourage her to talk and get a new medication order to control pain.

11/8 The increased medication order worked. I think Mrs. J and her family are beginning to trust me.

11/9 I reported on Mrs. J today. The supervisors and staff reassured me that I'm doing everything I can be doing for now and gave me some pointers to watch for the next step.

1/6 Mrs. J is dying. Strangely enough we're all ready, yet I wonder what the actual moment of death will be like. Maybe I should ask the on-call nurse to call me so I can be there at death

Late Entries

12/1 I guess I was trying to deny that such a nice lady would be dying soon

12/26 I'm beginning to understand that many symptoms can be controlled. I feel less afraid and helpless and more confident in how I can offer reassurance to patients.

1/8 I'm on call and Mrs. J just died. I made a visit and Mr. J was upset because he had taken the dog for a short walk and when he returned, she was gone. We talked about those last few minutes and how well he cared for Mrs. J. He feels OK about it now.

1/16 I did it — I really made a difference, but it was sure great to have the team behind me. I think I can help Mary Jane. Her patient is dying and is so angry that it's hard for her to remember how good it feels to know you've done your very best and really made a difference.

Journals need not be a requirement or regulation within the program. Keeping one should be strongly encouraged, however. Supervisors and colleagues can help staff members gain perspective from entries they care to share, to look for patterns indicating evidence of growth that a fatigued or discouraged worker may not appreciate about him- or herself, or perhaps to identify stress symptoms earlier. Naturally the key to this self-help journal method is honesty and trust enough to share entries as frequently as necessary. It is not at all unusual for strong insights gained a year or more later to be added to the right side of the page. Journals are useful to experienced as well as novice staff.

Group Staff Support   The experience of hospice programs with group conferences designed specifically for staff support has been variable. Many programs have found such meetings extremely helpful. Others have not been favorably impressed with their value; they have made the staff support function a by-product of conferences whose primary objective is education or patient care. Regular in-service education programs that update staff members' knowledge can help reassure them that they have done all they could as caregivers. If meetings for the specific purpose of staff support are held, they should be planned and organized with extreme care.

Support is a vague term and usually means different things to different people. Stressed individuals have a tendency to narrow their perspective as a coping mechanism. If this occurs, it is even more difficult to satisfy their identified needs since they are less open to new ideas and insights. The leadership should be selected thoughtfully and the program monitored carefully to be certain that problems are properly identified, that content is appropriate, and that individuals with special needs can be referred to qualified counselors, instructors, or clergy. Counterproductive results occur if unskilled leaders cannot guide the group properly, lack understanding of grief responses and typical group dynamics, or try to meet therapeutic needs in a general meeting. Poorly planned or conducted meetings with conflicting agenda can be most disappointing to the team and most detrimental to effective functioning.

Work Assignments   It is usually advisable to assign hospice workers to regular shifts over a period of time. Periodic short breaks from work should be provided and vacations should be given and taken. When hospice staff members are away from work, their time off should be completely free of hospice responsibilities and concerns. Staff members should be encouraged in the development of outside interests. They should be instructed in the use of some distancing techniques that are compatible with hospice care philosophy. It is important that they learn to use their colleagues effectively in the care of patients. Each hospice staff member must recognize that he or she is indeed a member of the team, does not individually need to provide all aspects of care to each patient, and can call upon teammates for help. This aspect cannot be over emphasized. It goes without saying that the physical structure of the environment is important in avoiding fatigue and frustration.

If the logistics can be worked out, it is often helpful to develop a system whereby hospice staff members can arrange temporary transfer or change of assignment to other types of work. This not only assists in avoiding staff stress, but also encourages cross-fertilization between the hospice program and other providers of patient care. Some programs have found it advantageous to have a regular rotation system. If this is not possible, temporary or permanent transfer should be made easy and graceful. At Church Hospital home care has developed a regular rotation system of "staff respite" whereby staff members have no hospice patients for a period of time.

With respect to staff stress, it is important to note that integration of hospice inpatients into a general medical-surgical nursing unit, as has been done successfully at Church Hospital, alleviates some of the stress problems related specifically to terminal care. Under this system each team member has responsibility both for hospice patients and for patients who will recover. In this environment staff stress problems more nearly approximate those of general medical-surgical care. Nurses, for example, may be frustrated by the end-of-shift feeling that because of time constraints they were not able to accomplish as much in the care of some of their patients as they would have wished. Some have been reluctant to recognize the role that other hospice caregivers can play for the patient who simply needs to have someone with him.

Although the sources of stress in this type of program tend to be more of a general nature than those related specifically to terminal illness care and death, the hospice team members are still thrown into intimate contact with the dying and their families. Therefore, they are subject to the individual sense of loss in specific cases that is a feature of all hospice care. Nonetheless, it has been our impression that the overall effect of the integration of hospice patients with general medical-surgical patients has been to diminish staff stress problems.

Recognition and Treatment of Staff Stress Syndrome

Both for the individual team member and for the hospice team as a whole, it is difficult to draw a clear-cut line between a healthy, creative stress response and a frankly abnormal or pathological state. *Extreme* stress in the individual and the team can be recognized by the disintegration of function. However, next to prevention of harmful stress reaction, *early recognition* and *prompt treatment* are the optimal means of preventing serious difficulty. Each hospice program should develop its own mechanisms for the rapid and appropriate diagnosis and treatment of stress. The team members, for example, should understand their responsibility to report their signs of stress to the supervisor.

In the individual team member, symptoms of harmful stress reaction include fatigue, sleep disturbance, appetite changes, somatic symptoms without organic basis (e.g., headache and diarrhea), paranoia, and withdrawal (Patrick 1979). Depression, anxiety, and irrational anger may occur. The use of depersonalizing and derogatory terms for patients is frequently seen. Errors in observation and recording, together with decreased concern about mistakes, may be a symptom of unfavorable stress reaction.

Treatment of staff stress syndrome in a team member must be highly individualized. In some instances simply a little informal counseling by another appropriate individual such as the head nurse or chaplain may be the wisest choice. More formal counseling may be necessary for others. Sometimes staff stress symptoms in the individual will respond to relatively minor modifications in assignment, routine, or schedule. Occasionally, temporary or permanent transfer out of the program provides the only solution. The decision as to whether or not to employ psychiatric therapy for team members suffering from work-related stress must obviously be made on an individual basis.

Staff stress tends to be a communicable disease. A relatively minor degree of stress among individual team members may mushroom as the team interacts. Therefore, one must be alert to team symptoms as well as individual symptoms. No staff functions entirely smoothly at all times, but a sharp change in the level of intrastaff friction and frequency of personality clashes deserves the attention of program leaders. So does an unusual number of requests for transfer. Some observers have commented upon the fact that an increased pace of activity with an appearance of frantic bustle may be a sign of group staff stress. Increased use of sick leave for vague illness of short duration and habitual tardiness also can signal a problem. Generally all these symptoms can be categorized under the headings of irritability, unquenchable fatigue, and decreased productivity.

Once the early symptoms of an unfavorable staff stress syndrome are recognized in the hospice team at large, treatment consists fundamentally of amplification of the preventive measures. Potential causes of unhealthy stress reactions should be sought out and dealt with promptly. Sometimes such sources are physical factors in the environment, workload distribution, or institutional regulations. Sometimes an individual team member is a source of team stress; stress is indeed contagious.

Beyond eliminating, insofar as possible, the causes of team stress, everything should be done to facilitate the capacity of staff members to help each other. The regular staff meeting schedule should be examined to determine whether the frequency and quality of the meetings are adequate. Some consideration may be given to the development of special programs for staff support, although, as noted earlier, these must be developed carefully, not casually. Scheduling breaks and vacations and the easy opportunity for temporary or permanent transfer must all be looked at.

There is no simple, totally effective treatment for staff stress either in the individual or in the team. The important points are as follows: It can be more easily prevented than treated. The potential for occurrence of staff stress should be recognized, and the program should be designed and operated to minimize the opportunity for it to develop in individuals or the team as a whole. However, because prevention is not uniformly successful, the mechanisms for early detection and treatment should be established.

References

Benjamin WW: Healing by the fundamentals. *N Engl J Med* 311:595, 1984.

Benson H: *Relaxation Response*. Avon Books, New York, 1975.

Brallier L: *Transition and Transformation: Successfully Managing Stress*. National Nursing Review, Los Altos CA, 1982.

Brown, B: *New Mind, New Body Biofeedback, New Directions for the Mind*. Harper & Row, New York, 1974.

Brown B: *Stress and the Art of Biofeedback*. Bantam Books, New York, 1977.

Carrington P: *Freedom in Meditation*. Doubleday Anchor Books, New York, 1977.

Fawcett J: *Analysis and Evaluation of Conceptual Models of Nursing*. FA Davis Company, Philadelphia, 1984.

Flynn P: *Holistic Health: The Art and Science of Care*. Robert J Brady (Prentice-Hall Publications), Bowie MD, 1980.

Frankel V: *The Doctor and Soul*. Bantam Books, New York, 1946.

Kelsey M: *The Other Side of Silence*. Paulist Press, New York, 1976.

Korn ER, Johnson K: *Visualization: The Uses of Imagery in the Health Professions*. Dow Jones-Irwin, Homewood IL, 1983.

Krieger D: *Foundations for Holistic Nursing Process: The Renaissance Nurse*. JB Lippincott, Philadelphia, 1981.

Kübler-Ross E: *Death as the Final Stage of Growth*. Prentice-Hall Publications, Englewood Cliffs NJ, 1975.

Kurhts SB: Symptom control in terminal disease. *PA Journal* 7:189, 1977.

LeShan L: How to Meditate. Bantam Books, New York, 1974.

Mathew LM, et al.: Attitudes of house officers toward a hospice on a medical service. *J Med Educ* 58:772, 1983.

May G: *Will and Spirit: A Contemplative Psychology.;* Harper & Row, New York, 1982.

Orem DE: *Nursing: Concepts of Practice*. ed 2. McGraw-Hill, New York, 1980.

Patrick P: Burnout, job hazard for health workers. *Hospital*, pp 87 – 90, 1979.

Pelletier K: *Mind as Healer, Mind as Slayer*. Dell, New York, 1977.

Pelletier K: *Toward a Science of Consciousness*. Delacorte Press, New York, 1978.

Selye H: *The Stress of Life*. McGraw-Hill, New York, 1956.

Selye H: *Stress Without Distress*. McGraw-Hill, New York, 1976.

Shealy N: *Ninety Days to Self Health*. Bantam Books, New York, 1976.

Tolle SW, Girard DE: The physician's role in the events surrounding patient death. *Arch Intern Med* 143:1447, 1983.

Chapter 7

The Volunteer as Team Member

Lucy B. McBee and Maureen Mason

Probably no other form of health care welcomes and involves volunteers as much as hospice programs. Volunteers are an integral part of virtually all the hospice activity in the United States. Besides carrying the spirit óf hospice, these are dedicated people who provide the added advantage of cost effectiveness. They make it possible to offer many services not otherwise available and in so doing, have actually made some hospice care for the terminal patient financially feasible. Volunteers are of immense value in meeting the needs of the dying patients, their families, the home care team and the hospital itself. They are naturally caring, willing and hard working and serve to complement all the others who maintain health care in the hospice setting.

In the proper use of volunteers, the fundamental word is *balance*. There must be a very careful balance between professional care and volunteer services. Since the patient is dependent upon both, it needs to be a shared contribution. Volunteers have to earn the trust and confidence of their professional co-workers by demonstrating their commitment and responsibility; professionals should be willing to respond to these efforts and be ready to advise and help. Balance also counts heavily in the amount of supervision given to volunteers. Between the supervisor and the individual, harmony is required for the common purpose. Too much supervision can be stifling and discouraging for the volunteer, but a free rein and inadequate direction are neither safe nor sound. Since all are pointed toward a distinct goal, team work is the effective method, the busy professional making an extra effort to encourage and enable the volunteer to contribute his or her own special skills. Finally, a rich dividend for patient and family, the physical and emotional benefits derived from a well coordinated hospice team.

The difference in function between hospice and other forms of health care is generally greater for volunteers than for other team members. For medical staffers most of the change is in degree and emphasis. But the volunteer is introduced to direct patient care and contact in an area that carries an enormous increase in responsibility. The nature of the hospice program not only permits this heightened role for its members, but encourages and capitalizes on it. Hospice can meet immediate, basic needs with its voluntary resources, such as providing physical comfort for patients. Naturally, the program must be selective as to whom it assigns bedside functions. A proven rule of thumb is to pick volunteers who can safely and productively perform those chores. They can be used in cleaning and bathing of the patient, in back rubs, getting the patient into a chair, bed changing, Foley catheter care, and certain aspects of charting, such as intake and output records. Using volunteers for such duties creates time for the nursing staff to extend to its charges services not otherwise available and permits a measure of flexibility in ward routine. For example, it might be difficult for a nurse on duty to supply a bath for the patient who wants one at 2:30 in the afternoon. Enter the volunteer. The patient, perhaps infirm and difficult to move, gets bathed, and the nurse is relieved for more pressing matters.

In utilizing volunteers, particularly for physical care, the preferences of the individual volunteer are paramount. Such work may not appeal to some volunteers, and no amount of training and supervision can change this. There also is an appreciable difference in the need for bathing and other such services on day and evening shifts. Assigning the right person to the right time and place is vital to the hospice program. Appropriate supervision means an awareness and consideration for the volunteer on a par with treatment of the patient. In addition to physical considerations, the hospice volunteer finds in day-to-day contact with the patient that he or she is making a unique contribution. As the program is meant to do, the volunteer is providing a psychological service. It appears to be most effective when there is direct involvement in the patient's physical care. For someone who is dying, the volunteer can be a friend, to listen, share thoughts, and serve as a conduit to the professional members of the hospice team. The volunteer may assist in taking walks around the hospital, visiting the garden or chapel, being nearby as death approaches, and being a part in the provision of bereavement support.

By virtue of their status as nonprofessionals, volunteers are often in a better position to offer direct patient services, acting as a bridge between the personal world outside the hospital and the impersonal routine within. Without interfering with the discipline and procedures of the nursing unit, a volunteer can sometimes soften the edges.

The volunteer, as an unassuming layman, may be perceived by the patient and family as someone outside the normal health care delivery system, someone to whom the patient can convey thoughts and feelings not expressed to medical personnel. The volunteer's freedom from other hospital responsibilities permits talking and listening at length, particularly at a critical juncture when a patient wants to unburden him- or herself.

These are large demands for an individual: to meet a stranger whose life is ebbing away and to summon up the necessary patience, compassion, and sensitivity to sustain that person. So the initial step of volunteer recruitment is as important as all the other subsequent phases. Hospice has to find the right people.

In an era when volunteerism is supposed to be declining, most hospice programs are encountering little trouble in filling their rosters. Potential volunteers seem to sense that their work will be interesting and rewarding, especially when the hospice volunteer director lays emphasis on the responsibilities and values ahead. The appeal is to all age groups, although older individuals retired from busy careers are a particularly fertile source of volunteer strength. Others who have suffered family losses bring a special empathy to their duties. The Church Hospital program includes a number of nurse-volunteers (see Chapter 8,"Outpatient Hospice Care") and one retired physician.

Some of the newcomers were brought into our program by the traditional recruitment methods: newspaper articles, church bulletins, local periodicals, and referrals by staff employees. Others were attracted to the program by talks given by the hospice staff and active volunteers, part of the campaign to seek out groups interested in working with the terminal patient.

Hospice volunteers don't just come aboard. When an interested person reports for the first interview, the director of volunteers puts in motion a carefully considered selection process. Selection and screening are the groundwork that will produce a successful addition to the hospice tream. The director exerts every effort to know the applicant, to discern and assess motivation, and to determine what special skills that individual might have to enrich the overall hospice performance. Each applicant is interviewed one or more times by the director and at least one other staff member. For the volunteer with a professional background, there is further screening by staff members from that particular discipline.

In our program, we have only four rigid criteria:
1. A high school diploma is the minimum educational requirement.
2. Prospective volunteers are asked to commit themselves to the program for a year.
3. It is our policy not to accept anyone who has experienced the death of a close family member within the past year.
4. Volunteers must satisfactorily complete the training program and 20 hours of probationary inservice.

Obviously, intangibles and subjective considerations figure in the evaluation of a prospective volunteer. Instant assessment is not a practice of hospice management, but the director and other interviewers are alert to read certain characteristics in their prospects; they can make an accurate prediction of an individual's performance. Basically, hospice looks for evidence that the applicant has the ability to communicate, feel compassion, show sensitivity and understanding, accept responsibility, and display a capacity for growth. A sense of humor is a definite asset, the sharper the edge on it the better. Flexibility is essential, with the expectation of dealing with patients and families of a different cultural and religious heritage.

On the negative side, the director and staff try to detect foibles and attitudes that are not welcome. Preoccupation with death and a morbid or immature view of dying are most undesirable. Personalities that may conflict are turned away. The very subjective type who tends to impose personal values on others, the insecure, the erratic, and impatient—they will not make the hospice team.

Uncovering these various traits may be a simple matter in some cases, very complex in others. And since the judgment of interviewers can only be imperfect, volunteers are appointed on a trial basis; their performance is carefully monitored during a probationary period. From the start, great emphasis is put on volunteer's understanding of just what is expected of them. When that is clear, trainees and staff are able to establish a relationship of mutual trust, the foundation of a strong support system from within. Lectures, class discussion, and outside reading—all are employed. Once the "on the job" training period has covered the essentials, the new members of the hospice team are initiated on the nursing unit. The training program lasts 26 hours and includes the following:

1. hospice concept and philosophy—senior volunteer.
2. disease processes and effects of therapy—hospice physician.
3. symptom control—nurse-practitioner.
4. inpatient hospice care—head nurse.
5. listening skills—bereavement coordinator.
6. volunteer role—senior volunteer.
7. social services in hospice care—social worker.
8. hospice home care—home care director.
9. grief and loss—bereavement consultant.
10. hospice bereavement program—bereavement coordinator.
11. spiritual evaluation of hospice patients—chaplain.
12. nursing procedures and hands-on care—unit nurse.

Once the training and the probationary period on the unit are completed the volunteer is rated by the director and hospice staff; all feedback on performance is taken into account. The volunteer then may elect to stay in the hospital or take further orientation and become part of the home care or bereavement team. The new member begins to attend a regular meeting of volunteers, which affords the working team educational opportunities and communal support, and is encouraged to sit in on regular staff sessions relating to patients and policies.

The hospice volunteer is now a full-fledged, assigned, and valued addition to this new, innovative calling in health care. The volunteer is a member of a team, in balance with professionals and sharing their concern for patients and families. Thus it is the full measure of the volunteer spirit.

Chapter 8

Outpatient Hospice Care

Kathleen A. Roche

If "a man's home is his castle" during life, it should remain so as he faces death. Traditionally, people were born and died at home — often the same one. They were cared for by people they knew, loved, and trusted in this familiar environment. They maintained control over their domain.

The modern trend in health care has been hospitalization of patients so that the high technological advances of the last decade can be applied to the fullest extent. High technology, however, cannot replace the human caring that is so vitally needed as earthly life draws to an end. Home care most frequently meets the needs of the dying person who has family willing to provide care. Additionally, it provides the opportunity for the family to anticipate the loss of a member and to interact in an intimate and satisfying way. The proverbial house can be put in order, business finished, and peace made as necessary (Jivoff 1979). This period of shared grief tends to enhance the bereavement period .

Home care is the option frequently chosen in today's economic climate with the emphasis on shorter hospitalizations. In the last five years, home care expertise has grown to the extent that more health care can be provided in the home setting than ever before. Although the benefits of home care make it superior to other available options for both patient and family, it is a difficult commitment to make; it requires deliberation and careful planning. Home care is not a panacea effective for everyone. The choice must be made by the entire care-providing group; most especially, the patient must participate in the decision. Other very basic considerations are the availability, capability, and health of the caregivers. Elderly hospice patients frequently have elderly spouses caring for them who are sick themselves. Although perfect health is not a prerequisite, conditions such as spinal arthritis, orthopedic, cardiovascular, and psychiatric diseases need careful assessment and extra support. For middle-aged patients, one cannot assume that spouses can provide care because of their need to work. The threat of employment loss to the well spouse is often as stressful as the terminal illness of the patient is to the couple. These needs cannot be ignored by the hospice team.

The hospital-based home care program is perhaps the ideal system of hospice care because of its flexibility and continuity. Both emotional and physical support can be provided whether the patient is in the hospital or at home. Even in the home setting, the health care team has the resources of the hospital on which to rely if necessary.

In general, home care serves the patients' medical, social, economic, and spiritual interests by extending health care to their residence. In addition to providing continuity of care, the home health program shortens the length of hospital stay and in some instances obviates hospitalization. This in turn promotes appropriate utilization of beds and other hospital facilities and reduces health care costs. Home care provides the opportunity to continue or to modify patient teaching begun in the hospital. With shorter hospital stays and the possibility of avoiding hospitalization, the home care staff finds that it must do more teaching. This in turn can lengthen the visit or necessitate more frequent visits for a period of time. The staff must be alert to recognize early those factors in the home environment that may interfere with high-quality patient care so that they can be corrected. Frequently, adjustments are needed to make patient care more convenient for those providing it. Any labor-saving ideas that will save the family unnecessary work will prevent or forestall exhaustion. In our experience families who have not managed well in home care prior to coming on the hospice program are most reluctant and anxious about attempting it again. They need much planning and reassurance.

The home care program serves as an excellent setting in which students and health care professionals can be taught holistic family care and hospice philosophy; they can test their clinical skills with supervision (Church Hospital 1984).

The whole population benefits from humanistic health care practices. Because the patient and family are an intereacting system, holistic practice dictates that they be treated as a single unit. Each member affects the others, as does any change in family status. Thus an adolescent son may experience crisis when his father's terminal illness forces him to sacrifice or delay college education to assist in the provision of care or to supplement the family earnings. The entire family's strengths, weaknesses, resources, and responsibilities must be taken into consideration as care plans are devised. Too often only one individual's wishes are taken into consideration. Usually this is the family leader or most verbal member. The best hospice care will be sabotaged by a frightened or angry family member who has not been taken into consideration in the plans.

Reimbursement for home care in general and hospice in particular has been a complex specialty in administration itself over the last five years. The specifics will be addressed in a later chapter. In general, within the last two years there have been many standards developed for hospice care. There are those established by the Joint Committee on Accreditation of Hospitals. Many states also have developed standards in collaboration with state or regional Nation Hospice Organization members. While standards define hospice care and help to ensure its quality, they also reflect the state of the art, which is young and immature now.

The designers of various models of hospice care (hospital based, free standing, coalition, rural, and urban) anxiously peruse standards, and federal and state regulations with an eye toward equality. However, these models are not "equal" because they are designed to meet the population they serve. The objectives of care-intensive programs, even though less costly and more appropriate than high technology, frequently conflict with health care cutbacks and cost-saving mechanisms. Reimbursement is *sometimes* denied by "letter of the law" determinations.

Compliance with various regulations and standards together with ensuring our own high quality and priorities of hospice care keep home care in a constant state of audit. As mentioned previously, paperwork and audits are stress for which hospice staff members, like all other health care workers, need to be prepared today. Because hospice grew out of tender loving care does not exempt it from the rigors.

The problems are complex ones involving ethical issues such as the allocation of relatively scarce resources and health care dollars. The answers to these questions are difficult, but dying patients are a minority group whose rights and needs deserve attention.

The Church Hospital Home Care Program

The Church Hospital home care program was originally developed as a public health nursing experience for the students in the hospital's school of nursing. Although the school closed several years before the hospice program officially opened, home care remained viable and was under the direction of Helen Fowler, registered-nurse, until her death. By this time, the home care had progressed to the status of a full-fledged department within the hospital structure. The preliminaries of certification were well under way when a new full-time home health director was hired. In January 1979 the program was certified for Medicare and Medicaid and additional nursing staff was hired.

At the present time the staff is composed of 10.6 full-time-equivalent (FTE) registered nurses, some of whom "float" and are used only when needed; three home health aides, one administrative secretary, one secretary, one billing clerk, one medical social worker, 0.5 FTE bereavement coordinator, one head nurse, one registered-nurse home care director/hospice coordinator, and two registered nurse-volunteers.

To date we have not been able to accept into the program certain patients whose physical needs have been greater than could be met by staff or volunteers. These include people who have insufficient caregivers to provide round-the-clock care or who require more than five visits a week on a prolonged basis.

In the past a medical social worker served the home care patients by contractual agreement. The cost of indirect services, however, became prohibitive; it represented about twice the time involved for the actual visit and was nonreimbursable by third-party payers. A method of having one hospital social worker assigned to home care was developed. This plan not only reduced cost, but also provided greater continuity as well. Regulatory changes may necessitate alteration of this arrangement.

Our experience with physical therapy was just the opposite. Serving the home care patients proved too great a burden on the department. A contractual agreement has worked out much more effectively. Speech therapy and occupational therapy are required for less than 5% of the home care population, and it has been most satisfactorily provided through contract.

Because the program is hospital based, each of the hospital departments can serve the home care patients. Thus pastoral counseling, nutrition therapy, respiratory therapy, and the like are all available when needed. Therefore, in serving patients at home, the home health department does not have to duplicate personnel already employed by the hospital.

Durable medical goods and pharmacy services are also provided by contract. The pharmacist is an integral member of the team. He or she not only monitors the drug profiles carefully and stocks the specialty items but also frequently makes up special suppositories for use when patients can no longer swallow. This service often makes it possible to keep patients at home; their families are not traumatized by having to administer injections. The pharmacy delivery service is much more than a convenience, it saves human energy and relieves the nurses of the temptation to assist families by bringing the drug themselves. For safety reasons it is wise for the staff not to acquire the reputation of transporting drugs (especially narcotics) or otherwise controlled substances. Nurses should not risk personal harm unnecessarily.

A letter of agreement with a large local ambulance company ensures continuity of care should hospitalization become necessary. City and county ambulances will transport patients only to the nearest hospital. It is imperative that the patient return to Church Hospital rather than to another where that individual and hospice care are both unknown. Thus traumatic, aggressive or invasive treatment, and drug withdrawal are avoided. Ambulance drivers are alerted if a hospice patient is to be transported so that they will not initiate resuscitation.

The Concept of Primary Nursing

The primary nursing concept is utilized by the home care department. Each nurse carries a caseload of patients and plans their nursing care in collaboration with the attending physician. Since one nurse is responsible for each patient, long-

and short-term goals can be well planned and accountability issues are clearer. The department is open only Monday through Friday, 7:30 AM-4:00 PM; there is a nurse on call every day. This means that each nurse not only has the responsibility for a caseload (usually 12 to 17 patients, with approximately 20% being hospice patients), but also must become familiar with the total population. To accomplish this there is a weekly meeting on Thursday morning, during which time each nurse gives a complete report on each new admission and an update on the rest. Occasionally, the primary nurse will form a special relationship with a patient and family and choose to be notified by the on-call nurse if this patient's death is imminent. Because all nurses experience such a relationship, they understand the request and do not feel their competence is threatened. Rarely does a primary nurse or patient request a change of assignment, even during long or repetitive admissions to home care. Changes of assignment usually require sensitive handling for all parties concerned to avoid or deal with feelings of inadequacy or abandonment. As mentioned previously, periods of respite from hospice care are being encouraged within the department on a seniority basis. Respite periods are perceived as a well-earned rest.

In the early period of the program, it was estimated that nurses spent 50%-100% more time during the hospice visit than for other types of visits. This amount of time is often required, particularly during crisis periods. In general, there are more bases to cover in a shorter period of time because of the shorter life expectancy. Patients and families simply cannot and should not be unduly rushed during this period of crisis. Admission visits for *all* patients generally require double the usual visit time, since the patient care plan data base must be obtained on the initial visit.

The Church Hospital program extends its general home care boundaries to serve a greater area for hospice patients. It is important, however, not to require of the staff more than 20 to 30 minutes driving time. Clustering visits saves staff time and reduces cost of travel. A recent management study revealed that RNs spend an average of 82 minutes each visit performing direct care for hospice patients and 48 minutes for regular home care patients. This would represent a 70% increase in direct care for hospice patients, despite the observation that nonhospice home care patients are now more ill than they were in 1977, due to earlier hospital discharge. Hospice patients may also consume a greater portion of social work and nursing time in indirect care, telephone contacts, on-call situations, and family meetings. No difference was observed in the time spent by home health aides who visit both categories of patients. Both RNs and home health aides spent approximately 13% of their day in travel.

To summarize, the average home health/hospice RN's typical day was spent as follows:[1]

direct patient care	33.7%
paper work and telephone	31.2%
travel	13.4%
meetings (including family meetings)	11.5%
on-call direct patient care and other associated indirect activities	3.3%
personal (including emergency car repair, getting gas, meals, etc.)	6.9%

One of the strongest features of the Church Hospital program is the guarantee of a bed for a justifiable emergency hospice admission. Families are less fearful of attempting home care if they have the back-up support of an inpatient bed. The home care nurse's anxiety is reduced by the awareness that there are standing orders to be followed should management problems be observed that cannot be successfully dealt with at home.

Advantages and Disadvantages of Hospice Home Care

Home care is nothing new on the health care scene. In this era of high technology and impersonal health care, it has been rediscovered and newly appreciated. The following advantages of home care should be noted:

- The cost is considerably less than that of institutional care and is reimbursable either in part or totally by health insurance plans when care is skilled, intermittent and the patient is homebound.
- The family and patient have the opportunity to fully experience the final days as a family together without any restrictions except those they wish to impose.
- The patient and family retain much more control over the situation; feelings of hopelessness and helplessness are greatly reduced.
- Invasive life-prolonging (or death-prolonging) procedures are unavailable in the setting but can be obtained if needed. They are less likely to be inappropriately used in a crisis.

1. C.Boyne, 1985, Productivity in home health — a management proposal (unpublished data). This study was conducted excluding the medical information forms now required by Medicare. By fall of 1985 the percentage of paperwork could increase to 35%, thus reducing productivity.

- Food and activity can be geared toward usual life-style or preference.
- Hospice staff can help teach a family how to care for the ill person, monitor progress, and be available for problems or questions.
- Hospice staff, entering into the family system, has the opportunity to effect positive change in the patterns of communication and guide the family toward resolution of conflict.
- Trust and relationships with the hospice team are generally well established prior to the patient's death, making bereavement follow-up a continuation of care rather than the intrusion of a stranger.

There are also disadvantages to be considered:

- Families often do not understand how demanding the 24-hour care of a person can be; they can become exhausted.
- Reimbursement of cost is often to some extent uncertain.
- Families may feel abandoned by the health care system and improperly pre-pared for the task of home care. Emergencies can trigger overwhelming anx-iety.
- Unless the care is planned, the bulk of nursing responsibilities may fall upon the shoulders of one person, who becomes drained (Roche 1979).
- If the patient's condition stabilizes, care no longer may be considered skilled and therefore would not be reimbursable by third-party payors. Alternative plans must be provided.
- The regulations with which home care agencies must comply are often con-fusing to families, who then may call the hospice program into question when they do not qualify for certain services.

The critical consideration is, however, that the care settings may not be as impor-tant as the caring that takes place within them. Home care should not be forced on anyone. Very apprehensive people may respond to the opportunity to meet with the primary nurse several times before they are actually placed under his or her care. On-call systems, readmission policy, and use of emergency staff visits should all be explained several times to allay anxiety.

Preparation to Return Home

Preparation for discharge from inpatient hospice care is really begun during the screening process before admission to the program. Rapport already has been estab-lished with the home health director or designees. Rounds are made fre-quently to check patient progress in anticipation of discharge to home care. Home health staff together with the physician, nurse practitioner, social worker, and dis-charge planner meet to discuss any equipment that might be needed. The options are presented at the family meeting.

Patient care is taught in the hospital by the staff and volunteers. Refinements are made in the actual home setting. Since there is constant communication between the home care department and the nursing unit, the initial visit at home can be scheduled the same day as discharge if necessary. Some patients realize that they are going to die very soon and want to be at home. These are times when discharge must be successfully completed very quickly to fulfill the patient's request. It is essential that the contracting agencies with which the hospice deals understand the priority nature of assisting the patient to get home. The family has to be well prepared and understand that the patient in such a situation may only live a few hours. If they are unprepared, they may fear that they caused the death prematurely because of their inexperience. The importance of alerting the on-call nurse to the discharge of such an ill patient cannot be overemphasized. The on-call nurse needs not only the usual appropriate clinical information, but also directions to the house by the quickest route.

Families are encouraged to keep a simple notebook "chart" on the patient. This is especially important if many caregivers are going to be involved with the patient. Sometimes it is appropriate to photocopy for the family the patient care plan from the home health record. Care must be taken to document the updates in the official record as well as on the family chart. Through this notebook the nurse can be kept abreast of changes noted by all family members, not just the one present during the visit, or can pick up on information that a single caregiver may forget to report. In addition, instructions can be written out, which can be helpful to the on-call staff. The most important point is to keep this notebook chart simple. If it is packed with medical and nursing jargon, the patient and family may be intimidated by it and not use it.

Many patients want to maintain as much independence and control as possible. Others become forgetful, confuse medications, and need help. In either case it is helpful to have a supply of small bottles into which the day's doses can be individually poured and marked with the appropriate administration time. Many patients set an alarm clock to remind them of their next dose. Pre-poured medications are a must during the night; they allow the patient to have the proper dose of medication without having to fully awaken and disrupt sleep.

The importance of bowel care cannot be overemphasized. It seems that many patients have to experience the discomfort of severe constipation and/or impaction to fully understand the need for prevention. All too often patients protest that they do not need stool softeners or laxatives that are ordered because they have never been constipated in their life. Analgesics, particularly narcotics, given in large quantity over a prolonged period quickly change usual bowel patterns . The care plan is not complete or effective until the patient maintains the right to refuse any medication or treatment.

Families often ask what they need to care for a patient at home. Most patients need very little in the way of major equipment. Many do need to rent a hospital bed so that they can be turned, positioned, and cared for properly once they are bedbound. Some patients remain ambulatory until death. Table 1 lists equipment together with its use as a guide for families. It represents an *optimum*. Where resources are limited, patients can, for example, be adequately cared for with two sets of sheets. Very anxious families often tend to overprepare and gather too many supplies (Roche 1979).

Baltimore City, like many other areas of the country, now requires smoke detectors in rental properties. We recommend their use in hospice care for several hospice-specific reasons. Although anyone can have a fire, families under stress can more easily forget to turn off a heater, iron, stove, or other house hold appliance. They are already greatly preoccupied, have numerous caregiving distractions, and are often sleep deprived to varying degrees. Additionally, a confused or wandering patient (perhaps suffering symptoms of brain metastasis) presents an additional threat of kitchen or appliance fire.

Many fire departments offer decals that patients can display in a conspicuous place to alert the firemen of a disabled resident in the event of fire. The use of these decals is controversial. People in high crime areas often fear using them: they feel the decal frequently signals thieves of their disability. This visible signal together with the storage of class II drugs may considerably increase their safety risk. It is our practice to advise families of their availability and to point out the negative and positive aspects of their use, but encourage them to make their own choice. The families are encouraged to keep their medications out of obvious sight yet handy for themselves. Windowsills, for example, are the worst place to store medications. The home health staff wear washable street clothing and carry tote bags rather than the conventional medical bag. These measures help to keep a low profile in the community. Staff is strictly forbidden to carry any type medication so as not acquire a reputation for handling pharmaceuticals.

The police department provides periodic education on street safety and offers an emergency number to be used if police protection should be deemed necessary for staff protection. Although police protection has been needed only twice in our eight-year history, the mechanism had to be in place so as to be available quickly if needed. Staff members must remember that no matter what the reputation of the neighborhoods they visit, their best protection is in their own hands. They must acquire a street wisdom and alertness based on constant observation and assessment. They cannot get caught napping and must not expose themselves to unreasonable risk. On the other hand, they would arouse much curiosity if they were to frequently request police protection. Any one who is extremely uncomfortable while out in the street should not be employed in home care. Undesirable neighborhoods and weather conditions are part of the job.

Table 8-1

Equipment	Use or Underlying Reason
1. Rented hospital bed with siderails	To allow for safe lifting and turning without back injury. If total care, consider an electric hi-lo bed; only the charge for a regular hospital bed will be reimbursed in most cases.
2. Bed care utensil set, consisting of plastic cup, denture cup (if dentures used), kidney (emesis) basin, bath basin, bed pan, soap dish, water pitcher, and tray	These items allow caregiver to have all items necessary for personal care readily available. Patients may take these disposable-type sets home from the hospital, since they have paid for them.
3. Five or six fitted bottom sheets[a]	The smoothness of the bottom sheet protects the skin from extra friction and wrinkles.
4. Two large pillows, two medium pillows, and one or two small ones wilth two changes of pillow cases[a]	Pillows are used not only under the head, but also to support the patient's back in a side-lying position. Pillows should also be placed where bony prominences rub, such as knees or ankles.
5. Ten flat top sheets[a]	These sheets can be folded in half and used across the middle third of the bed to serve as a turn sheet in moving the person, as well as to prevent bottom sheet from having to be changed should the bed become wet or soiled.
6. One bath blanket or large heavy towel	Use this to keep person warm during baths or procedures.
7. Six wash cloths, six bath towels[a]	To wash and dry patient when bathing.
8. Six hand towels[a]	To put across patient's chest and keep it warm while bath blanket is pulled down to hips to expose abdomen. Also used in feeding patient as a large napkin/bib.
9. Large piece of plastic	Use across middle third of bed and tucked under mattress *under* the turn or draw sheet.
10. Good lubricating massage oil; powder or talc	For use in skin care to prevent skin breakdown and for massage.
11. Tooth brush, tooth paste, mouthwash	For mouth care.
12. Small table (e.g., card table)	Care items used daily are placed on it for handy access.
13. Rented wheelchair, if necessary	To allow patient to sit up, get around house (if level), or go outdoors.
14. Comfortable chair and other chairs for visitors	To allow patient to be out of bed and also enjoy visitors.
15. One box flexible straws, spoons	Bendable straws permit easier drinking, since they adapt to the angle of the patient's head position in relation to the glass.

K. A. Roche, 1979, *Sharing the experience of death: a manual of family care* (unpublished manuscript).

[a]These numbers are estimates. If patient is incontinent, more bedding will be needed than for a continent patient or one with an indwelling urinary catheter.

Table 8-1 cont'd

16. One bag large disposable bed pads (Chux). Incontinent patients will use considerably more	Protects bed from soiling and cuts down on linen changes.
17. Large size disposable diapers (several boxes) for incontinent patient	To absorb urine; reduces skin irritation and protects bed.
18. All customary personal care items: brush, comb, deodorant, razor or other shaving equipment, cosmetics	The patient needs all the usual favorite products within easy reach.
19. Television, radio, or other favorite diversion.	Diversion helps people to relax and pass time more easily.
20. Spiral or loose leaf notebook with dividers	The patient's "chart." Handy for recording medications, progress notes, observations, and questions for the doctor. Categorize each section for locating information easily and rapidly.
21. Trash can with plastic liners and sealing wires	For sanitary disposal of waste. Extra plastic bags are used to contain soiled dressings, tubes, or other types of human drainage or debris.
22. Rented over-bed table or lap tray	For meal tray. This is not covered by most insurance.
23. Large tray on which complete meals can be served	To allow one trip to be made to bedside and all food to arrive at appropriate temperature.
24. Easy access to laundry facilities	This will permit linen to be washed in a way that is most gentle on patient's skin (use of mild detergents, avoidance of starches, double rinses if necessary, and use of fabric softeners).
25. Stubby thermometer, one bottle ethyl alcohol, cotton balls, lubricant	From time to time it may be necessary to take the patient's temperature. This thermometer can be used for oral, rectal, or axillary recording provided it is thoroughly cleaned after each use.
26. Rented alternate air pressure mattress and pump for bed patients,[b] or egg crate mattress and chair cushions[c]	In addition to frequent changes of position, this prevents or relieves constant pressure on skin, which could cause bedsores.
27. Smoke detector	Early alert of smoke/fire

[b]Great care must be taken in the selection and use of these items. Neither is a substitute for frequent changing of position and massage of the bony prominences, which are most vulnerable to skin breakdown. Their use sometimes creates a false sense of security that skin care is being accomplished "automatically." If there is mechanical breakdown, it is difficult to observe that air is not reaching all the mattress cells because it is concealed by the sheets. The motor may be functioning, but the mattress still may be ineffective due to punctures and leaks.

[c]Care must be taken with egg crate mattresses if they are laundered because this usually results in washing out their flame-retardant properties. Then there is greater vulnerability to bed fire if the patient or some one else smokes near the bed.

The Process of Home Care

It is the primary home care nurses' responsibility to plan and delegate or deliver high-quality care for hospice families in the home. This includes writing care plans, keeping accurate records, and assisting patients in attaining all the benefits to which they are entitled. These nurses coordinate care with consultants and teach and counsel the family caregivers. They must have the maturity and experience to work independently as well a interdependently, as necessary. The role is not easy, but is is most fulfilling.

During admission to home care, baseline data about the patient and family are obtained and assessments are made as to strengths and deficits. This is often done with the assistance of the social worker. Nursing assessments are carried out and problems are indentified. Teaching home care management of symptoms is continued from the hospital setting. The family is oriented to home care and instructed in how to contact the nurse. Most important, the nurse and family relationship is established. There is usually a short period of testing before trust is gained. The nurse wonders if the family can be trusted to call with questions before getting into a troublesome situation; the family may call the nurse with minor problems to test the effectiveness of the on-call system. This period is usually short, as all parties concerned are eager to work with each other when they see the positive rewards of symptom relief. The admission visit is often twice as time consuming as the maintenance visits. Much teaching about patient care is done on a regular basis on each visit as care plans are adjusted. Every effort is made to keep communication as open as can be tolerated and to elicit active patient and family involvement in care planning.

This relationship grows and extends to include the entire family and hospice care team. Families are taught the basics of home care of the patient and are prepared for changes in condition. Preparation is important so that unexpected events do not develop into crises and in order to keep staff and family stress as low as possible. Equipment and medications must be readily available. There is no sense in extending service to the home if the staff is left impotent in an emergency situation. Written instructions (a care plan) to follow are just as important as "orders" are for the nurse. There is always the alternative of admitting the patient to the hospital if this is the most appropriate measure.

Preparedness is based on clear communication. Time spent together during the death trajectory is of little value unless it is used well. This period of terminal care can be a time of growth, shared preparation, and relationship completion. Used badly, it can be a time of mutual destruction and can mar memories of relationships. Fear and grief, even if intellectually denied, remain physically active. Despite the presence of these strong emotions, traditional psychiatric therapy is of little value. People respond better to caring and understanding (Parkes 1978).

Researchers Weisman and Worden (1975) studied the positive effect that mutually responsive relationships had on length of survival. Clearly, the interaction between staff and patients is likely to play a major role in survival. Home care itself may motivate a patient (Sutton 1979). Similarly, Gielen and Roche (1979) observed that patients who were surrounded by supportive families had not thought much about suicide. Conversely, patients abandoned by support systems not only had suicidal thoughts, but also planned what situations they would act upon.

Clear communication is blocked by such obstacles as double messages and incongruency of body language and speech. Language can be thought of as a way of creating a representation of one's world together with one's perceptions, the means to convey to others the choices one sees, hears, and feels are available. Thus language is a kind of territorial map of a person's reality. A personal filter system can enrich or impoverish perception and therefore one's reality territory. Unclear images of the world block perception and therefore limit the choice available (Bandler and Grinder 1975). Those working with hospice families must be sensitive and alert to their reality maps. Imperative in the helping process is listening for words like "never," "always," "should," "ought," "can't," and "impossible." These, together with patterns of thought that generalize, distort, or delete information, tend to narrow the possibilities. Such clues to perception present the opportunity for gentle challenge to expand perception. For example, a cancer patient who makes the statement, "I want to die because it is impossible to live like this," can learn a whole new form of reality by involvement with the choices of hospice.

The role of the counselor is that of sounding board: listening and understanding, yet ready to reverberate with encouragement, comfort, and praise (Parkes 1978).

Outside support groups such as Make Today Count, Can Surmount, I Can Cope, Ronald MacDonald Houses, Compassionate Friends, and Dr. Jampolsky's National Childrens' Support Group are most helpful in complementing the hospice support. Most families wish to retain affiliation with their usual support groups. Unfortunately, as word of the patient's prognosis is spread, old friends and acquaintances often do not feel they know what to say or do; consequently, they distance themselves from the patient. A self-help group such as Make Today Count, composed of patients and families with whom there is a common bond, can be an uplifting source of help. Hospice volunteers are immensely important in weaving a fabric of instant, specialized support.

On-Call System

Used properly, on-call availability is one of the most important support systems hospice can offer to caregiving families. Many have experienced nightmarish situations in which they have felt helpless and afraid to the point of panic. Despite the fact that on-call is taken most seriously and every precaution is taken to avoid system failures, they can and will happen. For this reason families should be informed and reinforced that they should call the on-call nurse as soon as they feel it might be necessary, rather than waiting until they feel frantic and a full-blown emergency situation has arisen. In our program we attempt to avoid calling the community emergency ambulances and rescue squads because they have been instructed to use the nearest hospital, as well as to provide life support.

The on-call procedure involves the families calling the hospital telephone operator or home care office. After office hours the phone is switched over to the telephone operator who receives the call for help and takes the family's name, phone number, and a brief message. Because these caring hospital employees understand the hospice concept, they frequently calm the anxious caller and reassure that they are notifying the nurse immediately. All nurses carry beepers during the working hours and the nurse on call leaves hers on. At times we have used longer range beepers for the on-call nurse. Once the page is answered, the nurse and caregiver can discuss the problem and take whatever action is appropriate. We attempt to accept patients who reside within a half-hour's driving time of the hospital. On-call staff may have to travel longer distances from their own homes. Families should understand this right from their initial orientation to the program. If possible, it usually helps to give the family an estimate of the amount of time it will take for the nurse to arrive. This prevents recalls while the nurse is en route which only delays her arrival. In our program the director or head nurse are also on call for supervision and consultation as well as back-up should the on-call nurse's beeper fail. Back-up is an important function.

Frequently the family is calling to report that the patient has died, or if they do not realize that death has occurred, they may only report unresponsiveness.

It is imperative that the primary nurse report any change of condition so that the on-call nurse can be aware of even subtle changes that the family may report. This not only helps the on-call nurse to be more responsive, but also to be prepared by anticipating the appropriate equipment and supplies to have on hand as needed. Lack of available supplies or medications could necessitate a hospitalization that is unwanted and could otherwise be avoided.

Inactive Patient Status

There is a final "gray area" in which a few patients each year experience remission or slowed disease progression. Once symptoms are under control, their conditions are stable and the need for skilled nursing becomes difficult to justify or nonexistent. During this period the main need is monitoring of medications and supplies. Our program has named this period "inactive status." It means the patient remains on our census but is discharged as far as insurance providers are concerned. Occasionally, if the dose of analgesic medication can be tapered down or stopped, the patient may choose to be fully discharged from home care and enjoy a well period without being reminded by the presence of staff that things are not really as good as they seem. Everyone will be in agreement that one phone call is all that is necessary to resume care. (Of course the appropriate orders and paperwork will be obtained.)

For most patients who cannot be fully medically independent, the primary nurse will call periodically and our volunteer RNs will make visits as often as is necessary to maintain continuity and rapport. Because the visit is by volunteer staff, there is no charge to the patient and the cost to the program is greatly reduced. Appropriate clinical documentation continues by the volunteer RNs, who are under the supervision of the director. When the patient's condition deteriorates, the volunteer RN may wish to remain involved and continue to follow the patient as co-manager with the primary nurse. In this situation the primary nurse who works full time may actually provide back-up for the volunteer RN who works less than full time.

In periods of high census, our volunteer RNs have served as primary nurses and even have been available for emergency care. Naturally these professional volunteers are as competent and dedicated as the full-time staff. Their communication and relationship with staff is noteworthy. All in-service programs are open to them and they are in full compliance with regulations.

Discharge from Hospice

A brief note is in order regarding the types of discharge from hospice. The most frequent and obvious is, of course, by death. There are others, however, such as by referral. This category would include situations in which the patient goes to live with an out-of-state relative or wishes to resume aggressive treatment. Similarly, refusal of service or noncompliance with treatment occurs. While these are relatively rare, they do happen.

The Home Death

Few experiences in life are more significant than death. Many families, believing that the event will be awful and traumatic, do not consider seriously the option of the patient dying at home. Through the whole process of the hospice concept of care, many families choose to have the patient die at home. Fear and anxiety are reduced as people realize death is more a gradual process than an unanticipated sudden event.

Families are encouraged to communicate with patients as to their wishes about burial arrangements. Funeral directors have been most helpful and understanding when they were consulted in advance of the patient's death. They have policies and procedures regarding home death from which they are prepared to deviate with hospice families. They must be assured that the patient has been under the care of a physician who can sign the death certificate. Funeral directors tend to remove the body of the deceased quickly in home deaths because so often families, completely shocked by a sudden death, do not feel comfortable otherwise. By contrast, however, the hospice families tend not to view the death as an emergency to be dealt with immediately and want to call extended members back to the house for one last goodbye. They often wish to bathe or groom the body, sit in silence or pray together, and there is no reason the request should be denied.

Even with preparation by hospice care, the event cannot be fully anticipated in advance. In fact, the family may expect to avoid grief or mourning through having cared for the patient. No matter how adequate the coping, few people expect the death *now*, at this moment. It always comes as a surprise. An advantage of preburial planning is the avoidance of having to function at a high level while in a state of shock (*Preparing Today for the Eventual Tomorrow* 1979).

Often the hospice nurse is present at the time of death or shortly thereafter, having been called by the family. His or her role is to guide the family through previously made choices, not to assume functioning for them. The ritual of burial and its planning and preparation are necessary to begin the healing process. Often the first task is to assist the family in the disposal of the patient's medication and equipment. The process of their disposal is symbolic of the recognition that the suffering process has ended. Clothing and mementos can be handled at a later date. If a special relationship has developed between staff and family, closure might be effectively accomplished by the staff member's attendance at the funeral or wake.

In closing, it must be recognized that hospice care is a unique kind of caring. It is specialized and by now is in possession of its own philosophy and theory. It is, by its very nature, demanding of staff. Much of what hospice is about is giving of the self, especially when there is nothing more medically to be offered. The staff members in our program have chosen to work in hospice care. They continue their commitment for varying lengths of time, fully aware of the risk of emotional pain they may feel. There is also the awareness that the honor of helping a fellow human being complete his or her life brings satisfaction and fullness into their own lives in a way few other career choices can.

The Church Hospital program has been successful in its mission to ease the suffering of terminally ill cancer patients and their families. Both the hospice and home care programs have grown tremendously over the last few years. This chapter would not be complete without being dedicated to the staff, who through their dedication, quality care, and compassion made this option available for patients. The early leaders of the program had a vision of a better way, and they took the risks necessary to bring that dream into fruition.

It is perhaps best expressed by an unknown author who said:
        To laugh is to risk appearing the fool
        To weep is to risk appearing sentimental
        To reach out for another is to risk involvement
        To expose feelings is to risk exposing your
            true self
        To place your ideas, your dreams before the
            crowd is to risk their loss
        To love is to risk not being loved in return
        To live is to risk dying
        To hope is to risk despair
        To try is to risk failure
        But the risk must be taken because the greatest
            hazard in life is to risk nothing
        The person who risks nothing does nothing,
            has nothing, and is nothing
        He may avoid suffering and sorrow but he
            simply cannot learn, feel, change, grow,
            love, and live
        Chained by his certitudes he is a slave, he
            has forfeited his freedom
        Only a person who risks is free

References

Bandler R, Grinder J: *The Structure of Magic.*Science and Behavior Books, Palo Alto CA, 1985.

Church Hospital: *Church Hospital Home Health Policy Manual: Philosophy and Objectives,* ed 3. Church Hospital, Baltimore, September, 1984.

Preparing Today for the Eventual Tomorrow, National Funeral Directors Association, Milwaukee, 1979.

Gielen A , Roche KA: Death anxiety and psychometric studies in Huntington's disease. *Omega* 10:2, 1979-1980.

Jivoff L: *In Prichard E (ed) Home Care The Quality of Life.* Columbia Press, New York, 1979.

Parkes CM: Psychological aspects. *In Saunders CS (ed) The Management of Terminal Disease.* Edward Publication, Year Book York Medical Publishers, Chicago, 1978.

Sutton K: Hospice. *Make Today Count,* (Chapter Newsletter,) Montgomery County MD, p 4, January 1979.

Weisman AD, Worden J: Psychosocial analysis of cancer death. *Omega* 6:61, 1975.

Chapter 9

Inpatient Hospice Care

Marjorie M. Lamb

Diversity in the models of hospice care is widely recognized. From the inception of the integrated program at Church Hospital, it has seemed imperative to have a designated unit that houses our hospitalized patients. There are many reasons related related to selection of staff, enhancement of communications, expertise in symptom control, and understanding of needs specific to this patient population that reinforce this initial decision. This chapter addresses the dynamics of such a unit.

Nursing staff members in an acute care setting are not all privileged to experience the total spectrum of response to patients' needs that is part of hospice care. The opportunity to provide care and comfort to the patient and family who have chosen to stop aggressive treatment of the disease process does not occur in many clinical settings. The terms "hospice care" connotes to some the idea of "hand holding". To those who have participated in hospice care, it is readily recognized as a complex process utilizing the full range of nursing skills and abilities. When there is no further curative medical treatment to be offered, the primary consideration becomes the need to provide comfort, care, and consolation while achieving the highest quality of life for the patient and caregivers.

Response to Patient Problems

An integrated plan of care that incorporates all members of the hospice team and that is begun promptly becomes important and meaningful. At the first meeting with the patient and family, needs are fully assessed and identified problems are routed quickly to the appropriate experts. For example, financial and social concerns are referred to the social worker; nutritional problems, to the dietitian. Each member of the team becomes active in planning and implementing care promptly and intensively. However, many problems — achieving positions of comfort, preventing constipation, establishing feeding routines, diminishing anxiety, coping with urinary problems, alleviating respiratory distress, easing sleep disturbances, minimizing confusional states, and minimizing feelings of isolation and depression—can and should be dealt with primarily on a nursing level.

There are no set formulas for the care of hospice patients. Although there are some symptoms and problems that these patients share in common, each is a unique person, bringing all of the cares, concerns, and strengths that have characterized his or her life to date. The mandate of the hospice team is to assist each patient to achieve the highest quality of life in the time remaining.

"No resuscitation" is not assumed with hospice patients. This decision is thoroughly discussed with the family and when feasible, with the patient. When a decision is reached that this is acceptable, a specific order is written.

When hospice care was initiated, there existed some "we always . . ." and "we never . . ." rules of thumb. These have been largely discarded as the range of individual variation has been increasingly appreciated. As a source of discomfort is identified, the simplest and best palliation for that particular problem in that particular patient is initiated. Nasogastric tubes were at one time in the "we never . . ." category. To some patients with intestinal obstruction, vomiting fecal material is acceptable, to others it is not. Recognizing this diversity means that assessment of this aspect of the patient's physical and psychological comfort may lead to a nasogastric tube being utilized at times. If this enhances that patients' overall status, it is deemed appropriate. Small-volume blood transfusions may be used if this will increase mobility, improve respiratory status, or enhance cognitive function. These are two examples of the reasons why no therapeutic intervention is automatically ruled out; instead, whatever is appropriate to achieve true palliation for a particular patient is done. Psychological, physical, and spiritual comfort are the main concerns, and the energies of the hospice team are directed toward achieving these. Many patients need improvement of their diminished abilities to acquire the time and energy to complete unfinished business, about which they feel an urgency as death impends.

Hospice patients are subject to the same length-of-stay constraints as are other patients in the acute care setting. Rapid development of a comprehensive plan of care that will be appropriate to the patient at home is therefore mandatory. This is done with recognition that only during the acute care stay will there be the 24-hour presence of nurses to assess the patient, identify needs, develop a plan to meet them, and evaluate the effectiveness of the intervention.

Inclusion of the family and friends who will be caregivers at home is imperative to achieve a workable plan of care. The staff must be sensitive to the needs of the home caregivers. If skills and techniques need to be learned, the caregivers participate in providing care to the patient so they can become comfortable with these skills while the staff is there to support them. However, if the caregivers do not need new skills and are exhausted from previously caring for the patient, they are actively incorporated in the planning, but the staff provides the care to allow them respite and a chance to regain the strength to resume the care of the patient after discharge. Between these two extremes, the staff needs to be aware that some people are more comfortable participating in care rather than watching, whereas others prefer less involvement in the physical care.

Staff Selection and Protocols

How does this intensive process fit into the care of all patients on a general medical-surgical nursing unit? Some description of the nursing model and staffing ratios is indicated. Hospice inpatients are housed on a 28-bed nursing unit, which is one of 7 such units designated intermediate care to distinguish them from critical care areas such as the intensive care unit. There are no designated hospice beds. The inpatient hospice census varies from 0 to 12, with a usual population of 2 or 3. The remainder of the patients on the unit are the general mix of intermediate care medical, surgical, and gynecological patients.

The basic staffing numbers for this unit are the same as for other units. Distribution of pool staff on a daily basis is determined by the acuity of patient care needs as indicated by the daily classification of patients done by each nurse and collated by nursing administration.

There are two important components of the hospice unit staffing. One is that each staff member has an expressed interest in and commitment to hospice care. There was a recent opportunity to reassess this when the hospice unit and appropriate staff moved from a 50-bed unit to a 28-bed unit. There was an attendant relocation of personnel. Each staff member was interviewed to ascertain his or her feelings about staying with or leaving the hospice unit.

The desire to continue caring for hospice patients was the primary consideration for staff placement on the new unit. Seniority was the second consideration when appropriate positions were not available for all persons who wanted to remain on the unit.

The second and extremely important component is the pool of trained and dedicated hospice volunteers who become increasingly available as the hospice census rises. Without their talents and availability many goals could not be met. Their philosophy is invaluable in accomplishing our mutual purpose. They feel that any type of help to any patient or staff member on the unit enhances the care of each hospice patient. Therefore their tasks are many and diverse. In addition to their role and functions as described in Chapter 7, they are utilized in providing TLC for elderly, confused, or anxious nonhospice patients. They transport patients, specimens, and papers to other departments to keep the staff on the unit and readily available to the patients. They are an asset in helping to orient personnel to hospice concepts by demonstrating in action what can never be completely shared in a didactic manner.

The total patient care model is utilized in nursing practice. The ratio of patients per nurse is currently 5 to 1 on day shift, 9 to 1 on evenings, and 14 to 1 on nights. With the recent movement of staff and patients from a 50-bed unit to a renovated 28-bed unit, these ratios will be reviewed and will be subject to modification as the feasibility is observed. There are two nursing assistants per shift who are utilized in direct and indirect patient care.

The fact that it is socially acceptable for a staff member to ask for a temporary or permanent transfer from the care of hospice patients is periodically reinforced. Each member of the staff tries to remain sensitive to other staff's needs and to extend a helping hand to each other to avoid the emotional overload that hospice care can precipitate. The intensified relationship to the family and patient brings with it an involvement in the grieving process that is not common in other clinical situations.

It is interesting to observe the age range of the personnel who have constituted the inpatient staff. Newly graduated young nurses, as well as people with many years of professional and life experience, work well with hospice patients. There is a need for compassion and maturity; this is obviously not an age-related phenomenon but is more related to the value system of the individual staff member.

The staff must be aware of the issue of morbidity, both for patient and self. There is a need to see the many shades of gray that constitute the area between the black and white extremes that unexamined values can impose. People who are tied to the either/or way of perceiving do not cope well with hospice patients. The ability both to recognize where the patients are in the acceptance-denial spectrum and to accompany them at that point is imperative.

Because the patient population is drawn from diverse socioeconomic backgrounds, it is important that each staff member understands the customs and beliefs of each patient and avoids the imposition of his or her own values when planning and implementing care.

Fortunately, the nursing administration at Church Hospital recognizes that as patients have varying strengths, life experiences, and needs, so do staff members. This acknowledgment makes it possible to work constructively with staff members who need to transfer to other units. Because the emotional commitment to hospice patients can be taxing on either a short- or long-term basis, it is important to have administrative as well as unit level concern and recognition of this factor.

On a unit level the peer support available to date has been sufficient to obviate establishment of a formal support mechanism. This would be considered if the need were demonstrated or expressed.

One of the virtues of the mixed population of patients that exist on an integrated unit is that each staff member's patient load is composed of those who are being helped toward a gentler death along with those who are being assisted to achieve an optimal health status. Coping with nonthreatening illness provides a shifting focus, which helps the staff member maintain a balanced perspective.

Integration of Hospice and Nonhospice Patients

Location of an incoming hospice patient is determined by the charge nurse. If the patient is coming from another unit of the hospital or from our home health clientele, extensive data about the person is available. Referrals from outside facilities may include only sparse information about the patient and family initially. The bed assignment is based on as much as can be ascertained about the patient in relation to acuity of needs, alertness, confusion, and required equipment.

The status of the potential roommate and the acuity of needs of the other patients in a particular nurse's current assignment are other factors considered. The floor plan of the unit places some geographical constraints on patient placement for best utilization of each staff member's time and energy.

An effort is made to achieve daily continuity of care by assigning the same patients to the same nurse on a consistent basis. When this is not desirable, based on the patient's, family's, or nurse's preference, an adjustment is quickly made. There has been, in most instances, another staff member ready to step into the gap created by this situation. The total picture is analyzed before making the assumption that changing assignments is the best solution. An increase in support, enhancement of skills, or utilization of additional resources is considered first.

Private rooms are sometimes utilized for hospice patients. The patient's request for this accommodation is, of course, honored. If the family is staying with the patient 24 hours a day, a private room is sometimes indicated for the comfort of all of those involved. In general, it is desirable for most other hospice patients to be placed in semiprivate rooms to avoid segregation of the terminally ill patient and the related disadvantages of the attendant feelings of isolation. If the initial placement of the patient does not seem appropriate after the full range of needs is identified, transfer to a more appropriate room is easily arranged. There are few taboos in patient placement, but location of a newly diagnosed cancer patient with a patient in the very terminal stage of illness is avoided.

The dynamics of most roommates' interactions with hospice patients is interesting to observe. Much caring and support of the patient and family is seen by the nonhospice roommates and their families in the usual case. A brief explanation of hospice care is given to the roommate to achieve understanding of the special privileges accorded to the hospice patient. Hospice families are encouraged to bring food and belongings from home to create a more homelike environment for the patient. There are no restrictions of visitors to the hospice patient in relation to time of day, age, or species of visitors. (Pets are welcome as appropriate.) The roommate needs to know why the conventional rules do not apply. Because the staff and the volunteers provide many extra services to the hospice patient, the roommate frequently benefits. Common courtesy dictates that an unusual snack at an unusual hour, coffee for the family, use of a radio or an electric shaver, conversation with a volunteer who has time to listen attentively, and other like privileges will frequently be shared with the roommate of the hospice patient. Education of the public is often achieved by the demonstrated care that is observed. If a nonhospice patient does not feel receptive to this situation, relocation to another room on the unit is arranged.

Extensions of Philosophy

There are many extensions of hospice care that apply to other patients in an integrated inpatient unit. If one believes and actuates the belief that the patient and family are the integral unit of care in hospice, this concept is not discarded when dealing with other patients. This leads to recognition of the need to gather thorough data about all patients and their home environments to predict their needs after discharge and to initiate a plan to meet these needs early in the hospital stay.

Working closely with all members of the hospice team enables the staff nurse to recognize the range of resources and the ready availability of all departments to enhance the care of each patient. The right of the patient and/or family caregiver to control decision making causes the staff to recognize this right for all patients.

Although the criteria for acceptance into the hospice program limits the population to cancer patients, the staff recognizes that any patient with terminal illness has similar needs and may deserve similar response. There has been observed a more rapid response to the need for early and complete discharge planning. Family involvement is enhanced during the inpatient stay for all patients.

Team Approach

At weekly hospice team meetings, information on all inpatient and home care patients is presented by the nurses, and sharing as colleagues is developed. The patient's primary nurse at home is perceived by the inpatient nurse as a resource to be utilized in planning care, as are all other members of the team who contribute to this conference. Because all team members are represented, each leaves the meeting with an enhanced perspective of his or her role in relation to each patient's care. There is a consequent easing of each person's load as aspects of care are shared and specifically delegated to others.

One of the learning experiences for inpatient staff is the blending of roles that occurs with assorted members of the hospice team. Nurses and social service both handle the complexity of family relationships. Nurses and dietitians are both concerned with the diverse problems relating to nutrition. Nurses and physical therapists have like goals in maintaining appropriate mobility and/or achieving pain relief. Nurses and chaplains both work toward addressing the spiritual anguish of the patient and the family. Nurses and pharmacists each work toward the most efficacious and simplest medication for symptom relief. Prompt and continuing communication with the patient's physician is the only way for the nurse to achieve a rapid response to the need to modify the patient's medical therapy.

Working closely with all of the allied disciplines is the only way one can expedite relieving all of the controllable discomforts attending the transitional process that these special patients present. There is no sharp demarcation as to the specialist who will work with each symptom. It remains the nurse's role to integrate all of the potential services and resources for each patient.

Because there is a diversity of understanding among physicians who have patients in the hospice program, it is sometimes within the nurse's role to explain the resources available through the team and the philosophy of care that the program entails.

As a result of the close relationship that develops between the nurse and the patient in the hospice mode of care, it is frequently the nurse who tells the family that the patient has died if the family is not present at the time. In other instances this would usually be done by the on-call physician or the attending physician. However, having accompanied the family during the journey that has been leading to this event, the hospice nurse feels comfortable in being the person to share this news.

Need For Education and Research

It is important to have an ongoing critique regarding delivery of care. Three years ago an in-depth needs analysis was conducted because it was recognized that perceptions and understanding of hospice care by the members of the staff were diverse. Based on the findings of this study, a protocol for orientation was established. This procedure is followed with each staff member new to the unit. Some aspects included are an overview of the hospice manual, introduction to key members of the hospice team, attendance at weekly rounds, attendance at a family meeting, and direct care of a hospice patient. The findings of the study were also utilized in planning in-service programs concerning hospice care.

The inpatient staff contribute to orientation of new volunteers. One of our newly graduated nurses, who began her professional career on this unit, developed "Standards of Nursing Care for Hospice Patients," which is now a part of the hospice manual (Elder 1983). Staff members also respond to the need to meet with the community as outside speakers.

The concept of the interface of curative and palliative treatment and the gray area that exists as a patient moves from one to another require thorough understanding by all staff. This dictates a need for periodic discussions and in-service education on this topic. This is done both on a formal level during the monthly in-service meeting and on an individual level with unit staff and physicians.

Summary

While some hospitals scatter hospice inpatients throughout the hospital, there seem to be many advantages to localizing them on a designated unit. With the dynamics of staff mobility, adequate orientation of staff and maintenance of communication is difficult to achieve on a single unit, and this would be complicated further by utilizing multiple units. The need for a response to the emotional involvement of the hospice personnel is best met by a staff attuned to this recurrent need.

In the inpatient care of hospice patients, many of the nursing concepts that previously have been encountered on a theoretical level are actualized. One cannot function on a mechanical level of performing tasks but must utilize fully the nursing process to address the complexity of needs presented by the hospice patients and their family caregivers.

Reference

Elder C: Standards of nursing care for hospice patients. *Hospice Care Program Manual*, ed 3, p.10-1, Church Hospital, Baltimore 1984.

Chapter 10

Administration of a Hospice Program

Gloria R. Cameron

This chapter addresses the organizational structure, financial aspects, and staffing of a hospice care program. It is written from the perspective of a hospital-based program and draws on the experience of the Church Hospital hospice. While the advantages of a hospital-based program are emphasized, the success of other program models should not be ignored. The applicability and appropriateness of any particular delivery mode is contingent upon numerous factors that must be appraised in each community. Many of these factors are explored in the text that follows.

Organization

The Health Care Delivery System

Questions of how to organize and deliver hospice care in the United States frequently prompt controversy concerning its proper place in the existing health care delivery system. The organizational structure needed to support a hospice care program must provide for a very special integration of program components into this system. Whether this calls for an entirely new element within the system or adaptation of existing elements, or both, has not been determined.

In the early development of hospice care concepts, emphasis was placed on deficiencies of health care provided to the terminally ill. The emotional backlash to these deficiencies was such that the hospital setting was rejected outright by many hospice care proponents. The creation of a separate delivery system for hospice care was the dream of many. This dream was idealistic in its assessment of both the cost of care and the ability of a separate element to adequately fulfill the comprehensive needs of a hospice patient.

Continuity of care, which is essential to the hospice concept, is a major medical goal in this country. Growing economic constraints and the scarcity of the health care dollar have provided further motivation for enhanced continuity of care that emphasizes the nonacute setting. Changes in the organization of health care delivery are increasingly more compatible with the environment needed to support a hospice care program. New incentives encourage the prevention or delay of hospitalization, and less intensive use of resources in the acute care setting as well as increased use of home care, are rewarded. In a competitive arena, the personal comfort-oriented caregiver has the edge. Fortunately, many key features of hospice care are compatible with incentives in the changing health care delivery system.

Organization Within a Hospital System

Church Hospital chose to offer hospice service as a program of care integrated into its existing organizational structure. This approach began with analysis of the components of hospice care as they would relate to the hospital's mission, goals, and mode of operation. The approval and support of the board of directors of the hospital were procured early in this process.

A review of basic components of hospice care included recognition of the terminally ill patient and his or her family as the focus of care, the palliation of disease symptoms, supportive efforts in a holistic approach to health care, and an emphasis on home care. These characteristics do not preclude the provision of hospice care by hospitals. Although they are not necessarily typical of hospital care, there is no reason why they cannot be and many reasons why they should be. In fact, the ability of hospitals to coordinate health care resources enhances the potential for delivery of hospice care in this country. As a centralizing entity, the hospital is in a key position to foster continuity of care with efficient use of resources. It was from this perspective that Church Hospital developed its hospice care program.

The structure needed to manage and implement the program and coordinate the interdisciplinary team already exists in the community hospital. Hospital accreditation standards require the establishment of an organized medical staff with bylaws and a means of accountability to the hospital's governing body. A standing committee structure typically provides the mechanism for review and evaluation of medical staff practice and functions. These committees are also responsible for providing direct medical staff input and guidance to important medical functions within the hospital (e.g., pharmacy and therapeutics, blood utilization review, infection control).

This familiar hospital structure is an excellent vehicle to centralize the various hospice care components through formation of a standing hospice care committee. Such a committee derives its authority from the medical staff bylaws and is accountable to the medical leadership and, ultimately, the governing body of the hospital. Representation by responsible hospital management (i.e., administration and appropriate department heads or supervisors) taps the authority of the existing managerial hierarchy and utilizes effective channels of communication. The composition of such a committee will necessarily vary as dictated by the particular organization of services and functions in a given hospital. Representatives would likely include department heads from social work, volunteer activities, home care, chaplaincy, selected nursing supervisors, and the administrator responsible for program coordination. Physician members would typically include an oncologist, a family practitioner, and others with special interest or experience in hospice care. At Church Hospital the medical director of the program chairs the committee with other physician members, including representatives from the medical, surgical, and gynecological services and the medical director of home care. Responsibilities of the committee include initiation and review of policies, procedures, and forms, evaluation of program status, and planning.

Operational choices for hospital-based programs range from establishment of a distinct unit, to an integrated unit, to dispersement of patients throughout the facility with services provided by a consultative team. Hospice home care services may be provided by a hospital-based department or through formal liaison with an outside home health agency.

The alternative of a separate unit with designated staff normally presents a prohibitive expense to the typical community hospital. This model is more appropriate in a larger facility or university teaching hospital where institutional organization and patient volume may support the expense. The option of providing a consultant interdisciplinary team with patients dispersed throughout the hospital may not effect the desired changes in patient management. Although the concept is excellent, hospitals may find such a program difficult to coordinate; there may be insufficient impact upon the traditional curative environment. This alternative has been successfully employed in some hospitals; the roving consultative team can be an excellent means by which to introduce hospice care to the medical community and may be used as a first step toward the development of a more centralized program.

In the case of the hospice care program at Church Hospital, patients are admitted or transferred to a particular nursing unit in which the personnel specialize in the care of the terminally ill. Other medical-surgical patients are also located in this 28-bed nursing unit. Hospice team members relate to the unit and to the home care department, which is closely aligned with the program. The hospital opted to develop its own home care agency in order to facilitate continuity of care and ensure strong control and coordination of the hospice program. The home care department also serves nonhospice patients and meets other community needs.

Liaisons with independent home health agencies have been developed by other hospital-based programs but present a difficult management problem. Program requirements such as 24-hour on-call coverage are not always possible. Medical record keeping, orientation of home health staff, and effective and timely communication of patient care plans are more complicated. Familiarity of the patient and family with hospice staff may not be optimal.

Organizationally, the home care director at Church Hospital holds a key position, as this office acts as the clearinghouse for hospice inquiries and information. Initial admission screening is accomplished through this office, as is monitoring of continuity of care and maintenance of program statistics. Working in conjunction with .

the hospice medical director, the home care department and its corporate officer coordinate the administrative support for the program. It is important to assign day-to-day program coordination to a specific individual, whether it be the home care director, a nursing supervisor, or a person in a position created solely for this activity. Such assignment will vary according to the organizational characteristics of each program.

Further organization and implementation of the program is similar to that of other specialized patient care programs within the hospital, such as hyperalimentation or cardiac rehabilitation. Appropriate protocols and procedures are developed, physical facility or equipment adjustments are made, special training and orientation of personnel are conducted, and interaction among members of the health care team is coordinated. A component not necessarily typical of specialized patient care programs is the role of the volunteer organization, headed by a director responsible for this important service.

The structure of the hospice service at Church Hospital is an example of a "program management" approach that organizationally crosses several jurisdictional lines. This is not alien to hospital operations, in which separate department functions must effectively interact in the provision of patient care. A network is designed to shift the orientation of managers away from differentiated departmental patterns and toward an integrated concept of the program into which their particular contributions must fit. For this approach to be successful, a concerted effort must be made to ensure that program objectives do not conflict with departmental goals and operations.

Financial Aspects

In considering the financial aspects of hospice care, most attention is given to the question of reimbursement for services. With little known about the actual cost of hospice care, payment issues are poorly addressed. Determining costs is complicated in the face of disagreement over minimum and/or legitimate components of care. Third-party payors (most significantly the federal government and Blue Cross) have studied the cost of hospice care and its impact on the cost of health care in general. Demonstration projects designed for this purpose were initiated during 1979 and 1980 throughout the United States.

The variety of programs participating in the federal study was marked; participating programs were quite different in setting, organization, age, and geographic locations. Record keeping and accuracy of data were likely problems in drawing conclusions from the study. Blue Cross studies are continuing, and since this is the case, it is likely that savings may be in evidence. Hospice care, with its emphasis on home health, may be compatible with the financial strategies of the Blue Cross organization.

Standards

The determination of costs and the financial viability of any hospice care program should begin with a look at standards of care. Acceptable standards for hospice care are of utmost concern to the public and to those committed to implementing the hospice concept without compromising its philosophy. The National Hospice Organization (1979) has labored to produce standards that are intended for use in the accreditation process.

Since standards of care meaningfully prescribe resources necessary to characterize a program as hospice care, recognition and acceptance of minimum standards is a basic financial consideration. However, there is no present consensus on either minimal or optimal acceptable standards.

The Joint Commission on Accreditation of Hospitals (JCAH), in cooperation with the National Hospice organization, has developed a voluntary accreditation program (Joint Commission on Accreditation of Hospitals 1983a, 1983b). The JCAH standards are the result of over two years of study, conferences, and testing, and their development included the participation of varied groups with active interest in hospice care. By and large, these standards are the best available reference by which start-up and operational costs may be quantified.

The successful achievement of any standard for a contemplated or existing hospice program depends largely upon its available resources. Hospital-based programs will find themselves already in compliance with the most costly aspects of the JCAH hospice standards by virtue of their routine hospital accreditation process. Organizational costs implicit in the administrative aspects of the standards (e.g., the interdisciplinary team and the system for continuity of care) may be minimized through successful integration of hospice care into the existing hospital system. All aspects of patient care may benefit if hospitals use the ready means available to meet high standards in a cost-effective and efficient manner through program management. Fluctuating hospice census and varying intensity of services are managed with maximum productivity through program-oriented plans and goals superimposed over existing departmental structures. Developing hospice care as a separate entity within the hospital organization has the same costly ramifications as developing hospice services separately in the larger health care delivery system.

Planning

Financial analysis of hospice care is initiated in the planning process. Hospice program planning in the formal sense must identify hospice care as it relates to the organization providing the service, to those who would receive services, and to political and economic realities. This is a most difficult aspect of the program planning, since the product of such identification often presents the challenge of change to the system. Universal planning considerations include an analysis of need to be translated to demand and to projected program capacity and scope. The grassroots movement from which the hospice concept developed represented a response to an unmet need. Quantification of that need is essential to organize effectively the resources required to meet it.

There is no magic formula for measuring need. Planning professionals must utilize their knowledge of the many variables involved in a given community and logically piece this data together to project an estimated demand. Planning is at best an educated guess, since the factors considered may not interact in the expected manner and important influences may not be taken into account.

Before estimates can be made, some basic definitions must be established in order to limit and identify boundaries. This may include limiting the program to cancer patients who reside within the hospital's service area.

Church Hospital employed the following method to estimate demand:

Step 1. Determine areawide hospital utilization rate: 132.4 admissions per 1,000.

Step 2. Determine the year's medical-surgical admission projection: 9,288.

Step 3. The hospital's use-rate population base therefore is:
$$9,288/132.4 = 70.15 \times 1,000 = 70,150$$

Step 4. Approximately 50% of the hospital's admissions are from Baltimore City and about 50% are from Baltimore County and the four adjacent counties. City use-rate population base: 35,000; county use-rate population base: 35,000.

Step 5. Cancer death rates for the Baltimore area are city, 288/100,000; county, 196/100,000.

Step 6. To determine the annual number of cancer deaths from Church Hospital's use-rate population base, the following computations were made:
$35,000/100,000 \times 288 = 98$ patients from Baltimore City;
$35,000/100,000 \times 196 = 68.6$ patients from the four counties.

Step 7. The hospital estimates, therefore, that the hospital's present market share from its service area will provide approximately 170 admissions per year to the hospice program.

This method provides a baseline number from which to work. Other factors are subsequently analyzed and used to adjust this figure.

– Hospice care may not be appropriate or may not be desired by all patients.
– Program admission criteria such as a requirement that a caregiver be present at home excludes some patients.
– The proportion of cancer patients in any other hospital is affected by the specialty mix of the medical staff, services available at the facility, and medical referral patterns.

- The presence or absence of other hospice care providers can make a significant impact on referrals to the program.
- It may well be determined that a specific demand exists but that resources are available to meet only a portion of that demand.

Once program capacity is determined, institutional costs may be calculated on the basis of the number of beds involved and the associated overhead. Other considerations include the need to modify existing physical facilities (e.g., add private family lounges or redecorate rooms) and the impact of the program on hospital census. Will patients who would otherwise be admitted to curative care simply be reclassified as hospice patients? Will additional patients be admitted who otherwise would receive services elsewhere or no services at all?

Every hospital will answer these questions differently. Moreover, in the face of variables such as length of stay, physician understanding and support, and the mix of medical services provided in each hospital and its community, answers may change over time for each hospital. Because of the financial implications of these planning considerations, the option of developing a hospice care program based upon a "swing bed" concept and flexible use of personnel is attractive. In this way a developing program may still respond to community need and be allowed to gain momentum on its own strength.

Personnel

The need for a variety of competent personnel to comprise the hospice team is a critical cost and quality issue. The individual needs of patients and families encompass a wide spectrum of manpower resources. A formal program structure in a hospital setting provides the means to tap these resources for hospice care. Otherwise, staffing may be supplemented through contractual agreements in order to provide special services needed on an individual patient basis.

Although hospice care is labor intensive, much time is contributed by volunteers. Volunteers are essential to successful hospice care; the existence of organized volunteer services in hospitals facilitates recruitment and involvement in the hospice care team. Through volunteer support, program staffing expenses may be defrayed. This is especially true in the context of hospice care standards, where personal attention and time to spend with the patient and family must be readily available. Special services such as art or music therapy may be successfully provided by volunteers.

For volunteer support to be financially meaningful, it must be incorporated into program planning and consistently available. Otherwise, additional staffing expenses should be budgeted to maintain program standards. It is highly desirable, if not essential, to incur the expense of employing a volunteer director to maintain a stable and well-organized volunteer component.

Home Care

Whether provided through a hospital-based department or through contract with independent agencies, home care services are integral to a hospice care program. The feasibility of hospital-based home care in general may be a major financial obstacle. Reimbursement for hospice-type home care is further complicated since visits are typically two to three times longer than other home care contacts. Bereavement follow-up, liaisons with nursing homes and the inpatient unit, and other special services are not reimbursed at this time. On the other hand, coordination with outside home health agencies is often difficult and continuity of care issues are raised.

If a viable hospital-based home care department already exists, the prospect of increased staffing expenses must be reviewed. This includes not only the impact of the program on volume of visits and staff productivity, but the increase in administrative time needed to participate in the admission process, coordinate with the inpatient unit, and organize other home care resources. A hospital considering the addition of a home care service should evaluate the options of providing care to hospice patients only or a combination of hospice and other patients. The differences in volume, expense, reimbursement, and organizational requirements are significant, yet each is a viable alternative.

The financial aspects of home care are undergoing dynamic change due to the influence of new prospective payment systems in health care. Incentives for early discharge of hospital inpatients are encouraging development of home care services. Adequate financial control is significantly diminished when home care is not hospital based. Costs may be further controlled if the home health service is hospital affiliated by way of an organizational relationship (i.e., through diversification of services and organizational entities) instead of a division of the hospital proper.

Medical Support

The expense of formal medical input varies greatly and ranges from totally volunteered services to part- and full-time compensation for physician services. Unless key physicians understand, support, and actively participate in its development, a hospice care program will never get off the ground. Major educational efforts must be made with the medical staff in general and with individuals on a physician-to physician basis. At least one physician is needed to actively participate in program management, medical policy development, screening, and acceptance of patients and consultative services.

The method of reimbursement for physicians' services is influenced by the particular organizational structure of a program and its setting. In a program in which patients are transferred to the care of a hospice physician, fee-for-service reimbursement through billing of third-party payors is possible. However, reimbursement for physician visits to the home is not sufficient to encourage this service.

Physician payment under the new Medicare hospice option is limited within the overall per case payment limits. In any event fee-for-service compensation does not address the cost of physicians' services on an administrative level. Administrative overhead is further increased when the hospice physician acts as program consultant to the attending physician who continues to care for his or her patient. Depending on the nature of services and the average time involved, reimbursement for medicoadministrative services may take the form of a flat fee payable on a monthly basis. A salaried position is also an option for compensation. In a hospital where a salaried physician already plays a medicoadministrative role, it may be possible to include hospice care as one of the physician's responsibilities.

Payment for physician services from hospital rates should be supported by record keeping that establishes the nature and time involved in provision of such services. Otherwise, the legitimacy of physician services may be questioned by federal auditors or other third-party payors. The reasonableness of the physician expense component and its relationships to overall costs is an administrative determination.

Reimbursement

Once the projected expense of a hospice program is calculated, that expense may then be related to the reimbursement system. Funds received from grants, endowments, or other special trust sources are useful in underwriting start-up expenses but generally cannot be relied upon for continued operational support on a large scale. The resources of self-paying patients are sorely taxed by the costs of prolonged illness and/or the aggressive curative treatment that usually precedes hospice care. As with other forms of health care, third-party reimbursement in the form of Medicare, state medical assistance, and commercial insurance comprises the major source of operating funds.

Since this reimbursement system has categorized health care services according to levels, hospice care is reimbursed according to services approved under acute (hospital), intermediate (nursing home), or home care levels. These three categories offer a simplistic description of levels of care; a confusing and lengthy terminology exists, which describes levels of care from regulatory and medical viewpoints. It is not difficult to see how official reimbursement definitions and policies shape and influence the nature of health care services delivery. A program such as hospice care does not fit the mold. Paradoxically, hospice care takes issue with the reimbursement system while simultaneously courting its support. Lobbying efforts by hospice proponents resulted in legislative provisions for a Medicare hospice benefit in the Tax Equity and Fiscal Responsibility Act of 1982 (P.L. 97-248, Section 122). Proposed regulations attendant to this act were published in the Federal Register in 1983 (Department of Health and Human Services 1983a).

A review of the Medicare hospice benefit follows this discussion of basic reimbursement problems posed by the traditional payment system. Hospice care has not been recognized as a separate category of provider care. The continuity of care embraced by the hospice concept is disrupted by the reimbursement system, which strictly defines the circumstances and services for payment (i.e., conditions of participation). Third-party reimbursement at the skilled nursing home and intermediate levels of care is generally not sufficient to cover the labor-intensive expense of hospice patients. However, major components of hospice care do fall within reimbursement guidelines and provide a foundation for the survival of a program. At the acute level virtually all services are covered by third parties. Much less coverage is available for home care, and reimbursement guidelines are particularly restrictive in the hospice context. Usually absent is third-party reimbursement for program components such as bereavement follow-up, respite care, art therapy, and many professional consultative services. Nonetheless, payment for basic home care service is widely available although not always chosen by the consumer, including employers, when purchasing insurance coverage.

The aforementioned conditions of participation serve to monitor and control utilization as a safeguard for limited resources. Such guidelines are designed to combat fraud and abuse of the reimbursement system and to contain costs. Examples of requirements and exclusions that present and/or once presented problems to hospice care include:

- The requirement that, to be eligible for home care or skilled nursing facility services, the patient must have been hospitalized for at least three days prior to admission to the lower level of care.
- The requirement that, to be eligible for home care services, the patient must be homebound; that is, unable to leave home except for infrequent or brief absences to obtain services in another setting.
- The exclusion of drugs and biologicals provided in the home and self-administered.
- The exclusion of reimbursement for bereavement counseling to the family by a nurse or other qualified professional after the death of a hospice patient.
- Restrictions on reimbursement for visits made by the hospice team to hospice patients who have been reinstitutionalized.

It is against this background that a hospice program faces a now-too-familiar financial dilemma. If the calculated expense of a program exceeds revenues provided by reimbursement policy, a plan to handle the resulting shortfall must be developed. The nature and extent of deficits will vary according to the circumstances of a particular program. Several avenues may be pursued:

1. An increase in the degree of volunteer support.
2. The ability of the hospital to increase general overhead expenses to be justifiably allocated to other cost centers.
3. The possibility of coordinating liaisons with other agencies, health care providers, or private groups.
4. Special funding or grant monies.

Table 10-1 Comparison of Average Costs of Hospice and Comparable Medical-Surgical Patients

	Hospice Patient	Medical-Surgical Patient
Room	$1547.58	$1784.02
Pharmacy	$ 58.77	$ 294.60
Laboratory	$ 24.82	$ 405.12
Radiology	$ 29.89	$ 265.91
Respiratory therapy	$ 77.40	$ 73.07
Admission	$ 73.45	$ 73.45
Supplies	$ 64.97	$ 95.95
Electrocardiography	$ 8.41	$ 57.69
Physical therapy	$ 9.38	$ 30.14
Other	$ 26.27	$ 351.36
Charge per patient day	$ 173.94	$ 345.30
Charge per admission	$1920.84	$3431.35

Reproduced with permission from Breindel and Gravely (1980).

In the long run, if gaps in reimbursement are to be filled or special legislation passed to provide for hospice care, it must be shown that a savings to the health care system is possible and/or that other benefits outweigh the expense. Several reimbursement guidelines themselves serve as barriers to the cost containment opportunities offered by hospice care. The requirement for a new plan of treatment upon a patient's discharge following reinstitutionalization creates unnecessary administrative expense. Other requirements tying reimbursement to episodes of illness in acute care facilities force patients into the most expensive setting while those exclusions denying reimbursement for certain skilled and nonskilled supportive services restrict preventive health care measures.

The savings potential of hospice care is primarily a matter of providing an alternative to expensive acute care technology. It is unlikely that savings achieved from the preventive care aspects of hospice care can be quantified. Cost containment opportunities do exist in the avoidance of an acute level of care and, when hospitalization is indicated, in less expensive palliative treatment. Just how much less is the object of much speculation and likely to vary widely due to medical (case mix) and demographic (socioeconomic) factors.

Breindel and Gravely's (1980) study of Church Hospital's experience has shown that the total direct labor cost per patient day for the hospice patient is less than for the average medical-surgical patient. Although this finding is surprising, it is not unusual to find that hospice patients utilize ancillary services to a much lesser extent than the average medical-surgical patient. Breindel found that the average charge per patient day was 27% less than the average charge per patient day hospital wide and 50% less than the average charge per patient day when compared with other terminal patients with the same length of stay. Savings are more significant if one assumes that the alternative for many terminally ill cancer patients is an intensive battery of expensive curative measures more costly than those used by the average patient. A comparison of costs with comparable medical-surgical patients is shown in Table 1.

These findings accentuate the need for valid statistical measures, in-depth program evaluation, and accurate financial analyses to enhance payment prospects for hospice care. Although it is encouraging to find evidence of cost efficiency, it is of little value unless the program meets its objectives and standards.

New Payment Methods

The Medicare Hospice Benefit enacted under Section 122 of P.L. 97-248 (Tax Equity and Fiscal Responsibililty Act of 1982) offers an alternative payment method for hospice care. Prices are prospectively set for defined levels of care for each day. Daily prices are all-inclusive at each level of care (e.g., routine home care, continuous home care, inpatient respite care, and general inpatient care). There is a limit in the aggregate for each hospice patient served; any difference between the limit and charges incurred below that limit is not available to the provider as incentive for efficiency.

Additional coverage that is not offered by regular Medicare benefits includes fewer restrictions on types of home care services covered, outpatient drugs, and some counseling services. Some copayment provisions apply. Payment for physician services is handled as separate Part B charges but is included in the calculation of the cap amount when the physician is employed by the hospice.

The Medicare beneficiary may elect to use the hospice benefit in lieu of regular coverage and payment for medical services. The limit average (cap amount) has been disputed, with payment limits generally perceived as unrealistic and inadequate. This perception and the fact that hospitals are not required to seek Medicare certification of their hospices have resulted in few applications for eligibility. Nonfinancial aspects also strongly deter interest in this benefit since the organizational requirements of the regulations are inconsistent with effective management and in fact promote inefficiencies that increase expense.

Prospective Payment

Medicare implemented a prospective payment system (PPS) in October of 1983 for acute inpatient service. Payments are made for diagnostic-related groups (DRGs), with standardized amounts per DRG calculated according to a method adopted by the Health Care Financing Administration (Department of Health and Human Services 1983b) published in the Federal Register. These amounts are adjusted for a phase-in period, outlier (atypical extremes) payment, medical education, wage and salary indices, and other factors. There is continued legislative and regulatory activity shaping the prospective payment environment (Department of Health and Human Services 1984a; 1984b; see also P.L. 98-369, The Deficit Reduction Act of 1984).

This significant alteration in hospital payment has major implications for services such as hospice care. Strong incentives are created to decrease length of stay and intensity of resource use (e.g., ancillary services), and home health care is encouraged as a means for early discharge. Thus hospice care conforms with these new incentives. In addition, quality-of-care concerns brought about by attention to efficiency and economy are ameliorated by the commitment to the continuity of care found in a hospice service.

It is widely believed that if the federal prospective payment system is successful in reducing health care costs without undue deterioration of quality or access to care, other third-party payors will follow suit. If the change in practice patterns induced by the new economic incentives provides a boost to hospice care, it is coincidental, yet real nonetheless.

Competition

Another significant change occurring in the health care delivery system is the promotion of a heightened environment for competition. Again, if the expense of hospice care proves to be less than that of conventional treatment, there are incentives for providers to make such care available in the market. The attractiveness of hospice care from a marketing standpoint can also be an asset in a competitive arena. Consumer demand for palliative treatment and holistic medicine could encourage further growth of hospice programs.

Staffing

The heart of a hospice care program is its staffing. Proper staffing of the program allows it to realize its stated objectives, not only through the number of individuals involved and their professional credentials, but through their special commitment to the hospice concept. Staffing is also the heart of the expense of hospice care and should be analyzed to measure resources needed for the program and to compare its cost to other forms of health care.

Cost Accounting

Due to the nature of program integration at Church Hospital, it is difficult to segregate the expense of staffing for hospice care. No separate "cost center" exists to isolate costs; staff participate in the care of other patients, and their activities in hospice care vary with hospice census and the individual needs of patients in the program. Although program responsiveness and productivity are enhanced by the integrated structure, this advantage is lost if hospice-related expense is not monitored. The depth of professional disciplines and numbers of personnel are of no use to the program if other responsibilities conflict with hospice care. Consequently, program capacity, and therefore, expense, is directly related to the staffing needs of hospice patients.

To identify staffing expense, a study was undertaken using management engineering techniques to determine for each discipline the time spent providing care (Breindel and Gravely 1980). In a comparison with staffing required by the average medical-surgical patient at the hospital, it was found that the hospice patient received less nursing care from the nursing staff (3.9 hours per patient day) than a medical-surgical patient (4.4 hours per patient day). However, when nursing care supplemented by volunteers and family was taken into account, total time spent in hospice nursing activities was 7.3 hours per patient day. The findings underscore the role of volunteers and the general interaction with the family in maintaining a high standard of hospice care.

Other disciplines were found to spend more time with the hospice patient than with the average medical-surgical patient. They include physical therapists, dietitians, nurse-practitioners, social workers, and others. However, due to the "savings" in nursing time provided by volunteers and family, total labor cost per patient day for the hospice patient was less than for the average medical-surgical patient. The alternative of staff designated solely for hospice care presumed a caseload consistently large enough to justify the expense. This may be realistic for certain core personnel such as nurses and social workers, but it becomes less certain for other professionals such as physical therapists, dietitians, or respiratory therapists. Here it can be seen that the relationship between available resources, program standards, and estimated patient volume significantly impacts upon the proper mix of employees, volunteers, and contracted services that comprise program staffing.

With the advent of prospective payment systems such as that introduced by Medicare, cost accounting in hospitals is changing. Due to the nature of the payment system, it is now essential that diagnoses or "product lines" be individually costed out and related to the amount available for payment. This development will improve cost-of-care information available for hospice services as a component of the product mix of hospital and/or home health services.

Program Integration and the Hospice Team

The integration of hospice patients into a general medical-surgical unit and into the total workload of each hospice team member was intended for more than cost efficiency. Its aim was also to alleviate staff stress associated with caring for the terminally ill. This integration also aids in alleviating the pressure associated with participating in what is perceived to be a novel and pioneering program. Subjective feedback from staff at Church Hospital supports this approach.

A staffing consideration of special importance in an integrated program such as Church Hospital's is the establishment of the hospice team concept. Without the unifying force of active teamwork, coordination would break down, continuity would be lost, and personal stress would be magnified. Any cost efficiencies achieved would be impossible without the team effort; integration of volunteers into the working nursing unit and into the home care field is a prime example of this.

To have an effective hospice team, staffing should include a variety of professional disciplines to provide depth and expertise. Hospitals have excellent access to health care professionals and the means to orient and incorporate them into the hospice care team.

The Church Hospital team includes home care nursing, inpatient nursing, social workers, chaplains, physical therapists, dietitians, volunteers, nurse-practitioners, and physicians. Support is provided from the pharmacy, respiratory therapy, and all other hospital departments. Psychiatric services and other specialized personnel are available and ready to respond to an individual patient's need. Chapter 6 describes the components and coordination of the hospice team in the clinical setting.

Continuity of Care

The hospice concept strives to eliminate the fragmented health care that occurs when patients move from one delivery setting to another. Staffing patterns and responsibilities can be utilized to achieve optimal coordination of patient care plans and maintain familiar and secure relationships with the patient and family. At Church Hospital, key personnel who act to ensure continuity of care include home health nurses, the chaplain, social workers, volunteers, and the hospice physicians. This function is well understood by the staff involved and is an essential thread tying the program together and influencing interaction with other personnel. Patient rounds are alternated with team conferences on a weekly basis as an additional mechanism to ensure coordination and optimal patient care.

In a hospital-based program providing inpatient and home care services, continuity is jeopardized if for some reason the patient cannot be at home when he or she no longer requires acute care. This circumstance is controlled for the most part by admission screening criteria but cannot be avoided entirely. In the absence of affiliation with a skilled nursing home or intermediate care provider, hospice staff ordinarily maintain some continuity of care through volunteer efforts. The concept of continuity visits by hospice staff as a reimbursable service is being considered by some third-party payors but is not now a reality. Those patients who are not eligible for admission to a particular program due to the absence of a caregiver in the home are of concern to all hospice programs. In most states the free-standing hospice is not recognized as a provider category, and it appears that staffing requirements present a major deterrent to the nursing home industry in developing hospice care. The development of multi-institutional health care systems in the United States may create the network necessary to accommodate the levels of care required for hospice care continuity. Many hospitals are converting beds or purchasing nursing home (intermediate level) facilities.

Prospective payment systems and competition in health care are forces causing hospitals to diversify services and seek creative avenues to address decreasing inpatient utilization. Emphasis on outpatient services and less-than-acute inpatient care is a necessity. These developments will enhance continuity of care and should serve to promote the development of hospice services.

Reference

American Hospital Association: *Implementation of New Medicare Hospice Benefit*, (September 1, 1983) Memorandum. AHA, Chicago, September 1, 1983.

Briendel CL, Gravely GE: *Costs of Providing a Mixed-Unit Hospice Program*. Working paper, Department of Health Administration, Medical College of Virginia, Richmond, 1980.

Department of Health and Human Services, Health Care Financing Administration, Medicare Program: *Hospice Care Proposed Rule*. Federal Register, vol 48, p 38146, August 22, 1983a.

————: *Medicare Program: Prospective Payments for Medicare Inpatient Hospital Services*. Federal Register, vol 48, p 39752, September 1, 1983b.

————: *Medicare Program; Prospective Payment for Medicare Inpatient Hospital Services: Final Rule*. Federal Register, vol 49, pp 234-340, January 3, 1984a.

————: *Medicare Program; Changes to the Inpatient Hospital Services*. Federal Register, vol 49, p 27422, July 3, 1984b.

Joint Commission on Accreditation of Hospitals: *Hospice Self-Assessment and Survey Guide*. JCAH, Chicago, 1983a.

Joint Commission on Accreditation of Hospitals: *Hospice Standards Manual*. JCAH, Chicago, 1983b.

National Hospice Organization: *Standards of a Hospice Program of Care*. NHO, Arlington, VA, 1979.

Chapter 11

Public Perceptions of Hospice

Frederick T. Wehr

These are the observations and recommendations of the person charged with the public relations duties of an acute care hospital that was the first institution in its community, a major metropolitan area, to establish any kind of hospice service. They may not be applicable in another setting. What I know of Church Hospital's hospice service has been learned not only in the course of performing public relations duties but being witness to the care given to my first wife who died here of cancer in 1977 when the service was in its formative stages. In short, I am a beneficiary as well as an advocate, a fact that may color my conclusions.

Assuming that most of the readers of this short chapter will be people who will be engaged in the public relations aspects of a hospice service of some kind, I offer the following observations:

Unless your community is a particularly sophisticated one, most of its residents will not know what hospice means.

If your community already has an institution that calls itself a hospice but is something other than a place or service for the terminally ill, you have a problem. It is surmountable.

If your institution is a hospital that proposes to initiate a hospice service, some residents of your community will fail to grasp that you are not, in this instance, attempting to cure a disease but, instead, to palliate its effects. These people may assume that hospice offers a new kind of therapy.

Although hospice does not induce death, some people will conclude that it is a form of euthanasia.

Do not assume that all physicians know about hospice: they don't. Among those who do will be some who oppose the concept because of the strong antiphysician attitude taken by certain hospice advocates. This antagonism has done wonders in slowing the acceptance of hospice by the medical profession.

Some of the pharmacological aspects of hospice will be disturbing to physicians, as well as laymen, for society — or most of it — has been taught to dread morphine and addiction. In hospice, morphine and its cousins are often indispensable for cancer patients, and addiction is almost never a problem. Dr. Zimmerman has enlarged on this in Chapter 3.

Once the word is out that you are inaugurating a hospice service, be prepared to contend with all sorts of advocates who may or may not have a place in your organization. Hospice attracts some strong personalities with very firm opinions. You may welcome the personality and the opinion. But if you don't want it and can't convert it, send it elsewhere. Otherwise, it will undermine your work.

A suggestion: You will need a pamphlet to respond to the question "What is hospice?" A publication of 500 to 600 words can be sufficiently comprehensive to satisfy most people. Include a name and telephone number if the reader wants more details.

Since Church Hospital was one of the first in the nation to establish a hospice service, we received from doctors, nurses, social workers, and clergymen hundreds of inquiries, most of which were not addressed in detail in our pamphlet. So we obtained a grant from the A. S. Abell Company Foundation of Baltimore and published a 24-page booklet entitled *Toward a Gentler Dying*. Not only has it answered some of the more sophisticated questions, but it has been useful as a guidebook for our volunteers. Incidentally, copies were sent to every hospital in the United States in the hope of encouraging others to proceed as we had. Although the booklet has been helpful, most hospice institutions will probably not need anything so comprehensive.

There is, however, another kind of publication that may well be in order. We prepared a pamphlet of about 750 words entitled *About Hospice and Home Care* for the families of hospice patients who have been stabilized in the hospital and are about to go home. The pamphlet is candid. It starts with the words "You are now taking care of someone who is not going to live much longer." It goes on to tell the reader what to expect, how to cope, and what to do if the patient dies at home. Obviously, something like this should be given only to those who thoroughly understand the prognosis.

Regarding the media, although hospice is not the hot issue it was back in the 1970s, it is a subject that the press will find attractive, particularly if yours is the first in the area. Although reporters often hold some of the misconceptions and biases listed above, those who have visited Church Hospital have been both receptive and sympathetic. Usually they will ask for permission to interview a patient and the family. When the request arises, I suggest you ask the hospice nurses if they know of a patient who might want to talk to a reporter. Be sure the nurse understands that the reporter will be asking the patient about hospice and his illness and that neither the hospital nor the patient is under any obligation to grant the interview. If the nurse reports that the patient is agreeable, authorize the interview but tell the reporter that hospice patients sometimes reject what they have apparently accepted and may talk as if they expect, or at least hope, to recover. Warned of this possibility in advance the reporter can beat a tactful retreat if the interview takes this turn.

Without exception, the Baltimore reporters have been good with the patients. Some have been truly impressive. Nevertheless, it is our practice to be particularly protective of hospice patients and to discourage interviews when they might cause some emotional damage to the patient or the family. Remember, too, that a portion of the public may regard the interview — particularly if it is on the television — as an invasion of privacy, its effectiveness and the patient's willingness to participate notwithstanding.

Two questions come up time and again in inquiries from the public and the press. Although both are addressed elsewhere in the book, I believe it will be helpful to my counterparts at other hospice institutions to include them here as well.

The first is this: Do you tell the patient he is dying? The answer is that *if* he asks the question, you answer "yes" in the gentlest way possible. Usually, however, the question does not arise. Sooner or later, the patient will begin to indicate that he knows he is not going to recover. He may allude to things that he will never do again, to people he will never see again, to projects that someone else will have to finish. He and perhaps his entire family may make no direct reference to his dying in one another's company while demonstrating their acceptance of its imminence in a variety of ways. They seem sometimes to take refuge in the difference between "not going to recover" and "going to die." I hasten to add that a condition of admission to the hospice service is that one member of the family must acknowledge to us an understanding that the patient is terminally ill.

The second question: If someone is dying of cancer, for instance, how do you know whether he needs hospice care? Although one could reasonably argue that virtually any terminally ill patient would receive some benefit, albeit slight, from the service that hospice offers, there are certainly many patients for whom it is not necessary.

The extreme cases make the point. Mr. A is 78 years old; he is dying. He seldom complains of pain. When he does, it is readily controlled. His family is attentive and affectionate. He is sometimes quiet, perhaps depressed, but not for long. He gives no indication of needing spiritual support, and there are no money problems, no loose ends. Mr. A is dying well and, as far as can be told, easily. He does not need hospice.

At the other end of the spectrum is Mrs. B. She is 40 and terminally ill. Her pain and depression are severe. She has been in the hospital for two weeks, and her husband has yet to visit her. Her children visit occasionally but stay only for a few minutes. She knows she is dying, and she is frightened. Mrs. B and her family need hospice.

It is obvious that there is a continuum here. Obvious, too, is that many patients need only one or two aspects of hospice care, usually symptom control and little else. Furthermore, not everyone will accept what hospice has to offer, particularly in the area of emotional and spiritual support. A comprehensive examination of hospice in its continuum will be found in Chapter 14, "Hospice in the Matrix of Medicine."

One final observation: In my fourteen years here, nothing at Church Hospital has attracted so much favorable attention or drawn such appreciation as the hospice service, this in spite of the fact that all we can promise is that we will work toward making death as easy as possible for the patient and for the family. Over 1000 patients have died to date under hospice care here. Some of these deaths, our best efforts notwithstanding, have been wrenching. Yet even in these cases, thanks and grief flow together. Contributions from hospice families and their friends — all of them unsolicited — far outnumber any other form of gift we receive. The hospice concept may be controversial elsewhere. It has not been controversial here.

Chapter 12

Hospice: The Spiritual Dimension

The Reverend Paul S. Dawson

The interpersonal relationships that develop in a hospice program are experienced at an intensely personal level, making it difficult to think in terms of ready techniques to draw out of one's satchel for day-to-day situations. I avoid the "stages" approach because of the linear or horizontal impetus that it implies; it is tempting in a clinical setting to follow such a structured sequence slavishly. A "how to" approach is often impersonal and can generate a false confidence derived from the current mystique of expertise.

Rather, I shall suggest some guidelines that have helped me in my work and have seemed to be helpful to others. The attention here is deliberately personal, subjective (hopefully in an informed way), and humble. Humility is applicable and possible when that to which one relates is regarded with sincerity, with reverence. The patient and/or family are always considered to be unique entities. Each individual is a fresh frontier, a field for discovery, an opportunity for mutual endeavor that is rich in resources for creative understanding. These resources are found not in textbooks or manuals, but in the soil of our common humanity and shared religious faith — a community of genuine concern. Concentration must be deep and intuitive and the climate, sensitive and intimate.

Hospice as Family: Some Considerations Concerning the Spiritual Dimension in Hospice Care

Mrs. C., 75 years old, was typical of forgotten people everywhere. Having had no children, she was quite alone in her one-room apartment in a municipal high rise for the elderly when she was found to have cancer of the bowel and bladder. After surgery, she came under the home care department at our hospital. She lived just one block away. Old, plain, ill, with no friends or family nearby, she was nevertheless a happy person. Occasional dress-up visits downtown were high points in her life; she window-shopped, moved with the crowds, fed the pigeons, and basked in the warm sunlight. Her health continued to decline; finally, she was admitted to our hospice program. As the limitations imposed by her illness closed in, she was happiest, she said, when she was asleep. Then came hallucinations and confusion. None of us likes to think about the Mrs. C's of this world, and that is precisely their tragedy: no one cares.

In Mrs. C's case, someone did care. In hospice, the number of people who noticed and tried to do something for her increased. She was able to tolerate her situation because she knew that she would receive care that would see her through to the end. One of the hospice nurse interns visited her three times a day during those last days at home to see that she took her medicine regularly; she tended to forget. On her last birthday the home care staff gave her a fine birthday party. They took her picture; she was definitely a person to be reckoned with. One of the hospice volunteers took her to have her hair done. During the last few weeks of life, in our hospital, the confusion and withdrawal continued, but she was surrounded by her beloved stuffed animals, each given a name. Close to the end she was visited by the nurse intern who had given her medicine at home. Her face broke into a strong smile for the last time. Then this impoverished old lady, with so little to commend her to the world, died as simply as she had lived.

A month or so before, the one relative of Mrs. C. who lived in the city had died. An elderly cousin some distance away was not able to assume any responsibility for Mrs. C.'s burial. There was no one even to claim her body. Then a very significant thing happened. The hospice staff mobilized out of an initial anguished reaction to act on her behalf as a family normally would. The few remaining dollars were used for her cremation. A funeral service was conducted in the hospital chapel; some 10 or 12 hospice staff persons and volunteers were present. Her ashes were buried in a lovely grotto at All Saints' Convent near the city. (The All Saints Sisters of the Poor are an Episcopal religious order for women. One of the All Saints' sisters, Sr. Catherine Grace, herself an R.N., worked from the beginning in effort to form and establish the hospice program at our hospital.) We all knew a great peace as the small box containing Mrs. C.'s ashes was lowered into the tiny neat grave, marked by a simple wooden cross; the sisters at the Convent had prepared the site. Dr. Yukna, our hospice physician, stepped forward and gently covered the grave with fresh earth. One of the nurses had brought a beautiful, hardy chrysanthemum to plant at her grave, but we found that the grave was in a shaded, protected area unsuited for such a plant. At first the suggestion was made that we get another plant that would thrive in the shade. But we agreed that it would be more appropriate to let it remain as it was; nature would provide its own glory in that hallowed, humble place. There was a feeling of profound resolution that we all shared. Mrs. C. would be happy to know how things had worked out. We experienced there a profound intimacy that would never change, that we would never forget. We were all, including Mrs. C., a *family*.

It occurred to me then that hospice is, above all else, best typified as family. The psychosocial dynamic in hospice care is that of a family looking after its own, whether this is said of the staff in relation to the patient, to his or her family, or to itself. I would like in the next few pages to try to explain what this means.

Family as the Basic Unit of Human Life

Family is an extension of the individuals who comprise it. In turn, the individual continuously receives the projection of the family, for better or worse, and is shaped and profoundly affected by it. Family has often been described as a microcosm of the community. As such, it is at once laboratory, classroom, oratory, playing field, battleground, and sanctuary. It is literally the matrix out of which community life emerges and in relation to which the community's value and viability are tested. Should family life disintegrate, the community is affected specifically. A healthy and loving family is often recognized as a model at the heart of the community, a witness to its own strongest purpose. The Judeo-Christian imagery for the community of faith is drawn from family life, and much of its moral sense is directed toward perpetuating healthy and responsible family life. It is through the family dynamic, beginning with the experience of the warm nourishing mother, that the child achieves that most peculiar characteristic of human beings, which is *self* and *other* awareness: the ability to reflect upon oneself and others as distinct entities capable of relationship, sharing, and mutual endeavor.

Spirit: The Vital Force in All Human Life Participation in family life and, by extension, community life promotes the emergence of spiritual awareness and, with it, the sense of abiding significance and purpose. It has been said that "by its nature spirit is the presence of being, that which first gives rise to history and meaning" (Rahner 1975).

Presence Bernard Tyrell (1975) states: "By losing himself in participation [man] finds himself as a 'presence.' Interacting with [the] other, whether object or person, one is made aware of oneself as a distinct entity." I am here, and I see that in relation to the typewriter beyond and in front of me, and the chair on which I sit. The subject-object polarity can be a trap in which one's own sense of presence exists painfully as an inescapable reminder of isolation and estrangement from others. Our society tends to inhibit the experience of intimacy in which persons are deeply present to one another. The pain of such estrangement can be unbearable; it is a terrible form of suffering.

The communication that can emerge from persons being significantly present to one another is one of the most profoundly moving and meaningful occurrences in human experience. I have seen people transformed almost before my eyes from withdrawn, diseased, tense cripples to persons full of hope, peace, and healing power. This has happened particularly in those instances before surgery when persons have opened up and confided dark worries and concerns never revealed to anyone before. In these experiences the effect is miraculous and often the healing process is dramatically heightened and accelerated.

Perhaps there is no occasion when persons are more present to one another than when they are deeply in love. Henri Nouwen (1974) has said, "To care means first of all to be present to each other." Lovers share an intimacy that seems limitless. Such a relationship is profoundly spiritual. Inevitably, the lovers want to learn all about each other; they want to share history. As the relationship evolves, they want to make history together, and out of this mutual endeavor in which lives are shared and intermingled intimately, a profound and sustaining sense of meaning begins to take shape. Such shared meaning is rightly appreciated as one of the highest values in human life.

To be well is to have everything to live for. To possess a sense of well-being is also one of the greatest treasures in human existence. To be recognized as a valuable and appreciated presence in the community enhances and broadens one's personal horizons and permits the active development of personal potential.

History   Nouwen (1972) says, "The emptiness of the past and the future can never be filled with words but only by the presence of man." Time is important in hospice care. Opportunity may be once and for all. Need may require long periods of undivided attention from the staff. The development of themes that arise may require a great deal of effort from a great many people.

While engaged with another, one may not think very much about time, particularly the limits it seems to impose on our ordinary life. Time for most of us is a continuum moving along second by second, hour by hour, day by day. There is the illusion that this duration is open ended, that time repeats itself. "There's always tomorrow . . . I forgot, but I'll get it the next time around." Our past, particularly the painful, half-forgotten elements of the past, is assimilated slowly, dreamily. Even with the help of a skilled psychotherapist, coming to terms with the difficult areas of one's past takes time. The future seems filled with possibilities, renewed opportunities, "another chance"; the future is entered, also dreamily and expectantly. The present movement tends to be lost in the progression from the past toward the emerging future. Often we either lean back into the past, "living in the past," or project into the future, our "heads in the clouds."

Time in hospice care is focused much more insistently on the present. True, the patient and the family may be absorbed in the past, denying the present, or gazing nostalgically at the future, clinging to whatever wisps of hope for extended mortality might be available. But the staff must work always from the present and toward the present. They must ask, "What bearing does the past have upon the present situation . . . what future can one realistically expect out of the present situation?"

I remember a profound self-observation made by a Trappist priest, Fr. Stephen Usinowicz, who was talking about his own orientation in life. He said, "I have no past or future," and he went on to speak of the "gift of the presence of the moment." Of course, we all have past and future, but when we are absorbed intently in the present moment, with "presence of the moment," past and future are absorbed into the present. The *now* dominates experience as we move solidly planted in its growing edge. It is in the *now* that one finds the essentials for understanding and meaning, because it is in the *now* that one finds the incontrovertible certainty, vivid and tangible, of *life* .

I once visited an elderly Jewish woman who was scheduled for surgery. She was very frightened; I understood why when she revealed to me that she had spent years in a concentration camp in Nazi Germany. All of her family, except for a few of her relatives who were living in the United States at the time, were killed in the camps during the war. I have learned since that such persons are terrified by hospitalization, and particularly surgery, because the institutional experience is so reminiscent of the imposed controls of the concentration camp. We talked for a moment. My heart went out to her and she responded warmly to my concern. I asked if I could pray with her. I laid my hands on her head and prayed what I hoped would be an acceptable prayer. When I had finished, she took my hands in hers. Tears streamed down her face. Her eyes, filled with love, held mine; all the compassion of her suffering filled that moment. Slowly, her voice husky and tremulous with feeling, she prayed for me in Hebrew. It was one of the most intimate experiences of my life, in which this foreign Jewish lady and Christian priest were one. Our past and future melded into that moment.

One may find, wondrously, that in a few moments a problem is resolved, a disturbance cleared up, a confession made that would ordinarily take a great deal of time. One can observe in a patient or family the review of a lifetime accomplished redemptively in minutes. Sometimes a few words or a glance or a gesture may say it all. I remember another occasion when, fresh out of the seminary, I was beginning my ministry. Inexperienced and rather timid, particularly where crisis was concerned, I had been regularly visiting a woman in the parish who was a cardiac invalid. We grew close; I really looked forward to my visits with her. I left these visits nourished by her courage, grace, and faith. Finally, she was hospitalized with acute congestive heart failure. I visited her there and was appalled to find that she was fighting for every breath, her eyes wide, face contorted, chest heaving. She was a grotesque caricature of the woman I thought I had known so well. As I gazed at her, veiled behind an oxygen tent, I was horrified and paralyzed; there seemed nothing that I could do. She met my gaze, and for a moment her face relaxed, a look of radiant peace came into her eyes, and she smiled as if to say, "It's all right — it's enough for you just to be here." I knew immediately that she was all right in spite of her great suffering. Past and future meshed magnificently in that beautiful smile; the communion we experienced then was its own meaningful history and prayer. From that momentary glance, soon to dissolve again into the chaos of her suffering, we understood all that needed to be known, and I left with a strong feeling of peace and confidence in her ability to cope.

Concentration, sensitive listening, openess, caring, and commitment all contribute to presence of the moment. Fr. Stephen spoke of it as a gift. I soon realized in seeking his counsel that it was indeed in him an extraordinary gift. But it is a gift that all of us can acquire, at least in some measure, through discipline and practice. It comes through a willingness to share our vitality, freely given without the requirement that it be reciprocated. Regular meditation through which one aims at inner focus and "centering" is a basic prerequisite. This means to be in firm touch with one's own interior or inner core of being. So much of the time we fly off in all directions, our concentration flitting from one surface to another, never settling down, never really consolidating the spiritual resources we all have within us toward one particular area. "Centering" involves a quieting down inside, a single-mindedness, a clarity of motivation, the cultivation of inner peace. (One description of centering that has been helpful to me is to form an image of oneself rooted solidly to the ground, with concentration and focus of attention being mobilized around this rootedness.)

Centering can be difficult to achieve or maintain in a clinical setting, but it is not impossible; perhaps it comes down to priorities. There are two ingredients that must come into play once centering has been accomplished: compassion and intuition. One must care enough about the other to be truly *present* with him. One must also listen for and respond quickly to clues, cues, and themes that may lie almost hidden in the multilayered *presence* of the other, as well as in oneself. Sometimes an expression or phrase from the other will suddenly resonate with something within our own backlog of experience, and insight springs into consciousness. Intuition has been described as the apprehension of truth from a minimum of data (Westcott 1968). For some, intuition is second nature; for others, its use can present serious difficulties (Jung 1971). But just as one can learn to identify subtle nuances of sound, color, or touch when necessity requires (as in hearing loss or blindness), so one can learn to listen more effectively beyond the surface. It is most important to avoid jumping to conclusions or leaping ahead of the person to whom we are relating. To do so is to lose presence. Listening intuitively requires staying with the person to whom one is relating, not jumping ahead or anticipating his thoughts, at least vocally. The intuitive interchange is intimate and profoundly sharing when it is going well. It is a kind of co-pilgrimage in which two or more people walk together on the same ground, hand in hand, one step at a time. As one seeks to understand, one must ask over and over, "What does this say to me; what does my 'gut' tell me?" The intellect comes forward to sift and sort, to make sense of the information perceived.

Memories play an important part in the factor of time with hospice patients and their families. In fact, one's earliest memories provide strong clues as to the underlying philosophy, life-style, or personality tone that shape one's histoy. Alfred Adler suggests that earliest memories symbolize one's outlook on life and one's life-style, perhaps reflecting a dominant inferiority; the mode adopted to compensate for that inferiority often takes the form of an overcompensation or striving for superiority (Adler 1959). To use an imaginary illustration, the following early memory might speak for itself in indicating an attitude of life. "I remember when I was 5 or 6 years old, my father, in a rage, beat my mother. I was cowering in the corner, feeling helpless and frightened. Suddenly, he noticed me, and started in my direction. His eyes were cold and murderous. I thought he was going to kill me. My mother grabbed him and kept him from reaching me. I ran out of his reach. I both hated and feared my father." The important thing to remember in looking at such memories is that although they may or may not be the earliest memory or may or may not be entirely accurate, they reflect upon the general attitude of the person. The object of this exercise is to provide a quick and incisive clue to aid understanding. It should not be used dogmatically to psych out or rigidly categorize an individual.

I have asked for earliest memories of experience with death as an exercise for those who are preparing to work with the dying. This also can be helpful with those close to a dying patient who have a particularly difficult time dealing with death. Sometimes the memory betrays an incident or symbolizes an early experience or attitude that affects the person's reaction and response to death or dying generally. It will most likely reflect, if nothing else, a predominantly negative or positive feeling toward this subject.

The review and recapitulation of the past is seen in dying patients as they try to make sense out of what is happening to them and to discover meaning in a grasp of the whole, the *gestalt,* of what went before. This involves a distillation in which certain themes, incidents, and conflicts stand out, interplaying with others and with the present, they establish a kind of skyline that, when transcended, having been absorbed into the fabric of one's life, provides a background for dealing with present developments meaningfully. In this fashion the patient is able to control what is happening in him.

We are all victimized by our ignorance. Enlightenment, through the discovery of meaning, brings a stronger ability to cope with the immensity of the dying process. Another way of putting it is that much unconscious material comes to the surface for the dying in the form of nonverbal images and symbols, dreams, fantasies, and hallucinations. These materials can be brought into the consciousness and understood. Once assimilated into consciousness, feelings of disturbance, anxiety, fear, and perhaps of losing touch with reality disappear to be replaced by an increased strength and greater resiliency. Occasionally, psychiatric intervention is necessary to come to terms with this psychic turbulence. Usually, sensitive support from the staff or family can provide all that is needed to come through.

Carl Jung (1971) has indicated that the human lifespan is like a parabola, beginning in birth and ending in death. In the first ascending half of life, the emphasis is on establishing oneself, accumulating, and making a place in the world. The second half, which normally begins in middle age, represents a coming to terms with death, whose approach is intimated in the physical signs of aging, the slowing down that is characteristic of middle and old age. There is an increasing tendency to turn inward in reflection upon the substance of life already apprehended. Direction is toward completion and the achievement of wholeness. In the dying patient the promptings from within also urge toward completion, rounding out, wholeness; this is as true in the young as in those who are dying at the end of a normal lifespan.

Jung's concept of the "shadow" figures significantly in that descending portion of life (Jung 1971). When one goes with the whole-making process at that stage, one enters into what Jung called individuation: the articulation of the individuality that characterizes a human life. The shadow is an unconscious reservoir of undeveloped, neglected, and rejected elements in the psychic makeup of each person. There is a dark, threatening, rough, even evil character to this shadow, which is often represented in dreams by a person who threatens to hurt or kill the dreamer. Jung points out that the shadow contains psychic energy that, although repressed or suppressed, does not go away; because it is not channeled, it festers and rankles, seeking an outlet. If there is no room for the shadow to be expressed in one's conscious life, it becomes truly dangerous; it seeps through the cracks, finding expression in hidden, unexpected, destructive ways. Because it is unconscious, the shadow can be detected in dreams, fantasies, and projections. As Whitmont (1969) has pointed out, we can get a glimpse of our shadow, in the mirror as it were, by noting the type of person we instinctively dislike for no good cause or reason. In fact, when we meet someone who resonates with our own shadow, it is projected onto that person so that our dislike is a reflection of the repellent character of our own shadow. Jung indicated that the shadow plays an active part in a healthy attempt (individuation) to come to terms with the requirements of the second half of life. In order to be whole, there is need to become acquainted with the shadow (always carefully, as with a volatile and somewhat unpredictable roughneck) and even to assimilate some of its characteristics into our personality. We may end up being less neat but will certainly be more human. (There but for the Grace of God go I.)

In the dying person there is an increasing need to come to terms with and assimilate the darker, less developed side of his nature, which is brought to the fore in part because the individual is progressively becoming, in an unavoidable way, less attractive, weaker, and less independent. In working closely with such people, one sometimes finds the person's shadow projected onto oneself. When this happens, a creative response rather than a defensive reaction is indicated. Carrying another's projection, although painful, can help to clarify the issues, as long as one understands what is happening and listens so as to read the underlying message. I recall a visit to a patient who was about to go to surgery. As I entered the room, a stranger to this man, he turned to me in fury, eyes blazing, his face livid. I asked, "Why are you so angry?" He suddenly stopped and explained in desperation that he had just come into the hospital; he was due to go to surgery in a few hours and no one had talked to him about his coming operation. For all he knew, he would go to the operating room without anyone knowing who he was; could he even be sure that they would do the right surgery on him? He felt anonymous, cheated, and unrecognized. I listened to him and left immediately to talk to the head nurse on the floor. In a few minutes she came with me, sat down beside him, and explained exactly what to expect. He responded calmly and quietly. When I had first entered his room, I came not as a clinical person, but as a fellow human being, as vulnerable and nonclinical as he was. I received his projection and was able, through listening at a deeper level, to go past his hostile affront to hear his anxiety and fear and was thereby able to help him better understand his situation.

We, the staff, sometimes project our shadow onto the patient, the family, or even fellow staff members. When we are faced, in the other, with someone we unreasonably dislike or resist, we can assume that the shadow, our shadow, is in the picture. We must ask, "Is there anything in me that I see in the person before me; am I seeing that person as he or she really is, or am I looking at my own shadow image?" It is not easy to be clear about this, but the exercise of careful and honest assessment can help clear the air, and the experience of meeting and dealing creatively with our own shadow in others can be a growth experience for us.

Agnes Sanford (1947) presents an excellent exercise for healing the emotions or memories that, because they are painful or unresolved, poison and plague us, even though half forgotten. She presents this in the context of confession and forgiveness before God, but it can also be used as I suggest here. Relax with pencil and paper at hand. Divide your life into seven periods. Dealing with each period separately, try to remember any unresolved or uncomfortable memories from that time span. Write them down simply and quickly; after the list is completed put it aside. Allowing some time to elapse, go on to the next period and continue in like fashion on through the seven periods. Once this list is completed, one can deal with the significantly difficult and painful memories by using a device suggested by Dennis and Matthew Linn (1978), which is based on the five stages of dying enumerated by Elizabeth Kübler-Ross. These are denial — I don't admit I was ever hurt; anger — I blame others for hurting and destroying me; bargaining — I set up conditions to be fulfilled before I'm ready to forgive; depression — I blame myself for letting hurt destroy me; acceptance — I look forward to growth from hurt. Applying these stages to the significant memories listed helps to bring them into perspective and to bring those persons involved in the memories into clear focus. It can set us up for forgiveness, healing, and reconciliation. This exercise can be a useful tool for those patients and family members who are dealing with painful memories and particularly for those patients who are embarked on the recapitulation process.

Meaning   Existence without meaning becomes intolerable. Viktor Frankl (1963) has pointed out that when life is deprived of meaning, spontaneous death often follows. Such deprivation leads to death of the spirit and life simply ceases.

Perhaps this is what we dread most as we contemplate death or dying: the extinction of meaning, all the more terrible should awareness remain. There is, then, literally nothing to live for.

We all long for a time and place when our spirits have found a home, where history and meaning are shared deeply and where the members of the fellowship in which such sharing takes place are deeply present to one another in love. Much of the appeal of the Church as God's family stems from such longing. Heaven, as a condition of heightened existence free of conflict and mortality in which one is present with loved ones, resonates with that same longing. To be at home in the universe, free of the limits of time and space, in a climate of love and peace, is integral with the deeper spiritual experiences that mark every human life. I'm speaking of those moments when time is forgotten, is in a sense unimportant, and when the limits of our existence as mortals seem to fall away and our own existence is experienced as one with all that is.

The Hebrew word "shalom" comes to mind. Among the rich meanings of this word is completeness, in the sense of rounding something out; it is the finishing of an ongoing process, not so much as an objective gained than as the achievement of wholeness and completeness. There is also a social sense of the word. It is often used as a term of greeting in a social setting, as if to say, "May you and I participate in wholeness and the kind of completion that bespeaks not just harmony and the cessation of strife, but brotherhood — a family unit." The word suggests a unity-in-diversity, the lion and the lamb lying down together and the sword recast into a plow blade that can be used together for our mutual benefit. Shalom is used many times in the Bible. It announced the birth of Christ: it was used by the angels as they addressed the shepherds in the fields. It was used by Christ with his disciples after his crucifixion in the resurrection appearances. Here it resonates with the terrible event just past and at the same time opens out into the future. Peace, that awesome serenity, holy and powerful, sometimes can be seen in persons close to death. It is peace in the midst of, and achieved through, great suffering. Its power is all the more impressive because there is well-being in it, a kind of victory in spite of all hell. To be able to die well is to make a magnificent witness to the indestructability of the human spirit. It is a great hymn of hope and victory to those of us who look often into the face of death.

Clearly, history and meaning do find their source in that presence of being that is spirit, realized in individual and communal life. Being well means being complete and whole and fully alive.

In dealing with dying persons, it is important not to confuse being cured with being well. In terminal illness, cure may be out of the question. However, paradoxically, one can be increasingly well as death draws near. Some of the most power-fully healthy persons I have known have been so immediately before death. Their *presence of being* seems to extend beyond the limits of mortality. This is not to imply that they have achieved a *perfection* of being; it is rather a *completeness* of being at that particular moment. One might wish to say, "This person is completely whole, even though it is clear that there is much left for him to accomplish were he to live." Michael K. Bice (1978), in a fascinating article titled "The Healing of the Dying," quotes Erik Erikson who, speaking about the final stage of ego develop-ment, says, "It is the acceptance of one's one and only life cycle as something that had to be and that, by necessity, permitted of no substitutions . . . In such final con-solidation, death loses its sting." Bice goes on to quote a doctor whose patient had died well, close to her family: "What was not lost was an intact person, and, it is to be hoped, an intact and functioning bereaved family." Bice comments: "That is true wholeness. That is dying healthy."

Family Matters The goal in good hospice care is to provide excellent clinical pal-liative care and to promote well-being in the patient and in his or her family. Family here refers not just to the *family* of the patient. as emphasized by the discussion above, *family* refers to the milieu generated by and within the hospice staff as well. Sometimes this means simply that the hospice staff assumes the role of surrogate family, but it can and should mean too that the staff functions in its own right as a family, a kind of model witnessing to and enablng healthy family life as a matter of principle and *raison d' etre*. Should this family sense be jeopardized, the staff suf-fers and disintegrates; the program loses its meaning and itself dies spiritually, how-ever disciplined and effective it may be clinically.

The level of concentration and intensity in hospice work is unusually high. People who work in such programs are subject to all the stresses, burnouts, and de-pressions that have come to be recognized as a chronic threat to those engaged in the helping professions. Breakdown has much less to do with the spectre of death hov-ering over such work than with emotional and spiritual depletion. Depletion can be controlled as long as we function as part of a larger whole. The drain on one person working alone can be exhausting. When the investment of energy is shared with other members of the staff so that the burden is lessened, the depletion factor is not quite so significant. The nourishment received from the hospice family provides a resource that makes the difference between a burnout and a good workout. Admit-ting the families, volunteers, and patients themselves into this community of con-cern and mutual support means that no one person is left alone; no one person is drained dry.

One must act upon an opportunity as it occurs; there rarely is another. An unex-pected crisis or pressure related to private life can be the straw that breaks the camel's back. In our experience the staff instinctively rallies like a family in re-sponse to trouble with one of its members. The sensitivity, caring, and nurturing attention that characterizes the staff's attitude toward patients and their families are then directed toward the trouble spot. The results are extraordinarily positive. Those on the staff especially skilled in counseling make themselves available. At such times the teamwork that is so vital a part of any hospice program is revealed in its deeper, family-like dimensions.

Mrs. H., the bearer of a European title, was a woman of vivid and great achievement. Beautiful and exciting in her youth, she lived life to the brim. Married several times, she sometimes left the children of each marriage with extended family as she undertook new adventures. She was much chastened when she came into our hospice program. Having lost her beauty, her youthful vitality, and her fortune, she was dependent upon her children and her last husband for spiritual and sometimes financial support. Her disease was such that she was faced with the real possibility of a catastrophic hemorrhage or closure of the throat. She begged to be able to die in the hospital; it was learned that she feared that she would hemorrhage or choke at home without the necessary clinical resources to help her. For one reason or another, all of her children but one were alienated from her and from one another. The hospice staff decided to try to call them all together in hopes that their differences might be put aside so that they could support their mother. The prospects for success were not good. To our surprise all of the children with their mates were present for the meeting, ostensibly to discuss the mother's condition. Suddenly, they began talking to one another, listening to one another; they began to function as a family. A schedule was established to enable them to take turns being with their mother around the clock until her death. She was able to let go and found a strong measure of peace as her family rallied at her side. One son who had been particularly estranged leaned close to his mother at one of his visits, kissed her, and said, "Mother, I love you." Her face beaming, she said to one of the staff, "I never thought I would hear those words from him ever again." The family learned to communicate, to relate together again as a *family,* perhaps more intimately than had ever been the case before. Mrs. H. died, as she wished, in the hospital, in peace, with her family at her side.

Elsewhere, I have referred to guilt as the failure (or estimation of failure) of love and/or responsibility (Hamilton and Reid 1980). Guilt thwarts the very process that will heal it, which is reconciliation and restitution. Insofar as injustice was involved in this failure, anger (as the reaction to injustice) fuels guilt as it veils the shame that makes encounter with the offended party so difficult. Nowhere is this more vividly exemplified than when a patient or family experiencing the loss of a loved one becomes alienated from God. "Why does God allow this to happen? Why am I/are we being punished? Why has God abandoned us?" Anger wells up against God. Behind this anger one often finds old guilt from past failures of love and responsibility toward God. This guilt is heightened as the anger toward God increases.

One must regard this as a family problem. This is clear when one acknowledges the many references to the Fatherhood of God in Holy Scripture. If God is as a father to us (in the most familiar sense, *Abba,* as Christ would have us believe), then in his infinite wisdom and love, he must be a *consummate* father to us whom he regards as members of his own family. Surely he must be able to understand our anger at such a time. Indeed, as an exceptional father he will help us toward restoration of a healthier relationship: a reconciliation based on fresh understanding, a new level of maturity, and loving support of our own best interests.

Anger is dissipated most effectively by working toward restitution of the injustice, or perceived injustice, that precipitated it. Guilt dissolves when reconciliation occurs with the loved one, when loving communication is restored and mutual responsibility for the terms of the relationship is again assumed.

This, however, does not eliminate the problem of suffering. Cicely Saunders (1978) has pointed out the many faces of suffering; it has not only a physical characteristic, but social, spiritual, emotional, and mental significance as well. There is no area of human experience that is more difficult to understand, that so mysteriously eludes management. Suffering can only be understood in relation to human freedom, the catapult to awareness and the ability to transcend that distinguishes human beings. Humans have the capacity to select from alternatives, to make choices and contemplate the ramifications of those choices, to discriminate, and to judge. The effects of wrong or counterproductive choices, as well as the happier type, are imprinted upon our character, personality, destiny, and community. When one speculates upon the age of human civilization, the implications of human choice become staggering. If we recognize that the individual is constricted, scarred, and perhaps even crippled by the poor choices and stretched, ennobled, and fulfilled by the positive choices made throughout a normal lifespan, we can begin to appreciate the cumulative effect on humankind of the myriad decisions of its members throughout history. In exercising our freedom we have to consider not only our own field of possibilities and limitations (genetic equipment, cultural conditioning, etc.), but also our race, the background of human history, our own social circumstances, and the like. Should we try to take all of this into account whenever a significant decision has to be made, we would be paralyzed. All too often we are faced with a choice in which neither of the alternatives is preferable. We live with our own mistakes and those of our race. We are all victimized by the mistakes others have made.

Inevitably God receives the blame for much human suffering that "does not make sense." If he is a just and loving God, how can he tolerate the pain and the injustice about which we are speaking? Perhaps we cannot find happy answers to that question, particularly if we ask the question out of our own great suffering. But if, indeed, we are free agents within the obvious limits of our animal mortality, and if our Creator respects that freedom primarily as a necessary condition for loving response, then he cannot continuously rescue us from painful or tragic situations without reneging on our human freedom. A *deus ex machina*[1] may be appropriate for robots, the existences of which are completely determined, but not for free agents. If God is love and wishes to be loved by the one segment of his creation that is capable of intelligent relationship, then he will try every means available to heal and save his broken and spoiled creation within the terms of freedom and shared responsibility. For Christians the wonder of Christ is that he opened a way to God from within human history in such a way that human freedom is not compromised or circumscribed but brought into its most creative possibilities for sound human evolution.

In conclusion, just as a model human father has the capacity for great wisdom, patience, forbearance, and loving concern for his children, never really giving up on them, so no less and much more must be expected of the heavenly *Father*. The author of the 23rd Psalm understood this supremely well.

Summary

If we are to be of help to those who suffer, we first must be present with them. This is impossible unless we allow our own pain and suffering to resonate to some degree with theirs. "I am where you are, and I know what it is like." It must be admitted that what the other is experiencing is unique; that must be respected. But there is a surprising resource of human affinity, much of it programmed into our racial memory. Our intuitive powers enable us to empathize through imagination; this helps when the sufferer begins to know that we *want* to understand, to share the burden of suffering. There is no room in such sharing for maudlin sentimentality.

I'm reminded of John Macquarrie's (1966) explication of the Christian conception of love: agape. He calls it "letting-be," in two senses of the word: respecting the privacy and independence of the other, granting him the prerogative to be his own unique self, and at the same time enabling him to be, pulling for him and for well-being.

Sharing history is important in maintaining presence. Opening one's life experience, one's life story to another requires trust and a kind of open intimacy that is typical of a sound family interrelationship. Meaning is spun out of this kind of trusting fellowship or profound meeting, which, if motivated by caring love ("letting-be"), brings out the best in the other.

Martin Buber (1965) speaks to this communion, one with another: "Man exists anthropologically not in his isolation, but in the completeness of the relation between man and man; what humanity *is* can be properly grasped only in vital reciprocity." He goes on to say, "The dynamic glory of the being of man is first bodily

---

1. A device used in Greek drama, whereby a deity would appear to resolve a complicated or impossible situation. The actor impersonating the deity would appear above the other actors, sometimes descending into the scene by the use of a mechanical apparatus.

present in the relation between two men each of whom in meaning the other also means the highest to which this person is called, and serves the self-realization of this human life as one true to creation without wishing to impose on the other anything of his own realization." In a healthy family the members know when to let go of one another so as to foster independence and growth. This can be painful. It can mean terminating a mutually nourishing relationship. It can mean taking the risk that the other can make it on his own and *needs* to make it on his own. It can mean being displaced, not being needed any longer. I remember a situation in which I had spent several months relating well to a woman who, as she approached death, was depressed and withdrawn. I had been able to bring her the sacraments, and we had long, significant talks together. Overall, her response was dramatic. She regained her sense of well-being as death drew near. I had met her family only fleetingly. At the last, I was called late in the evening and was asked to visit her at the hospital. The family was there: two sons, and a niece (who was an employee of the hospital). She was semicomatose and sinking quickly. I was sure she would not make it through the night. The family clearly appreciated my visit. I had come to feel very close to this lady and was prepared to wait at her bedside with the family through the night. After an hour or so, I was approached by the niece who explained that the family was all right now and I needn't stay. My reaction was a mixture of hurt at being "dismissed" and impatience with myself that I had not read the situation and left earlier. Upon reflection, I came to see that this was much less complicated than I was making it. The patient to whom I had become attached was all right; the support that I had given right after my arrival was all that was required. The family needed to be alone together. The niece's approach was a correct and appropriate one; she did not feel that she had to play games with me, and she felt free to be honest. This is how it is in a sound family. We can be honest with one another and speak simply and directly without fear of being misunderstood. If we appreciate this point, we begin to learn the limits of our involvement and the degree to which we can contribute creatively in a given situation. Knowing how to "finish" is a fine and necessary art to be cultivated by hospice staff, as in any family in which some may be less needed than others at a particular time.

There is a temptation in hospice work to feel that nothing less than resolution and/ or meaningfulness is acceptable. Some patients and families pass through our program without evidencing an extraordinary need beyond the caring, clinically competent attention that is basic for hospice care. Others come to the close of our experience with them as problematical as when they began. This may reflect on the inadequacy of our skills, but it also may stem from a condition that is normal for that particular family. The most we can do in such an instance is be available in an open-ended way.

Families are torn and crippled by the loss of a loved one, whether the climate in that family has always been cohesive and close or not. As the patient dies, it is as though an essential part of the family organism dies as well. It can seem as though life is impossible for the future. A great abyss, empty and frightening, is left in the family and the lives of the individual members. When staff is intensely involved with the patient and family, they are affected as well. This is the cost of investing ourselves in the lives of others. In spite of this devastation, normally, the total person begins to respond to such loss in a creative and unexpected way. Eventually growth occurs that might not have been possible except for the loss experienced. We are never previously aware of our inner capacity for growth and adaptation or our potential for creative response in the face of a dreaded threat to our equilibrium. We are never the same after such a loss, but we find in retrospect that there are compensations. New possibilities present themselves for the sound completion of our lives, our destinies. Communal or family support is necessary if we are to respond to the challenges loss and change present.

It is typical of such a time that everything appears to be different and strange. There is a "fluorescence" that at first is frightening and confusing in its promise of new directions and possibilities. Gradually, signposts emerge from that sea of new frontiers, and the configuration for a new way commands attention, often urgently. In a real sense, all that opens out afresh comes from the soil of the relationships that had existed before the significant loss. One does not necessarily jeopardize the memory and the tradition of the lost one but begins to integrate, to assimilate all that was meaningful from that relationship into the developing future.

Death as Birth

Finally, a word about death itself. The family often yearns to be assured that death is not the ultimate end of a previous relationship. "Will I ever see her, be with her again?" There are specific religious answers to this question, but I believe that we humans share an intuition that life does not end with death, that the spirit does not simply evaporate when breathing ceases, that the essentials of one's unique individuality are not obliterated. For some there is the comfort in realizing that one lives on in one's children, one's family, one's work, and the genetic continuity passed on from parents to children.

I would like to share my own strong sense that death is analogous to birth. We tend to attach little significance to birth or the gestation period that precedes it. This is significant because I intend to compare our conscious lifespan to the life of the fetus in the mother's womb. The nine months of fetal life do not seem impressive in comparison to the normal lifespan. But when one considers that the entire story of evolution on this planet is recapitulated in that brief period, the fetus passing from one evolutionary stage to another in telescoped succession, that nine months tells a wondrous story indeed. We are not clear whether the fetus possesses at any time before birth a mental state that approaches what we know as consciousness. It is not too outrageous to assume that as birth draws near, some premonition or sensation of a catastrophic event, imminent and irreversible, might affect that tiny individual. It may exist only as a primitive feeling, differing perhaps from previous instances of shifts and changes of position in the mother's body only in the steady, accelerating progression toward the final trauma, of which the earlier adjustments had been simply a foretaste.

There are many little deaths in our lifetime. Each opens out to a new threshold, a new beginning, the birth of new worlds one after the other; all are simply a foretaste of the final trauma of death. Is it unreasonably speculative to assume that as before — so many times before — a new world begins at a new level, a new plane? Is it not possible that death as we know it is the trauma of birth into a new, unforeseeable, larger life? One is reminded immediately of the imagery so universal in near-death experiences. Even more dramatically supportive is the abundance of material in religious lore, particularly in Christian scripture and tradition. We must die eternally to live eternally. Baptism, the sacrament of initiation into Christian experience, is regarded as new birth into another order of being fully realized only after death. I remember that when my own father was dying, he spoke of long-deceased family members all around him; he talked and even sang with them. Hallucination? Perhaps. In terms of "normal" conscious experience, most certainly. But I see this to be significant testimony, not so strange in the light of a faith that promises reconciliation with those that have gone before. If nothing else, it is a beautiful, curiously appropriate possibility. It is somehow inconceivable that an entity so inherently complex and yet pitifully undeveloped as is the "mature" organism when regarded from a spiritual point of view should simply evaporate to oblivion. It is my belief that family as we know it is comparable to the form of communal life that lies beyond.

Reference

Alder A: *What Life Should Mean to You*. Putnam, New York, 1959.

Bice MK: The healing of the dying. *J. Religion Health*, p 188, July 1978.

Buber M: *The Knowledge of Man*. Harper & Row, New York, 1965.

Frankl VE: *Man's Search for Meaning: An Introduction to Logotherapy*. Washington Square Press, New York, 1963.

Hamilton M, Reid H: *A Hospice Handbook*. William B Eerdmans Publishing, Grand Rapids MI, 1980.

Jung CG: *Psychology of Types*. Princeton University Press (Bollingen Series XX), Princeton NJ, 1971.

Linn MSJ; Linn DS: *Healing Life's Hurts: Healing Memories through Five Stages of Forgiveness*. Paulist Press, New York, 1978.

Macquarrie J: *Principles of Christian Theology*. Charles Scribner's Sons, New York, 1966.

Nouwen HJM: *The Wounded Healer*. Doubleday & Company, New York, 1972.

Nouwen HJM: *Out of Solitude*. Ave Maria Press, Indiana, 1974.

Rahner K (ed): *Encyclopedia of Theology*. The Seabury Press, New York, 1975.

Sanford A: *The Healing Light*. Macalester Park Publishing, St. Paul MN, 1947.

Saunders CM: *Management of Terminal Disease*. Edward Arnold Ltd., London, 1978.

Tyrrell BJ: *Christotherapy*. The Seabury Press, New York, 1975.

Westcott MR: *Toward a Contemporary Theology of Intuition*. Holt, Rinehart & Winston, New York, 1968.

Whitmont EC: *The Symbolic Quest*. Princeton University Press, Princeton NJ, 1969.

Chapter 13

Bioethical Considerations in Hospice Care
Jack M. Zimmerman

It is evident that there are important ethical aspects to the care of the terminally ill. Recently there has been increased interest and attention to the topic of biomedical ethics. This has been so not only among health care providers (Culver 1984; Siegler 1982), lawyers, and academicians, but among the general public as well. A number of reasons underlie this heightened concern with moral issues. Ethics are, in a sense, intrinsically controversial and thus fascinating. However, modern technology has brought with it a plethora of new, complex, and urgent problems. The changing social environment with its associated political and legal concomitants has played its part. Media coverage of graphic cases has illustrated vividly the practical realities of abstract concepts.

Much thought and discussion has resulted in an abundance of written material relating to biomedical ethics. In 1979 Congress established and the President appointed a commission to study a wide range of bioethical problems (President's Commission 1982).

In this chapter we will deal briefly with some issues in biomedical ethics that pertain particularly to hospice care. The vantage point is that of a physician, not of a lawyer or moral philosopher. Our scope will be limited. We will not cover in detail basic ethical principles and theories nor will we attempt comprehensive coverage of the subject matter of bioethics. These are available from other sources (Beauchamp and Childress 1983; Fletcher 1954; Pence 1980; Ramsey 1970; Torrey 1968). We will not provide clear-cut answers to moral dilemmas; neither will we present algorithms to follow in dealing with specific ethical questions.

Certain issues in the field of medical ethics do not arise, or occur exceedingly rarely, in the care of the terminally ill. Genetic engineering, artificial insemination, psychosurgery, abortion, and definition of death are examples of such matters. Other topics arise relatively frequently in hospice care but do not present questions that are greatly different from the form they take in other settings. Confidentiality, informed consent, clinical research, continuity of care, and professional competence are examples of subjects in this category. "Truth telling" does have some features which are unique in dealing with the dying, but the basic considerations are much the same, and the special characteristics have been covered in our discussion of patient understanding in Chapter 2.

A bioethical issue of immense general and long-range importance is the allocation of limited medical resources, e.g., the question of how much should be spent on dying patients (Bayer et al. 1983). Cost considerations in the care of individual patients is a related but separate matter. These topics are vital and deserve careful attention. However, national resources allocation is not an immediate concern of individual hospice programs, and although the economic dimension of cost of individual patient care is a daily reality for hospice, the ethical dimension usually arises only in the context of choices of aggressive or life-prolonging treatment.

It is the matter of decision making with respect to mode or place of treatment that is the source of the most frequent and pressing ethical questions arising in hospice care, and it is this area which will be the focus of our attention.

General Considerations in Bioethics

The field of ethics, or moral philosophy, deals with the study of the ways in which one may go about answering the question "What ought to be done?"

There are a number of approaches to ethics. *General normative* ethics deals with ethical theories, and *applied normative* ethics encompasses the application of general ethical principles to the resolution of specific moral problems. *Descriptive* ethics involves the observation of moral behavior and belief and the way in which these may vary from society to society and from time to time. *Metaethics* analyzes the meaning of terms such as "right" and "virtue" and explores the logic of moral reasoning.

Over the years numerous ethical theories have developed. For the most part they may be classified as either *deontological* or *utilitarian*. Deontological theories are based upon the concept that right and wrong is, to some extent, independent of the consequences of the act. Utilitarian theories determine the rightness of the act from its results.

As we speak here of ethics, we are *not* discussing established principles of behavior and codes of conduct that are uniformly agreed upon and are at the core of medical and nursing practice as we know them. These matters, which include the responsibility of health care providers to be fully qualified and compassionate and to accept fees only for services rendered, for example, are of great importance, but they don't require the study of ethics nor the involvement of an ethicist to teach them. They *do* require our continuing commitment to enforce their practice.

The scope of ethics as we have defined it is, however, very broad. As can be seen from the topics mentioned above, the subdivision of biomedical ethics is extensive in its coverage.

Ethical considerations in these issues clearly interlock with other fields such as medicine, economics, etiquette, and law (which can be viewed as the formal enforcement of certain ethical principles). It is important to note in this connection that *none* of the subjects with which the field of ethics deals is an *exclusively ethical* issue.

The relationship between ethics and other fields is an often complex one. For the most part, codes of conduct incorporate principles that have been generally agreed upon by the groups who adopt them. From these principles specific rules governing particular actions are formulated. Law, developing from legislation or court decision, may also simply reflect generally agreed upon principles. However, law sometimes represents an effort to resolve controversy between conflicting principles, preferences, and attitudes. Such laws naturally tend to be less stable. Of course, they may simplify ethical decision making where there are disagreements. However, although they may make the decision easier, they clearly constrict the options. Robertson (1983) has provided a review of the legal rights of the critically ill.

There are certain fundamental moral *principles* that have a bearing on decision making in medicine. These are

1. sanctity of life
2. autonomy
3. beneficence
4. nonmaleficence

5. truthfulness
6. contract keeping
7. confidentiality
8. justice.

A detailed consideration of these principles is far beyond the scope of this book or the capacity of the author. It is important, however, to understand that there are differences of opinion about the definitions of some of these principles (e.g., sanctity of life), that under certain circumstances some of these principles will come into conflict with each other (e.g., sanctity of life versus beneficence), and that there are deep-rooted conflicts about the relative importance or priority of the principles. Each of the principles is not isolated, of course; many are interrelated and some derive from others.

Certain *paired terms* appear frequently in discussions of the ethical aspects of selection of treatment methods.

Voluntary/Involuntary: Voluntary indicates volition on the part of the patient, by request or by action. *Involuntary* suggests an expressed wish on the part of the patient for contrary action but in actual practice is usually employed to designate the absence of prior indication. These terms are frequently used with respect to euthanasia. The distinction between voluntary and involuntary is not uniformly clear. Does voluntary, for example, only apply to a current request in a specific situation, or does it encompass also an earlier request or one that dealt with a similar situation or a general category?

Active/Passive: Active designates the undertaking of positive steps, whereas *passive* indicates absence of action. Both terms are subject to differences in interpretation. For example, is the cessation of an existing modality active or passive? These adjectives are also frequently applied to euthanasia and are paired with the terms voluntary and involuntary. By and large, ethics and law have looked more favorably upon voluntary-passive measures than they have upon involuntary-active ones, which are frequently viewed as murder.

Ordinary/Extraordinary: These have been very frequently employed terms, but their usefulness is open to serious question because of lack of agreement on definition. In addition, in today's technological society the *extraordinary* very quickly may become *ordinary*.

Direct/Indirect: A *direct* result is one with no intervening events, whereas an *indirect* result is one whose relationship to the cause is less proximate. These terms are usually employed to describe the effects of an act with respect to motivation or intent. Once again, distinctions are not always clear.

Not Starting/Stopping: Over the years clinical decision makers and the public at large have accepted these two types of actions as being of different ethical significance. Some, including the President's Commission (1983), have found no moral distinction between the two.

These paired terms are pointed out because of their frequent occurrence in discussion on biomedical ethics. Ethicists have differed sharply over the usefulness of each of these distinctions. Those of us involved in the day-to-day clinical decision-making process and concerned with its moral aspects must be aware of the terms, their common meanings, and the reservations about their use.

We have emphasized the amount and degree of controversy in biomedical ethics. It should be pointed out, however, that there is a broad consensus on certain points. For example, there would be little disagreement with the view that care provided the dying should prolong their living, not their dying, or with the position that competent patients have a right to withdraw from treatment (Callahan 1983a). Disagreements persist in part because a substantial percentage of the critically ill are *not* competent.

Decisions Regarding the Mode of Care

Many would reject the application of the term euthanasia to hospice care. Certainly hospice has nothing to do with inducing death by active means. In fact, although its aim is not to prolong life, it is to prolong *living*. Thus, as the term is customarily used, euthanasia is at cross-purposes with hospice.

However, in the literal and broad sense, *euthanasia* means easing the process of dying. In this sense, and in ethical considerations, hospice care has a great deal to do with euthanasia, particularly voluntary-passive euthanasia. Unquestionably, to the extent that euthanasia implies providing comfort, hospice is closely related to it. As will be seen, in certain situations hospice care cannot be completely divorced from the issue of mercifully hastening death.

Our concern here is, of course, with the terminally ill patient and his or her family. Euthanasia in this context presents somewhat different configurations than it does with other groups for whom its use has been suggested: the chronically ill and infirm, the demented, individuals in a persistent vegetative state, seriously deformed babies, and the like.

Because of its commitment to the entire family unit, hospice care presents some particular ethical challenges. The patient's preferences with respect to type or place of treatment may conflict with those of the family. Decisions in this regard are made more difficult when the patient's capacity for rational decision is impaired, and by the nature of terminal illness, patients usually will experience some decrease in their decision-making capacity. The monograph *Decisions in Hospice* (National Hospice Association 1985) provides a comprehensive review of the ethical and legal considerations in making these decisions.

Not all of the choices regarding mode and place of treatment are related to issues of euthanasia. For example, there may be conflicts between patient and family about whether or not a period of hospitalization for respite care is warranted. Similarly, there may be differences of opinion between hospice staff and patient over the appropriateness of home care. From an ethical as well as legal standpoint, competent patients have a right to make decisions regarding their medical care, and it is only in unusual circumstances that these can be overriden. Obviously, when differences of opinion occur, group discussion among those involved should be undertaken, and additional medical consultation should be requested where this would be appropriate.

For the competent patient the situation is no different when the matters at issue are of a more pressing nature with respect to their effects on hastening death. Ethical and legal views are congruent: refusal of life-prolonging treatment is not regarded as suicide if the patient's death is the result of an underlying condition that is not self-inflicted. Refusal of amputation and mechanical feeding devices and requests for removal from respirators and dialysis equipment by competent patients must be honored. Exceptions to this principle are rare and seldom apply in hospice care. Treatment against the wishes of a competent patient are appropriate for example, when a healthy individual attempts suicide or the patient is responsible for the care of dependent children and can be restored to health through a straightforward treatment modality.

A much more difficult ethical problem arises for the patient with diminished decision-making capacity, and this is relatively common in hospice care (Suber and Tabor 1982; Wanzer et al. 1984). Competence may be diminished by the physicial effects of advanced malignancy, by psychological factors related to the illness, by the effects of treatment, or by any combination of these. Determination of competence may range from straightforward to exceedingly difficult. It is of importance, however, that the determination be made with reference to the *specific decision* at hand. Many patients with diminished mentation are competent to make certain decisions regarding their medical care. As long as patients are deemed capable of understanding the options and of making and communicating a decision among them, they may be regarded as competent for that particular situation. A decision that appears irrational does not *per se* establish incompetence. Psychiatric consultation and legal advice may be required in difficult cases to determine competence.

Once the patient's incompetence is established, it must be determined *who* shall make treatment decisions for the patient and *how* those decisions are to be arrived at.

As a general rule the question of *who* shall make the decisions for the patient presents no particular problem if there is a single, indentifiable individual or group of individuals who, by virtue of their relationship with the patient, can speak for him or her and if there is no conflict of any kind. Thus the caregiving spouse of an incompetent hospice patient who wishes hospitalization for respite care of the patient, with concurrence of the hospice staff and no objection from other family members, has clear-cut authority to make this decision. The same would apply even if the familial and caregiving relationship were not so clear-cut, provided there was no conflict and the patient had, by statement or behavior, indicated that person as the decision maker.

In the presence of conflict or disagreement of any kind, the issue may be resolved in one of several ways: written directive made by the patient prior to becoming incapacitated, state law or court decision, or institutional policy. Of course, conflict can arise in a number of ways and from a number of sources. For example, there may be disagreement between family members or between the family on the one hand and caregivers on the other. Sometimes there is conflict between family and caregivers on the one and institutional policy on the other.

Written directives are, for the most part, of two types: *living wills* and *durable powers of attorney*.

In a sense living wills cover not so much the issue of *who* is to make the decision but rather *what* decision is to be made. Fundamentally, a living will is a document signed by the individual while healthy, specifying that in the event of hopeless illness, no extraordinary treatments are to be utilized. The moral impact of a living will is, of course, real. Caregivers are likely to take it into serious consideration in making decisions. The legal status of such a document, however, varies according to state law. In 1984 eighteen states had passed natural death acts (National Hospice Organization 1985). Such acts, also called "right to die" and "death with dignity" laws, usually provide protection to the health care provider from civil or criminal liability for withholding or withdrawing life-prolonging treatment. Many actually state that failure to follow the patient's instructions constitutes unprofessional conduct. Living wills are not without their problems (Eisendrath and Johnsen 1983). Definition of what constitutes "terminal illness" or "extraordinary treatment" may not be completely clear. It is difficult for a living will to cover in advance all possible circumstances and this may lead to ambiguity. For example, it may not be clear whether an individual signing a living will considers provision of nourishment through a nasogastric tube an ordinary or an extraordinary treatment. Also, it may be difficult for caregivers to predict the chance of response to therapy and thus to determine whether the patient meets his or her own definition of terminal illness. As noted, the legal status of living wills varies from state to state.

These problems with living wills have led to increasing popularity for the durable power of attorney. In contrast to a conventional power of attorney, which expires when the person creating it becomes incompetent, this document is designed specifically to provide proxy consent in health care decisions for the incompetent patient. It designates one or more persons to make decisions on the patient's behalf (Steinbrook and Lo 1984). All but two or three states have legislation permitting the creation of durable powers of attorney. *Decisions in Hospice* (National Hospice Organization 1985) contains a current listing of states with natural death acts and durable power of attorney statutes, as well as sample living wills and durable powers of attorney.

In the absence of a written directive, hospice workers must turn, if there is conflict of any type, to state law governing proxy consent. Naturally, these laws vary. They may or may not for example, specify who is authorized to give consent. In any event, each hospice should have written policies covering the way in which decisions are to be made on behalf of incompetent patients. These policies should of course be in conformity with state statutes and court decisions.

However it is determined *who* shall make decisions for the incompetent patient, the question of *how* that decision is to be made must be addressed. As noted, a living will covers this matter at least in part, even if it is not completely specific.

In the absence of this type of written directive, decision makers must come to a conclusion as to the most appropriate choice. For this there are two available standards: what the patient would have decided, or what is in the best interests of the patient. These may be called the *substituted judgment* and the *best interest* approaches, respectively.

Throughout our discussion it has become increasingly evident that, among the ethical principles listed early in this chapter, a very high priority is given to *autonomy* in decisions regarding selection of therapy in terminally ill patients. Consistent with this is the fact that, both ethically and legally, substituted judgment takes precedence over best interests. If there is any means of establishing what decision the patient *would* have made, this must be the standard for decision making. If there is insufficient information reflecting what the patient most likely would have decided, the decision has to be made in accordance with the best interests of the patient. At this point the process may become complex and difficult. *Decisions in Hospice* outlines a *benefits-burden approach,* reviewing the way in which various factors can be taken into consideration.

An ethical issue that has received great deal of attention recently is the provision of enteral or intravenous fluids to the dying patient (Callahan 1983b; Lynn and Childress 1983; Micetich et al. 1983). In the face of conflict among family members of an incompetent patient with no written directive, this can be a most vexing matter.

The difficulty in resolving this issue is reflected in the fact that on occasion no suitable decision can be reached without resort to the courts.

In addition to thoughtful and considerate use of the benefits-burdens approach, there is another technique that is very helpful in dealing with tough problems in biomedical ethics: the *medical ethics committee* (President's Commission 1983). Hospitals and hospices are turning to the creation and use of such committees. At this point there is a great deal of variation in the way in which such committees are organized and function. It is probably safe to say that there is no single best format because local environment will shape the need for and the capacity of such committees.

As a medical ethics committee is formed, a number of decisions must be made. The first step is probably the creation of a broad-based study group to decide such matters as how the committee will be formed, the nature of its composition, its line of responsibility in the institution, and the scope of its function, as well as the matter of who will have access to it and how that access will take place. In addition, decisions must be made about what types of biomedical issues will fall under the jurisdiction of the committee and whether committee decisions will be binding or advisory. How it will protect confidentiality, whether or not patient and family will be permitted to participate directly, the use of outside resources, and conformity with legal requirements must all be taken care of (Maryland Hospital Association 1984).

The American Hospital Association (1984) has recommended the formation of hospital committees on biomedical ethics and has suggested some guidelines. The National Hospice Organization (1985) has recommended that hospices establish interdisciplinary committees and has reviewed certain aspects of their function.

It must be recognized that medical ethics committees are not a panacea, but simply a tool to help institutions and individuals deal with troublesome ethical problems (Levine 1984). From the first it must be recognized that medical ethics committees do not provide a "right" answer acceptable to all. They carry with them certain hazards. As with all committees they may be dominated by one or more members with very strong convictions. Also, committees have a tendency to diffuse responsibility and thus leave no one responsible. Breaches of confidentiality are possible. Finally, such a committee might place inappropriate pressure on the patient and family or infringe upon the legitimate prerogatives of the patient, family, or caregivers.

Conclusions

Hospice workers must recognize the potential for and the nature of ethical problems they may face. Some of these may be general issues that face hospices as a whole, whereas others are immediate concerns of the individual hospice program. Although a thorough familiarity with ethics, or even biomedical ethics, is not essential for each hospice worker, an awareness of the fundamentals in making moral decisions is important. It is particularly important that hospices create the framework within which ethical conflicts can be settled as efficiently and as effectively as possible. We have tried to present here some of the tools necessary in building that framework.

Reference

American Hospital Association General Council: *Guidelines — Hospital Committees on Biomedical Ethics*. American Hospital Association, Chicago IL, 1984.

Bayer R, et al.: The care of the terminally ill: Morality and economics. *N Engl J Med* 309:1490, 1983.

Beauchamp TL, Childress JF: *Principles of Biomedical Ethics*, ed 2. Oxford University Press, New York, 1983.

Callahan D: Book reviews. *The Pharos*, p 44, Fall 1983a.

Callahan D: On feeding the Dying. *Hastings Cent Rep*, October 1983b.

Culver CM, Gert B: Seminars in neurology — Basic ethical concepts in neurologic practice. *Semin Neurol* 4:1, 1984.

Eisendrath SJ, Johnsen AR: The living will. *JAMA* 249:2054, 1983.

Fletcher J: *Morals and Medicine*. Princeton University Press, Princeton NJ, 1954.

Levine C: Questions (and some very tentative answers) about hospital ethics committees. *Hastings Cent Rep*, June 1984.

Lynn J, Childress JF: Must patients always be given food and water? *Hastings Cent Rep,* October 1983.

Maryland Hospital Association Advisory Committee on Medical Ethics: *Committee Report*. Maryland Hospital Association, Lutherville MD, 1984.

Micetich KC, et al.: Are intravenous fluids morally required for dying patients? *Arch Intern Med* 143:975, 1983.

National Hospice Organization Ethics Committee: *Decisions in Hospice*. National Hospice Organization, Arlington VA, 1985.

Pence GE: *Ethical Options in Medicine*. Medical Economics Company, Oradell NJ, 1980.

President's Commission for the Study of Ethical Problems in Medicine and Biomedical and Behavioral Research: *Making Health Care Decisions*. US Government Printing Office, Washington DC, 1982.

————:*Deciding to Forego Life-Sustaining Treatment*. US Government Printing Office, 1983.

Ramsey P: *The Patient as a Person — Explorations in Medical Ethics*. Yale University Press, New Haven CT, 1970.

Robertson JAA: *The Rights of the Critically Ill*. Ballinger Publishing, Cambridge MA, 1983.

Siegler M: Decision-making strategy for clinical-ethical problems in medicine. *Arch Intern Med* 142:2178, 1982.

Steinbrook R, Lo B: Decision making for incompetent patients: Designated proxy. *N Engl J Med* 301:1598, 1984.

Suber DG, Tabor WJ: Withholding of life-sustaining treatment from the terminally ill, incompetent patient: Who decides? *JAMA* 248:2250, 1982.

Torrey EF: *Ethical Issues in Medicine*. Little, Brown & Company, Boston, 1968.

Wanzer SH, Adelstein SJ, Cranford RE, et al.: The physician's responsibility toward hopelessly ill patients. *N Eng J Med.* 301:955, 1984.

Chapter 14

Hospice in the Matrix of Medicine

Jack M. Zimmerman

An important thesis of this book is that both medicine in general and hospice care in particular will profit if hospice is an integral component of medical care. Although hospice has some features that differentiate it from other aspects of medicine, much is lost whenever hospice is viewed as or becomes a separate entity.

This chapter deals with the relationship between hospice as a part and medicine as the whole. That relationship is still developing and is not always smooth and comfortable.

However, hospice draws from and contributes to the rest of medical care. As can be seen in Chapter 6, hospice team members come from a variety of fields, bringing their particular expertise to it. For example, the physical therapist generally employs for hospice patients the same techniques used elsewhere, but for somewhat different goals. Many of the methods of rehabilitation oncology (Dietz 1981) are applicable to the palliative as well as to the curative setting. Some of the critical elements of hospice care, such as dealing with the patient and family as a unit and the effective use of a multidisciplinary team, can be employed to advantage in many nonhospice situations.

In fact, none of the cardinal principles of hospice care described in Chapter 2 are in any way incompatible with the remainder of medical care. None of them are even unique to hospice. For example, when we look at the territory within which hospice functions, it is evident that medicine has dealt with the incurable before and will continue to do so and that not all terminally ill patients require hospice care.

The relationship between hospice and the remainder of medicine should then be complementary, contributory, and supportive — in other words, a positive association.

That relationship, however, has a somewhat troubled history. A sign of this is perhaps the observation that death and dying are not high-priority topics in most academic medical centers. But as one perceptive hospice worker (A.M.Brooks, 1984, personal communication) has put it, "death is not an elective." This discrepancy may be part of what Lewis and Sheps (1983) call "the mismatch between the overall thrust of these centers as they shape future medical care and the daily health needs of the public." If definitions of hospice in medical dictionaries and sections in major medical textbooks (as described in Chapter 1) may be taken as an index, it would appear that perhaps some of the breach is being closed.

Nonetheless, there are obviously potential sources of friction between hospice and nonhospice care, and it would be unrealistic to ignore these. In fact, at the risk of being negative, we will here approach our study of this relationship from the perspective of *problems* at the interface between hospice and other medical care.

Sources and Consequences of Problems

Hospice and nonhospice care may, of course, come into conflict because the matters with which they deal overlap. We will be looking at some of this "shared turf." As we shall see, difficulties here are inevitable but not necessarily irreconcilable.

It must be remembered that medicine is an inexact science practiced by imperfect individuals with differing values, frequently under difficult conditions. Thus we often don't have precise or even consistent answers.

Proponents of hospice care have sometimes aggravated the natural tensions at the interface between hospice and nonhospice care by emphasizing the problems associated with conventional care. As noted in Chapter 1, terminal illness presents many challenges, but not all of the difficulties arise from inadequacies in the health care system. Knowledgeable but excessively harsh and vigorous criticism of conventional care, sometimes magnified by those preparing material for public consumption, has made physicians and other health care providers feel threatened. The result has been not only defensiveness, but sometimes confrontation and hostility or, worst of all, indifference.

As a result the acceptance and implementation of hospice care occasionally has been impeded. There has been failure to understand what hospice care involves. Also, where hospice has developed in an atmosphere of opposition or indifference, little of what it can contribute to the rest of medical care has escaped from the confines of the hospice program.

The ramifications of this are regrettable. The care of individual patients has been adversely affected. In addition, unnecessary stresses have been placed on hospice staff and others.

It is worthwhile, then, that we address problems arising from the relationship between hospice care and the remainder of medical care.

Problem Areas

It is convenient to divide problems in this relationship into those occurring at the curative-palliative *interface* and those occuring *within* the field of palliative care. This is an arbitrary and not totally satisfactory distinction but one that is useful in getting a handle on the issues. Other approaches can be taken (Adams 1984; MacDonald 1984; Zimmerman 1983).

Our brief, systematic analysis of this complex topic will draw heavily from our own experience. We will look at some of our cases, all involving cancer patients, that have illustrated specific examples of general problems.

The Curative-Palliative Interface

Is the Patient Terminally Ill? This question can certainly be a most difficult one to answer.

A 62-year-old male is found to have moderately well differentiated squamous carcinoma of the lung invading the mediastinum. The tumor cannot be removed. Radiation therapy is decided upon. Although heavy dosage is to be given in an effort to cure the tumor, the radiotherapist thinks the chances of cure are under 10%. The patient has rather severe cough with hemoptysis. His appetite is poor and he has lost 25 lbs in the last three months.

Naturally, if this patient rejects radiation therapy he can be dealt with as terminally ill. However, if he does accept radiation therapy, a decision must be made as to whether to enter him into the hospice program during his radiation therapy on the presumption that it is palliative, or to defer hospice entry until he shows evidence of recurrence of tumor following radiation.

The somewhat philosophical issue of definition of *dying,* as discussed in Chapter 1, may thus have practical applications.

A 76-year-old generally healthy male presents with adenocarcinoma of the proximal stomach, producing dysphagia. At operation there are extensive celiac nodal metastases and the tumor extends well up into the distal esophagus. Esophagogastrectomy with esophagogastrostomy is carried out, removing all of the gross tumor. Histological examination of the resected specimen reveals tumor at the proximal esophageal margin. Radiation therapy is recommended but is declined by the patient and his family. He convalesces slowly but reasonably well from the operative procedure, never regaining his premorbid strength or weight; he is able to function reasonably well. About three to four months postoperatively, he begins to develop increasing weakness and malaise and anorexia without dysphagia or other symptoms. Except for weight loss, physical findings are unremarkable, as is chest x-ray.

The presumption, of course, would have to be that the patient has tumor recurrence and that if so, he must be regarded as terminally ill. However, it is possible that his systemic symptoms of decline are due to some other factor such as depression or intercurrent physical disease. The question then arises as to the vigor with which tumor recurrence or intercurrent disease should be sought.

As it so happens, in this patient barium swallow and endoscopy revealed no evidence of tumor recurrence, and findings on computed tomography (CT) scan of the chest were equivocal regarding local tumor in the area of resection.

The patient, for whom the prognosis with respect to cure is uncertain, presents a difficult dilemma. One does not want to deprive the patient of a reasonable chance of cure, but one also does not want to subject him to exhaustive diagnostic and therapeutic measures that have little or no chance of helping him and may make him quite miserable.

We have available to us today a variety of antitumor therapies:

1. surgical excision
2. physical measures: fulguration, cryotherapy, laser
3. radiation: external beam, implantation
4. chemotherapy
5. endocrine manipulation: hormone administration, endocrine ablation
6. bone marrow transplantation

None of these techniques is really used exclusively for curative purposes. Most are used both for cure and palliation, but some forms of antitumor therapy are used exclusively or almost exclusively for palliation.

We feel that in making decisions about patient care, it is important to be as clear as possible with respect to the *objective* of antitumor therapy, i.e., whether it is being used for cure or for palliation. Unfortunately, it is often not possible to predict accurately the chances of cure from antitumor therapy. In this situation one must then examine carefully what effect the antitumor therapy will have on palliation if cure is not achieved. That effect may be quite positive in prolonging life and increasing comfort; on the other hand, it may have a negative impact through its side effects. We feel it is important that physicians and others providing care to the patient, as well as the patient and family members, understand as much as possible the trade-offs involved.

For each patient for whom antitumor therapy is contemplated the benefits must be weighed against the "burdens." For this purpose the author has found the following outline helpful in asking the proper questions:

1. Benefits
   a. Tumor related
      1) Percent of patients who get response (e.g., can be resected)
      2) Degree of response (e.g., amount of tumor debulked)
      3) Duration of response, including percent permanent
   b. Nontumor related: the feeling that "something is being done."
2. Burdens
   a. Physical (side effects, complications, etc., including duration)
   b. Social (e.g., repeated trips to the hospital)
   c. Financial
   d. Other

Obviously the benefits must be balanced against the burdens. For each patient this is an individual decision based in part upon objective physical factors such as the age of the patient and the nature and extent of the tumor, but also in part upon the values and preferences of the particular patient and family. In this connection caregivers should be generous in sharing their expertise but should avoid imposing their own values on patients and their families.

The process of selecting therapy can be very demanding. There are comprehensive (DeVita et al. 1982) and brief ("Cancer Chemotherapy" 1985) sources of information about the benefits and burdens of various forms of antitumor therapy. Two-way communication with the family is imperative.

Patient Rejection of Curative Treatment

A 68-year-old male who is a longstanding heavy smoker presents with a somewhat ill-defined four- to six-week history of slight malaise and anorexia combined with cough and hemoptysis. Chest x-ray and CT scan of the chest reveal a large right parahilar and mediastinal mass. Transbronchial biopsy reveals small cell undifferentiated carcinoma. Combination chemotherapy and radiation or chemotherapy alone are recommended. The patient, who is a widower with no living children, rejects treatment.

At this point it is worthwhile to mention our attitude toward the patient who rejects curative therapy that we feel a rational individual would accept. Although we are obligated to be certain that the patient truly understands what is involved in the choice, the fact that he does not choose as *we* would does not establish that he is incompetent or even in anyway mentally impaired. As discussed in Chapter 13, there are really very few limitations upon the right of mentally competent patients to refuse treatment. Beyond feeling that the patient must be demented, physicians sometimes resent the rejection of their advice and respond with anger. The point to be made is that when a patient makes a decision running counter to our own judgment, the proper response is not to dismiss him from medical attention but to offer him supportive palliative care.

Patient and Family Attitudes and Acceptance

A 48-year-old female underwent colon resection for carcinoma 18 months ago, at which time all of the tumor was removed. She has done well since and has had no sign of recurrent tumor. She presents now with a nodule on her scalp, which on biopsy shows metastatic adenocarcinoma consistent with a colon primary. She feels well, is asymptomatic, and physical examination is otherwise entirely unremarkable.

One must understand that the meaning of clinical developments may be different to physicians, other caregivers, the patient, and the family. These differences must be recognized and clarified if rational management is to follow. For example, for one reason or another — lack of knowledge or denial — the patient may not recognize the significance of a development. Conversely, for another patient the same event may be a shattering experience. For the lady described above no productive decisions could be made until we clarified for her the significance of her scalp lesions.

Differences Between Patient and Family

A 36-year-old male underwent resection of esophageal cancer six months ago. He is now found to have local recurrence without evidence of distant metastases. When the options of repeat resection, radiation therapy, or palliative care only are explained to him, he expresses a desire for entry into the hospice program. His wife urges that he undergo either reoperation or radiation therapy. The couple has two children ages 9 and 12.

Obviously for this patient the chances of cure were exceedingly small, but he and his wife looked at the same facts from opposite vantage points. Such differences of opinion are not uncommon and can obviously occur in the reverse direction from those in the case above. Also the differences can involve other family members. Obviously, to a large extent the resolution of such differences is a personal matter among patients and family, but physicians and other caregivers can serve as facilitators as these agonizing decisions are made.

Nonapproved Therapy

A 42-year-old male with a several-week history of weight loss and upper abdominal pain is found on exploration to have extensive carcinoma of the pancreas with liver matastases. Except for entry into an experimental protocol, no anti-tumor therapy is thought to be feasible. When the situation and the availability of hospice care is explained to the patient and his wife, she is anxious to have the patient entered in the hospice program. The patient totally rejects this approach and wants either entry in the experimental protocol or to try Laetrile. The couple has two children, ages 11 and 14.

This case, in addition to presenting the problem of disagreement between patient and family, presented also all of the issues surrounding entry into unconventional therapy, either scientific or nonscientific. It is sometimes surprising to physicians that cancer patients and their families do not always draw a sharp distinction between the type of scientific study conducted, for example, under the auspices of the National Institutes of Health and what most physicians regard as quackery. In fact, many of the terms used to describe each would apply equally to the other: *unproven, unorthodox, unconventional*. Even the term *unapproved* may have a dual meaning. In the author's mind the terms *deviant, unscientific, quackery*, and *cancer underground* are useful to designate departures from scientifically based treatment. At Church Hospital our attitude toward the use of deviant therapy by terminally ill patients has perhaps been relatively tolerant. It should be emphasized that this is not so for potentially curable patients to whom we are likely to be much more forceful in our opposition to the use of treatment such as Laetrile and Krebiozen. Holland (1982) has reviewed this topic.

In and of themselves, drugs used in an experimental protocal or even substances with no scientific basis for use are not totally incompatible with hospice care. However, there are some problems. One has to do with the attitude of the patient and family toward the objective and likely results of treatment. Hospice care is designed for those for whom there is no reasonable hope of cure, but participation in either an experimental protocol or in deviant therapy usually requires a mind-set bias toward a possibility of cure. This is not an unbridgeable chasm, but it is one that must be recognized.

Another area of difficulty has to do with the level and type of care required by such patients. In an experimental protocol there is often need for close observation and monitoring, with performance of a variety of diagnostic tests that are somewhat at cross-purposes with the techniques employed in hospice care. Ironically, many forms of quackery pose a similar problem to hospice care because they involve an elaborate set of activities including rigid adherence to a prescribed diet, the use of high colonic irrigation, and the like.

For the patient who either is rejected for curative treatment or rejects curative therapy because the benefit-burden balance does not seem reasonable to him, hospice care offers an alternative to involvement with unscientific methods, but it is not an alternative that is always accepted.

Within Palliative Care

Even after it is determined that the patient is incurable and the decision has been made to provide palliative care, there are a number of potential problems that may arise between hospice care and other facets of medical care. For the most part these deal with the application of various forms of medical treatment in the palliative context.

Antitumor Therapy for Palliation As noted earlier, the various forms of available antitumor therapy can be employed either to achieve cure or to provide palliation. Some of them, such as endocrine manipulation in breast cancer, are used primarily for palliative purposes. As in selecting antitumor therapy for cure, a careful analysis of the benefits and burdens must be undertaken, and that balance must be evaluated in the light of patient and family preferences.

> A 73-year-old female with diabetes, congestive heart failure, and emphysema underwent mastectomy four years ago. On routine follow-up she is now found to have multiple lung metastases that are probably asymptomatic. The patient lives with her 69-year-old sister who is quite healthy. A trial on tamoxifen is planned.

Naturally a major determinant in deciding whether or not to undertake antitumor therapy is the presence of symptoms. As has been pointed out in the chapter on symptom relief, the first step in dealing with pain due to tumor is to consider the role of antitumor therapy. On the other hand, for patients in whom asymptomatic metastases are found, one must weigh carefully what is to be gained by treating those metastases and what the costs of that gain will be. Answers are not always clear cut.

Furthermore, as in the patient just described, the role of the tumor in producing the symptoms that are present may be unclear. This lady was moderately severely short of breath due to emphysema and congestive heart failure, and it was unclear whether lung metastes were contributing at all to these symptoms. Fortunately for her, a form of antitumor therapy with minimal side effect was available and could be employed. Of interest is the fact that tamoxifen produced an excellent objective effect — near-complete resolution of the pulmonary metastases — without changing her subjective status at all. This does not necessarily mean, however, that the drug did not contribute at all to her care. Longevity may have been increased, and the patient may have had a longer period of freedom from symptoms due to tumor than she would otherwise have had. One simply cannot say.

Clearly there is need for clinical investigation of the effect of antitumor therapy on palliation (Silberman 1982; Storm and Morton 1979). Such research must include studies of the psychological, social, and financial impact of therapy (McArdle et al. 1981) and measurements of the quality of life (Spitzer et al. 1981).

Other Aggressive Diagnosis or Treatment Difficult decisions are sometimes required in selecting among various management options for terminally ill patients. For example, such patients may present difficult diagnostic problems. In such instances the question arises as to whether symptoms themselves should be treated or a search for the underlying condition should be undertaken.

> A 62-year-old male underwent colon resection for carcinoma five years ago. He developed pulmonary metastases three years ago and liver metastases two years ago. He has undergone a course of chemotherapy with no significant improvement, but the progress of his disease has been slow. He has been largely free of symptoms except for anorexia and weight loss. Without other change in his symptoms, he develops considerable nausea and vomiting, which he finds very troublesome. Physical findings are unremarkable.

For this patient a decision must be made as to whether to embark upon a series of diagnostic studies including x-rays and blood tests or simply to place the patient on appropriate medications for nausea and vomiting. There is certainly a possibility that he has a treatable cause for his symptoms (Aabko 1984).

Even when the cause of symptoms is clear, a decision often must be made with respect to the aggressiveness of their management. Modern technology has provided many possibilities. However, we must often learn to distinguish what we *can* do from what we *should* do. Many disorders occurring in the cancer patient are amenable to treatment, but that treatment may require a great deal of manipulation, discomfort, and other "costs." Metabolic disturbances such as hypercalcemia and hyponatremia, coagulation abnormalities, and hyperviscosity syndromes are examples. When a patient develops a pathological fracture, a decision must be made as to whether or not traction or intermedullary nailing will contribute to palliation.

A 60-year-old male underwent esophageal resection one year ago. Four months ago multiple pulmonary metastases appeared, but there was no evidence of local recurrence. The patient was mildly symptomatic with dyspnea and was placed in the hospice program. He did nicely at home except for the development of difficulty swallowing two months ago, at which time he was given a course of radiation therapy. This resulted in no improvement in his ability to swallow, and now he cannot swallow saliva. He otherwise feels well and is hungry. Insertion of an intraluminal esophageal tube, which will require general anesthesia and laparotomy, is recommended to the patient by the attending surgeon. The patient and immediate family are agreeable, but a family friend says, "I thought he was in the hospice program."

For the patient in a hospice program there is no "standard hospice treatment." What is best for the particular patient is utilized. Thus there is no *right* or *wrong* decision in a situation such as this. Once again, careful clinical judgment must be made, based upon the type and extent of the tumor, the nature of the symptoms, the likelihood of successful treatment, the side effects of treatment, and the preferences of the patient and family.

As with antitumor therapy, we simply do not possess all of the information we need. Appropriate clinical research may help cast some light on these matters.

Some choices must be made that involve combinations of antitumor therapy and other aggressive treatment.

A 48-year-old female underwent resection of an ovarian carcinoma a little over a year ago. Six months later a solitary pulmonary nodule developed and was resected. On histological examination a definitive decision could not be made about whether this was metastatic from the ovary or represented a lung primary. In the last few weeks she has developed some ill-defined abdominal pain, and CT scan and laparotomy have found extensive intraperitoneal recurrence, including a solid mass in the retroperitoneal area. Her creatinine is markedly elevated and retrograde pyelogram reveals bilateral ureteral obstruction. It is thought that chemotherapy may be successful in producing substantial regression of the tumor, including relief of ureteral obstruction. However, because the patient's creatinine is rising rapidly, it is felt that before chemotherapy is initiated, relief of ureteral obstruction would be advisable, either by passage of catheter via cystoscopy or by tube nephrostomy utilizing sonographic localization.

This case illustrates the complexity of decisions that sometimes have to be made in patients with advanced malignancy. It emphasizes the need for careful discussion with patient and family. It is easy to see that different people might select very different options under the above circumstances. It also demonstrates the way in which technological advance has opened up new avenues in palliation, both with respect to antitumor therapy and ancillary measures.

Several factors have contributed to the more liberal use of invasive measures in terminally ill patients. As hospice care has gained wider acceptance, such programs are seeing patients somewhat earlier in the course of their disease. As a consequence, aggressive forms of therapy may more frequently be an appropriate choice. Technological developments have permitted earlier diagnosis of metastases so that they may be treated before they produce irreversible symptoms. Finally, some invasive procedures, such as nephrostomy in the above case, have become less traumatic through improved technology. These factors may change the benefit-burden balance.

Among the most difficult decisions that have to be made at times are those involving the provision of nutrition and hydration of terminally ill, obtunded patients.

A 78-year-old female underwent mastectomy 12 years ago for infiltrating duct cell carcinoma involving 2 of 12 axillary lymph nodes. Metastatic tumor in the lungs appeared eight years ago, since which time the patient has been given various types of antitumor therapy, including hormone administration, chemotherapy, and endocrine ablation. She has had temporary response to some of these measures, all of which now, everyone agrees, have been exhausted. The progression of tumor has been slow but inexorable. The patient was entered in the hospice program about four months ago, since which time her pain has been well controlled. She has exhibited progressive general deterioration with anorexia and weakness. Three weaks ago she began to have diminished responsiveness and has now been comatose for several days. Her older daughter feels that she should be given fluids and possibly nutrition via either a feeding tube or intravenous fluids. Her younger daughter is strongly opposed to this.

Chapter 13 examines the issue of supportive care for the incompetent patient. As has already been pointed out, there are few restrictions upon the refusal of a competent patient to accept any form of therapy. For the incompetent patient the problem is more difficult, particularly if there is a difference of opinion with respect to management. The matter of nutrition and hydration carries some strong emotional overtones for family members. For this patient a living will might have been helpful, depending upon the way in which it was worded. A durable power of attorney also might have resolved the issue.

Prophylactic Palliation   Some symptoms are clearly dealt with better by prevention than by treatment. For some patients with the potential for such problems, the course is relatively straightforward. In other circumstances it may be difficult to decide whether to undertake antitumor or other aggressive therapy on a prophylactic basis.

A 64-year-old female underwent mastectomy three years ago. A year later she was found to have local recurrence and a few pulmonary metastases. She had an excellent initial response to endocrine therapy with subsequent recurrence and then a good temporary response to chemotherapy. She now has scattered bony metastases. These produce a few aches and pains. Her most persistent pain is in her midthoracic back. X-ray and bone scan reveal clear-cut evidence of a metastasis in the T-12 vertebra. The patient has no symptoms of numbness or weakness in her legs.

This patient is obviously at risk for the development of paraplegia. However, she has no sign of cord compression yet and has very extensive tumor.

As noted earlier, technological advances in diagnosis and therapy have had an impact on prophylactic as well as therapeutic palliation. Techniques for dealing with potentially disabling and life-shortening tumor deposits (e.g. Amirati et al. 1985; Young and Becker 1985) offer prospects for improving both the quality and quantity of life. They must be used judiciously, of course.

Good hospice care involves more than simply responding to problems as they arise. It is incumbent upon caregivers to anticipate problems and to make decisions regarding a reasonable course. This is part of what makes hospice care a demanding undertaking.

Full Acceptance of All Aspects of Hospice

A 46-year-old female was found at laparotomy to have extensive ovarian carcinoma, with deposits in omentum and throughout the peritoneal cavity. Following chemotherapy there is evidence of disseminated recurrence. No further antitumor therapy is thought to be feasible. The patient, her husband, and her 24-year-old daughter are agreeable to entry into the hospice program and the appropriate paper work is completed. At the final conference before the patient is accepted, the daughter learns that among the orders that will be written on the patient is "no cardiopulmonary resuscitation." The daughter does not feel that she can accept this restriction and the patient's husband will not override his daughter's decision. At this point the patient is responsive but quite obtunded.

Clearly, the patient is terminally ill and only suitable supportive care should be provided. The problem posed, of course, is whether or not, in the absence of full acceptance of all elements of hospice care, the patient should be accepted into a hospice program. Obviously, a great deal depends upon the reasons underlying her daughter's refusal of a "no CPR" order. This needs to be explored because that refusal may mask some misunderstandings or basic philosophical differences that could create trouble. As long as the underlying reasons do not pose serious impediments to the provision of hospice care, few hospice programs would reject this patient on the "technical" grounds that the family did not accept all features of hospice care.

Variations of this situation are confronted from time to time. Each must be dealt with on an individual basis. Although there should be no requirement that the patient and family accept each detail of hospice care, some patients may be better off under nonhospice care if, for one reason or another, there are basic conceptual problems preventing acceptance of fundamental hospice principles. Good care for the terminally ill patient should be available outside of formal entry in a hospice program.

Miscellaneous Problems There are various other difficulties that may arise in palliative care at the interface between hospice and the rest of medical care.

For example, just as patient and close family members may differ about whether or not treatment for cure should be undertaken, so there may also be differences of opinion about *what sort* of palliative care should be provided.

> A 42-year-old female, divorced with an 11-year-old daughter and a mother whose sole care she provides, is entered in the hospice program with extensive hepatoma that her personal physician, a surgeon, and an oncologist agree is incurable with very limited chance of significant response to antitumor therapy. Her daughter, quite distraught, urges that she get another opinion. The second oncologist recommends a course of antitumor therapy.

Among the most vexing problems that arise are those concerning the management of intercurrent conditions in the patient with advanced malignancy.

> A 45-year-old male underwent excision of melanoma from his chest wall two years ago. Within six months he developed evidence of scattered lymph node, lung, and liver metastases. These have not responded to any form of therapy. He has pursued a course of very slow but steady deterioration. However, he has been at home and has been working part-time as an accountant. Three days ago he developed fever, cough, and hemoptysis. On physical examination and chest x-ray, he is found to have extensive right lower lobe pneumonia.

Decisions must be made sometimes regarding the handling of patients for whom there is a reasonable prospect of prolonged remission. This occurs particularly with certain types of leukemia and in some patients with small cell undifferentiated carcinoma of the lung.

As noted, particularly difficult decisions are sometimes required with respect to nutrition. For the cancer patient who is undergoing rigorous antitumor therapy in the hope of cure, there is no question but that every effort must be made to improve that individual's nutritional status. At the opposite end of the spectrum, there is virtually universal agreement that nothing is gained by force-feeding a patient whose death is inevitable within a few days. However, between these extremes there occurs a continuum of situations in which there are no simple answers. As we have pointed out, for most hospice patients intensive efforts to correct malnutrition are not appropriate. However, for some patients consideration must be given to the advisability of nutritional support, either by the venous route (peripheral or central line) or by the enteral route, selecting from among oral feedings, nasogastric tube, esophagogastric tube, gastrostomy, and jejunostomy. For the terminally ill patient, these measures should obviously be used only if there is a reasonable prospect of some needed gain. In this connection it must be remembered that eating has a symbolic importance to the patient and the family. Family members may need help in discarding inappropriate instincts toward a normal adequate diet. Helping them substitute more realistic and fulfilling ways to serve the patient than an insistance on feeding can provide comfort to patient and family.

Chapters 4 an 5 have dealt in detail with psychosocial issues and bereavement care. These are clearly areas in which hospice has a relationship to medical care in general. The psychosocial problems grow both out of the illness (Sutherland 1981) and from the imminence of impending death (Krant 1982; Maguire 1982). Physicians have some important responsibilities to meet concerning these matters and are sometimes poorly prepared to meet them. Communication is of the essence. Strull et al. (1984) have produced some data emphasizing that physicians do tend to *underestimate* patients' desires for information and to *overestimate* patients' desires to participate in decision making.

A topic that has created confusion at times is the performance of autopsy. It is often assumed that for the patient with advanced cancer, there is little to be learned by performance of an autopsy and that request for permission to do one is an imposition on the family. It is the author's personal opinion that a sensitive and gentle request for permission to carry out a postmortem examination is in no way an assault upon the patient's dignity nor the family's privacy. It is generally true that there is little merit in performing an autopsy on the vast majority of hospice patients. However, it must be remembered that sometimes there are questions in the family's mind that can only be resolved through careful autopsy examination. Mott (1982) has pointed out that this is particularly likely to occur in the death of a child, in which parents may be left with "some doubts and uncertainties about the course and final progression of the disease and what finally caused death. . . ." and notes that these can be very disturbing to them. Those of us caring for the dying should remain alert for this type of concern and respond to it by requesting permission for autopsy. However, this is almost always done best by gently introducing the topic at an opportune time several days or even weeks prior to the patient's death. When autopsy is carried out for this or other reasons, a meeting should be arranged with family members a few weeks after death to review and discuss the autopsy results.

Considerations in Dealing with These Problems

It will be noted that very little information has been provided about the way in which our staff has dealt with each of the cited cases. This has been done deliberately to emphasize an axiom in dealing with problems at the interface between hospice and the remainder of medical care: there are no absolute answers. The most that can be done is to formulate some *guidelines*. Some of these follow.

There is obviously need for *individualization* as decisions are made. Many variables must be taken into account: nature and extent of disease, patient and family knowledge and understanding, the capacities of the individual hospice program, and the availability of the other facilities. The optimal decision will not necessarily be the same in one hospice program as in another or even consistent in a single hospice program over time. We simply have to live with the uncertainty that there is no one universally correct course to take in many of these situations.

Conversely, there is value in the individual case of making a *clear-cut decision*. It may be necessary that that decision will be based on incomplete information and on probability. Nonetheless, the fact that a decision has been articulated can assure that management of the patient will be a great deal smoother and easier. Lack of an agreed-upon course can seriously impede palliative care.

It is obvious that for optimal decision making, the hospice physician and the patient's attending physician must be *well-informed* regarding not only hospice care, but oncology and general medicine. Similarly, ample *consultation* can be invaluable. A tumor board approach, in which expertise from several fields can be pooled, has been particularly helpful in our hands. The role of nonphysicians in contributing to the decision can be most helpful. Nurses, physical therapists, chaplains, and other members of the hospice team may possess information and viewpoints that can contribute vital components to the decision process.

The need for excellent *communication* in all directions can be readily seen. This includes communication between physicians, among hospice team members, and between caregivers and the patient and family. Absence of such communication is perhaps the greatest barrier to good palliative care inside or outside hospice programs. For example, patient and family not only must have input in making the decision but a clear-cut understanding of what decision has been made and the reasons for it. Also, hospice team members can become frustrated or even demoralized when they do not understand what is being done and reasons for it.

As these decisions are made, a very high priority must be given to preserving the *patient's autonomy*. Therefore, it is imperative that patient and family comprehension be carefully examined and their preferences established. If mentally competent, the patient's decision is final.

It is important to remember that the threat of changing caregivers may impede a patient's or family's acceptance of a recommended form of care. This includes both entry into a hospice program and the use of aggressive antitumor or other therapy. Sometimes assurance that there will be some *continuity* can strongly influence a patient to make a decision that is in his or her best interests.

Problems at the hospice-nonhospice interface are minimized if physicians not directly involved with the hospice program have some *understanding* of its objectives and methods. This is an ongoing educational endeavor but one that pays rich dividends for patients.

Finally, it should be emphasized that we need the same attention to *quality assurance* and the same interest in *clinical investigation* for terminally ill patients that we have for other patients. Hospice care should be audited and subjected to the same quality assurance techniques as is other care in and out of institutions. Similarly, nonhospice care of terminally ill patients should be audited to assure that patients are not being deprived of optimal management.

In the care of dying patients we cannot stand pat. There is critical need for careful study of methods in palliative care; such studies must be directed at not only quantity but also quality of life.

Patient care in general and the care of the terminally ill in particular will be enhanced if hospice becomes an integral part of medicine. To properly fit hospice care into medical care will take some effort, but that effort should be rewarding. Continuous attention to education is essential: education of all hospice workers regarding medical care in general, and education of nonhospice workers regarding hospice. It is important that we avoid *two solitudes* (McDonald 1984). All hospice programs must work at their integration into general medical care. All can do it, but it is our conviction that the hospital-based program is usually in a better position to deal with this critically important matter. Chapter 16 explores the way in which hospice care merges with chronic or long-term care when it is applied to diseases other than cancer.

References

Aabko K, et al.: Surgical management of intestinal obstruction in the late course of malignant disease. *Acta Chir Scand* 150:173, 1984.

Adams AB: Dilemmas of hospice: A critical look at its problems. *CA* 34:183, 1984.

Amirati M, Sundaresan N, Lane JM: Technique of vertebral body resection and stabilization for the treatment of spinal metastes. *Surg Rounds,* p 12, March 1985.

Cancer Chemotherapy. *The Medical Letter* 27:13, 1985.

DeVita VT, et al.: *Cancer: Principles and Practice of Oncology.* JB Lippincott, Philadelphia, 1982.

Dietz JH: *Rehabilitation Oncology.* John Wiley & Sons, New York, 1981.

Holland JC: Why patients seek unproven cancer remedies: A psychological perspective. *CA* 32:10, Jan/Feb 1982.

Krant MJ: The adult with cancer: In preparation for death. *Resident and Staff Physician,* p 89. May 1982.

Lewis IJ, Sheps CG: *The Sick Citadel — The American Academic Medical Center and the Public Interest.* Olgershloger, Gun and Haine Publishers, Cambridge MA, 1983.

Maguire P: The personal impact of dying. *In* Wilkes E (ed): *The Dying Patient — Medical Management of Incurable and Terminal Illness,* p 233. George A Bogden and Sons, Ridgewood NJ, 1982.

McArdle CS, et al.: The social, emotional and financial implications of adjuvant chemotherapy in breast cancer *Br J Surg* 68:261, 1981.

MacDonald N: The hospice movement; An oncologist viewpoint.*CA* 34:178, July-August 1984.

Mott M: Caring for children with cancer. *In* Wilkes E (ed): *The Dying Patient — Medical Management of Incurable and Terminal Illness,* p 45. George A Bogden and Sons, Ridgewood NJ, 1982.

Silberman AW: Surgical debulking of tumors. *Surg Gynecol Obstet* 155:577, 1982.

Spitzer WO, et al.: Measuring the quality of life of cancer patients. *J Chronic Dis* 34:585, 1981.

Storm FK, Morton DL: Treatment of metastatic disease. *Adv Surg* 13:33, 1979

Strull WM, et al.: Do patients want to participate in medical decision making? *JAMA* 252:2990, 1984.

Sutherland AM: Psychological impact of cancer and its therapy. *CA* 31:159, 1981.

Young HF, Becker DP: Indications for resection of intracranial metastases. *Surg Rounds,* p 42, March 1985.

Zimmerman JM: Hospice Critics: Sheep in wolves clothing? *Md State Med J* 32:106, 1983.

Chapter 15

Experience with Hospice Care at Church Hospital

Jack M. Zimmerman and Kathleen A. Roche

Whereas other chapters have focused primarily upon general principles of hospice care, we will be dealing here with the specific application of those principles in a particular hospice program. Although, based upon its unique circumstances, each hospice program must design and implement its own optimal organizational structure and will accumulate its individual experience, it is often illuminating and instructive to examine what others have done. Our own structure has grown, of course, from the study of other programs and through an effort to learn from our own experience. It has been particularly helpful to observe changes over a period of time.

As will be seen, overall there have been few major structural alterations and little change in our clinical experience over the years. Personnel *have* changed. More importantly, the health care delivery system generally is changing in a number of ways, especially with respect to attitudes toward cost control. Also, additional hospice programs have begun in our community. Personnel changes from within and societal changes from without have therefore challenged our hospital and its hospice program to adapt.

Description of Program

The hospice care program at Church Hospital developed gradually over a number of years and continues to evolve and develop. The following is a picture of the current status of the program, which is devoted to patient care, education, and research in the treatment of terminal illness due to malignant disease.

Church Hospital is a private, 280-bed urban general hospital with an active medical staff of approximately 100 physicians. Its major clinical services are medicine, surgery, and gynecology. It does not have pediatric, obstetrical, or psychiatric services and offers no residency training programs.

The hospice care program at the hospital was first proposed by the hospital chaplain, Reverend Paul Dawson, who interested key members of the medical and hospital staff of various departments. This group studied the experience of hospice programs in the United Kingdom and North America; it became convinced that a hospice program at Church Hospital would meet a need and would be feasible. The concept was very carefully presented to the medical staff, the hospital management, and the board of directors to obtain their concurrence. A program specifically designed for Church Hospital was then developed and approved by each of these groups. The program was begun gradually by incorporating various features of hospice care, such as measures for pain control and the provision of emotional support, into the care of terminally ill patients. Subsequently, the decision was made to place all hospice inpatients in swing beds on one nursing unit. It is from that move in December of 1977 that we date the formal initiation of our program. Because even today there is no designated hospice area on that unit, our hospice is a program, not a place, and the date of its true beginning is difficult to pinpoint. By the very nature of the state of the art of terminal illness management, it is a developing program. The hospital's home health program, which handles both hospice and nonhospice patients, was certified in the spring of 1979.

The Church Hospital hospice program, which is a hospital-based program without a discrete physical facility, is under the direction of a medical staff committee that establishes policy and oversees the program. The committee is composed primarily of physicians. The author is chairman of the committee; the hospice physician is a member, as are three additional physicians from the medical staff who have no other immediate connection with the program. There is representation from the other disciplines involved in the hospice program, including nursing and social work. There is cross-representation on the home care committee, which oversees the home care program.

The committee meets regularly and reports to the medical executive committee which in turn is responsible to the hospital board of directors. The hospice committee has drawn up, and periodically makes appropriate revisions of, the hospice care program manual. This manual contains, among other items, a statement of the purpose and philosophy of the program, guidelines for admission, a description of referral and admission procedures, the elements of medical care, standards of nursing care, and forms pertinent to hospice care, and it reviews team function and the components of inpatient and outpatient care, bereavement follow-up, and education.

In essence, the organization and implementation of the hospice is similar to that of other specialized patient care programs within the hospital, such as hyperalimentation and cardiac rehabilitation.

The hospice physician, whose background is in oncology, is employed part time. She supervises the day-to-day operation of the program and serves as the attending physician for many of the patients in the program. In her absence the chairman of the hospice committee or one of the other physician members of the committee takes over her duties.

Hospice care at Church Hospital is designed to serve patients of members of the Church Hospital medical staff. A few other patients referred by physicians in the community or by physicians on the staff of the Oncology Center at the Johns Hopkins Hospital, located one block away, are accepted. On rare occasions patients are accepted into the program on their own initiative or that of their families without physician referral. Although there is no rigid limit on the number of patients in the program at any one time, the demand for hospice services is considerable; at times it is necessary to accept patients in accordance with a priority listing.

Guidelines for admission to the hospice care program are as follows:

1. The patient must be terminally ill from a malignant disease. Terminal illness is defined as that situation in which antitumor therapy does not offer a reasonable possibility of cure, as determined by the patient's attending physician in consultation with the hospice physician
2. Life expectancy should be more than five days but in most instances less than six months.
3. It is desirable but not necessary that the patient be referred by a physician and the patient's attending physician give consent for entry into the program.
4. The patient must reside within a reasonable distance of the hospital and must have at least one involved family member or friend who will accept responsibility for giving care. An exception is made if, on the basis of the disease, there is no reasonable prospect that the patient will ever be suitable for home care and if life expectancy is short.
5. Patients and their families are accepted into the program only with the full understanding and acceptance of this mode of treatment.
6. Corollaries
   a. Patients with severe symptom control problems shall be given priority consideration.
   b. Admission to the inpatient unit is limited to patients whose needs are such that they cannot be met by home care.

From the first the Church Hospital hospice care program was, for practical reasons, open only to patients terminally ill from advanced malignancy. It was recognized that the demand for a hospice program would be substantial but that our capacity would be limited. The experience and interest of our medical staff in malignant disease were the principal factors in making the final decision to limit the program to such patients. Malignancy is defined broadly and includes all neoplastic diseases.

Although there might be disagreement in some instances as to whether a particular patient has reached the point where antitumor therapy offers a reasonable possibility of cure, as a practical matter this has seldom been an issue for our hospice program. There is obviously an element of self-selection in this; by the time the attending physician refers the patient, he or she already has reached the conclusion that the patient is terminally ill. Over the years since the program began, physicians have tended to refer patients at an earlier stage of terminal illness. As this has happened, we have seen more patients for whom there is some question whether all curative measures have been exhausted. Church Hospital has an effective, functioning tumor board in which internists, surgeons, pathologists, oncologists, and radiation therapists participate. Its recommendations, although not binding, are very helpful to the attending physician in determining whether or not there is a reasonable possibility of cure for the patient.

Even though duration of life in most patients with advanced malignancy is impossible to predict with any degree of accuracy, a guideline relating to life expectancy is included in order to distribute the limited resources of the program among those patients with the greatest prospect of benefiting from it. Patients who live only a day or two after entry into the program gain little from it, and the extent to which their families can profit is limited. Most patients with more than six months' life expectancy are relatively free of symptoms and are able to cope with their situation satisfactorily without all of the features of hospice care. Their admission is deferred until they become symptomatic. Recognizing the vagaries of predicting life expectancy and the fact that some with life expectancy outside the designated limits will benefit materially from the hospice program, guideline 2 is often relaxed.

Circumstances do occur in which a patient makes direct application for entry into the program without referral from his or her attending physician. If it seems that the patient is otherwise a candidate for the program, every reasonable effort is made to secure the attending physician's agreement to entry. If, however, this cannot be obtained and it appears, on the basis of available evidence, that the patient would profit from the program, the case is considered on its individual merits.

Ours is, of course, a hospital-based hospice with a home care program. At present we do not have access to a sufficient number of suitable intermediate care facility (e.g., nursing home) beds to permit the admission of patients who are likely to require this type of care. Consequently, patients with a life expectancy of more than several weeks and the prospect of being sent home ordinarily are not admitted to the program unless they reside within a reasonable distance of the hospital and have identifiable caregivers in the home. This clearly places a limitation upon the types of patients that can be accepted into our program, as, does the restriction of the program to patients with malignant disease. However, guideline 2 is relaxed in special circumstances; in such instances an effort is made to continue as much hospice care as possible through appropriate individual arrangements with a nursing home. We hope at some point to fill this gap in our hospice care program through the development of a formal on-going relationship with a nursing home facility. This would open our program to certain patients who are now excluded, as it would assure the availability of hospice measures at all three levels of care: acute in-hospital, intermediate, and home care.

Although our screening process has permitted us to admit only patients who are unlikely to need care in an intermediate facility, unexpected developments, such as changes in family structure due to illness, may *change* the situation dramatically. Accordingly, we developed an agreement with a local skilled nursing facility. Appropriate initial orientation and opportunities for on-going education were arranged for the nursing home staff, and a senior supervisor nurse was designated as liaison with the hospital. Under this arrangement the home care primary nurse continues follow-up in the nursing home, and the hospice medical director either serves as a consultant or as the attending physician. Our experience with this practice is described in the next section of this chapter.

The matter of what constitutes "full understanding" of the situation and the issue of informed consent are delicate, complex, and highly individualized problems. The general considerations that underlie our decisions with respect to specific cases are described in Chapter 2. There is no substitute for seasoned judgment based upon the particular circumstances.

Referrals to the hospice program are handled in accordance with a process outlined in the hospice manual.

Referrals from Members of the Church Hospital Medical Staff: Informal inquiries regarding suitability of the patient for the program are usually directed to the clinical nurse-practitioner or physician's assistant (CNP/PA) for inpatients and to the home care director for outpatients. If the patient is considered to be likely to meet the criteria for entry in the program, the referring physician completes the hospice application and the home care referral forms (Figures 15-1 and 15-2). An appropriate medical summary, including pathology report, must be available. This information is reviewed by the home care director, who is hospice care coordinator, the CNP/PA, other team members, and the hospice physician. Formal notification of acceptance is documented in the hospital chart for inpatients; the attending physician is notified for outpatients. In all instances a decision is made regarding whether the referring physician will continue as the attending physician or the patient will be transferred to the care of the hospice physician.

Other Referrals: Whether the patient is at home or hospitalized in another institution, inquiries are directed to the hospice coordinator in the home care office who will determine whether or not the patient falls within the guidelines for admission to the hospice program. If so, *calls from referring physicians,* or from social workers or registered nurses serving as agents of physicians, are directed to the hospice physician, who makes a decision regarding admission of the patient. If it is decided that the patient will be admitted, the referring physician completes the hospice care application and home care referral forms and forwards these together with medical summary, including pathology report and such other information as may be appropriate, to the home care office. When the caller is a *a patient or family member,* he or she is asked to discuss hospice care with the present attending physician, and if that physician is agreeable to referral, the physician is asked to contact the hospice physician and the procedure outlined above is followed. If the current attending physician is not agreeable to referral for hospice care, the caller is directed to contact

CHURCH HOSPITAL

HOME HEALTH DEPARTMENT

100 N. BROADWAY

BALTIMORE, MD 21231

Name_____

Address_____

Phone #_____

Insurance #_____ Date of Birth_____

Copies of the following should be sent to the Home Health Office:

1) Medical Summary   2) Pathology Report   3) Social Service Summary

Diagnosis_____ Date of Onset _____

_____

Primary site_____

Metastatic sites_____

_____

List surgical treatments   Date

List radiation sites   Amt.   Date

List cytotoxic drugs   Amt.   Date   Response

Is patient currently on any of the following:

Analgesic _____ Amt. _____

Steroids _____ Amt. _____

Hormones _____ Amt._____

Tranquilizer or
Sedative _____ Amt. _____

Other _____ Amt. _____

_____ Amt. _____

Does patient have any drug idiosyncrasies or allergies?

_____

List most distressing symptoms/problems and pain

_____

_____

_____

_____

_____

_____

Mental status_____

Activity level_____

Estimated life expectancy in weeks

What has patient been told about his/her

a) illness

_____

_____

b) prognosis

_____

Does family understand:

a) the patient is terminal _____

_____

b) its role in continuing to care for patient at home

_____

Additional comments

_____

_____

_____

I understand the principles of hospice care for this patient and am in agreement with care plan.

Physician's
Signature_____

Date_____Phone #_____

Address_____

504

1-08038 (New 6-83) W.P.   **HOSPICE APPLICATION FORM**

Figure 15-1

Phone: 522-8357

CHURCH HOSPITAL
100 N. BROADWAY
BALTIMORE, MARYLAND 21231
REFERRAL FOR HOME HEALTH SERVICES

If no phone,
# of neighbor
for emergency use

Patient's Name				Soc. Sec. #			Phone No.		Birth Date		Age	Sex	Race	M/S

Street Address		.	City		State	Zip Code	Regis. Date	Health Plan Estab.			Started Care	

Service	P/T **H**	F/C	Payment Source		Religion	

Primary Care Taker		Relationship	Phone No.	Address	

Next of Kin		Relationship	Phone No.	Address	

Guarantor		Relationship	Phone No.	Address	

Name of Qualifying Institution	Address		Verified Adm. & Disch. Dates	

Other Ins. Plan & Policy #		Group No.	Effective Date	Expiration Date	Name of Policy Holder		P/H Birth Date

Medicare No./Health Insurance Claim No.		Medicaid Number		Date of Issue	Expiration Date	

Attending Physician		Phone	Other/Specialty Physician		Phone No.

Medical Alert		Prognosis	

Diagnosis		Related to Employment?

Secondary Diagnosis		Estimate of Inpatient days saved

Visits per week _____

Est. of patient's need for Services — Weeks _____ Months

Services: Skilled Nursing ☐   PT ☐   ST ☐

Ancillary: SW ☐   HH Aide ☐

Physician's Orders and Treatment:

Medication ordered: (Specify dose, route of administration and frequency)

Therapeutic Goals:

Diagnosis known by patient   Yes   No

Diagnosis known by family   Yes   No

Activities: Bed rest _____   Acitivity Limitations
Chair _____
Stairs _____
As tolerated _____

Diet _____
(Type)

Copy to Patient   Instructed

Supplies/equipment

Baseline Vital Signs

Assessment: Nursing, Physical Therapy, Social Services

Other Orders, Treatments

Discharging Nurse's Signature   Date

Medical Supervision at home provided by

Name _____
(Physician or Clinic)

Address _____

Phone _____

DPN obtained preauthorization for the following:

CERTIFICATION AND RECERTIFICATION STATEMENT: I certify that the above-named patient is under my care, is homebound except when receiving outpatient services, requires skilled nursing care or therapy on an intermittent basis as specified in the established plans of care and is periodically reviewed by me.

Physician's Signature   Date

Home Health
1-08036 (Rev. 7-84) 1M W.P. 7-84

CHART COPY 505

Figure 15-2

the hospice physician who, on the basis of discussion with the family, makes a decision regarding acceptance of the patient into the program.

Ordinarily, at least a tentative decision can be made within a few hours of referral of any patient, and a definitive decision can be made as soon as the application form and supporting material are received. If appropriate, the patient can be placed on a priority list.

It should be mentioned that the decision to utilize this sequence in dealing with applications for admission to the program was based strictly upon the personnel and support facilities (such as secretarial assistance) available in the hospital. This point simply illustrates the need to adapt a hospice program to local circumstances.

Sometimes, when an attending physicians suggests entry into the hospice program, patients and their families are uncertain or reluctant. There are a number of reasons for this. It may be a manifestation of denial, the patient and family may be coping well with the situation, or there may be uncertainty about the nature of hospice care. In such circumstances the patient and family are given an opportunity to discuss the hospice program thoroughly with members of the hospice staff; following this discussion a decision can be made. One decision may be to defer entry into the program. Occasionally patients who enter the program while quite ill will improve enough so that they and their families do not feel the need for ongoing, full-fledged hospice care. In that situation patients are placed temporarily on inactive status, and their cases are reactivated when the situation warrants.

Once the patient is formally accepted, it is understood that the care given will be symptomatic and palliative, in accordance with hospice care objectives and philosophy. Antitumor therapy will be utilized only insofar as it contributes to palliation. The patient and family are provided with an instructive brochure entitled *About Hospice and Home Care,* which has been prepared by the hospital development office and which contains useful general information and a place for recording the names and telephone numbers of staff members whom the patient and family may wish to contact.

Being a hospital-based program designed primarily for patients of members of our own medical staff, a large percentage of those accepted into the program are already hospitalized at Church Hospital. Patients hospitalized elsewhere are promptly transferred here. It has been our practice, insofar as possible, to *admit* to the hospital for a brief period all patients who are at home at the time of entry into the hospice program. We have found that this facilitates the familiarization process between hospice staff and the patient-family unit and makes the transition into hospice care smoother and better. For the most part, patients and families have liked this arrangement, although some are initially a little resistant even to a short period of hospitalization. However, cost containment and utilization stringencies may limit our ability to employ this useful approach in the future.

A specially designed hospice order sheet (Figure 15-3) is used to initiate orders on hospitalized patients in the program.

←

CHURCH HOSPITAL
BALTIMORE, MARYLAND

ORDERED		DOCTOR'S ORDERS AND SIGNATURES	Pt. Teaching Author- ized	CARDED BY	ORDER COM- PLETED
DATE	HOUR	HOSPICE ORDER SHEET			
		1. STANDING ORDERS			
		NO BLOOD WORK OR RADIOGRAPHS			
		NO I.V. FLUIDS			
		NO NASOGASTRIC TUBES			
		FOLEY CATHETER AS NEEDED			
		DECUBITI PREVENTION			
		TURN q 2 HRS. _____ EGGSHELL _____			
		K-PAD PRN _____			
		NO INTAKE AND OUTPUT			
		DEFER WEIGHTS			
		VITAL SIGNS B.D.			
		2. ANALGESICS _____ DO NOT DISCONTINUE			
		AWAKEN FOR DOSE YES _____ NO _____			
		3. ANTIEMETICS			
		4. TRANQUILIZERS			
		5. ANTI DEPRESSANTS			
		6. SEDATIVES			
		7. BOWEL STIMULANTS			
		PRN SS ENEMA _____ FLEET ENEMA _____			
		CHECK FOR FECAL IMPACTION q WEEK			
		8. EXPECTORANTS			
		9. VAPORIZER YES _____ NO _____			
		10. OXYGEN THERAPY _____ LITERS PER MIN.			
		11. DIET			
		12. ALCOHOLIC BEVERAGE YES _____ NO _____			
		13. ACTIVITY			
		14. OTHER MEDICATIONS:			
		SIGNATURE			

DOCTOR'S ORDER SHEET
1-00108 (Rev. 12-80) 1M W.P. 2-84   **HOSPICE ORDER SHEET** 509   **CHART COPY**

Figure 15-3

Very soon after a patient is accepted into the program, a *family meeting* is scheduled. The purpose is, of course, the exchange of vital information in both directions. The hospice team needs to learn as much as possible about the patient: physical problems, psychosocial dimensions of his or her status, family makeup, needs and expectations of the family, and other critical material that will be utilized in designing an optimal care program. This is an opportunity for the family members to be briefed on the patient's medical status, to learn about hospice, to meet team members, and to have their questions answered. The conference is usually held two to three days after therapy has been initiated because at this time the physician and nurse-practitioner are able to assess its effectiveness and to outline a plan of treatment at home if this is appropriate. Patients are invited to participate, and if they do so choose, the hospice staff requests an opportunity to meet alone with the family initially. The patient already has had ample opportunity to speak with key members of the team and to have input into the various treatment options, and this initial part of the meeting gives the family a chance to catch up. The hospice team gathers information about family members who are not present, and a member of the family group is identified to pass along information to those who are not present. It is made clear that the hospice team is available to such family members who may wish to call. The following team members attend the family meeting: CNP/PA; primary care nurses, both inpatient and home care; social worker; home care director; and such other individuals as may be appropriate to the particular situation. A systematic, comprehensive approach is used, summarizing past care, present status, and future plans. Questions and verbalization of feelings and concerns are encouraged. As the team, patient, and family share, the plan for home care is finalized. Specifics such as family schedule, the location of patient, needed equipment, and special problems are covered. Our experience confirms the observation that children often benefit greatly from having the opportunity to voice their concerns and to ask questions in the group setting (Kübler-Ross 1984). Some families, especially if they are large, benefit from opening and closing the meeting together as an entire unit, while breaking into adult and child subgroups, each with an experienced hospice team member, for part of the meeting. As it is difficult for one facilitator to deal with all the important issues, at least two experienced members of the hospice team should be present for a family group meeting. Facilitators should be comfortable with the normal emotional expression that often accompanies the discussion of such painful situation as the loss of a family member. Although specific stages are not necessarily individually identifiable, those facilitating a family conference should be familiar with Dr. Kübler-Ross' five descriptive stages of dying (Kübler-Ross 1969). The meetings usually last about one to one and a half hours and are a critical part of our hospice care program.

For those patients who are referred to the program from outside the Church Hospital medical staff, the hospice physician becomes the patient's attending physician in the hospice program. An important feature of the Church Hospital program, however, is that members of the medical staff of the hospital who refer a patient to the program have the *option* of turning the patient over to the hospice physician or of continuing as the patient's attending physician, utilizing the hospice physician as consultant. In either event all of the facilities of the program are available to the patient and family. This approach has the advantage of making the program appealing to different types of physicians. A referring physician who has known and followed the patient for many years is able to retain that relationship. On the other hand, a referring physician whose contact with the patient has been relatively limited is able to refer the patient to an environment where he knows the patient's needs will be met. The potential problems in such an approach are evident. It is theoretically possible that an attending physician with little knowledge of the principles and practice of hospice care can elect to retain responsibility for the patient. In actual practice a fine balance of diplomacy, education, and perseverance on the part of the hospice staff has kept this from being a serious or frequent problem. The value of providing this option for referring physician should not be underestimated, since it can aid in gaining medical staff acceptance of the program and in controlling the work load of the hospice physician.

All hospice patients are placed on one 28-bed general medical-surgical unit, which consists of one- and two-bed rooms. Within this nursing unit there are no beds set aside for hospice patients; such patients are more or less randomly distributed in accordance with bed availability. In other words, a bed occupied today by a hospice care patient may be occupied tomorrow by a nonhospice patient; within any two-bed room, there may be one hospice patient and one nonhospice patient. Thoughtful selectivity, based upon a variety of factors, is used in room assignments.

The staff on this nursing unit consists of the usual nursing staff found on a general medical-surgical floor: head nurse, assistant head nurse, CNP-PA, staff nurses, aides, and clerical personnel. A total patient care model of nursing practice is employed for all patients on this unit. Hospital departments such as social work and physical therapy assign staff members to serve this nursing unit as they do to serve other units. All of the personnel have been specially trained in hospice care and participate in continuing education programs related to such care. However, on any given day all of them are providing care for both hospice and nonhospice patients. For the reasons identified in Chapter 10, the level of staffing on this nursing unit is essentially the same as that on the other nursing units of similar size.

On the basis of a needs analysis survey, a hospice orientation protocol for inpatient nursing staff was designed. Each new nursing service employee serving on the unit with hospice patients spends one full day on the unit during his or her orientation period. This day is specifically for orientation to hospice concepts and practices. It occurs on the day of the weekly hospice care conference. The orientee meets with each member of the hospice team, discussing a prescribed list of appropriate topics, and also spends time with a peer observing the day's activities and routines. For example, the new employee covers topics such as the role and function of the home health staff with the hospice coordinator and items such as the team concept with the head nurse or assistant head nurse. Each orientee also attends a family conference and one monthly in-service educational session.

In addition to the normally assigned staff on the unit, there is a cadre of carefully selected and trained volunteers who work primarily with hospice patients.

On this unit standard hospital policies and regulations are relaxed for hospice patients. For example, visiting hours are unlimited and patients are encouraged to keep favorite personal items at their bedside and are allowed to have pets visit them. There is a special visitor's lounge for families of hospice patients; this includes sleeping facilities. Chapter 9 describes in greater detail the organization and function of the nursing unit in which hospice inpatients are located. It also describes the implementation of nursing standards of care for the hospice patient.

One of the first steps taken at Church Hospital when the decision was made to initiate a hospice program was to strengthen the existing home care program and to gain the necessary state approval for this improvement. This home health department, the organization of which is described in Chapter 8, operates a very active home care service for all hospital patients who qualify for the service. In other words, it serves both hospice and nonhospice patients. As noted earlier, one of the criteria for acceptance into the hospice program specifies that the location of the patient's home and the home situation will permit home care.

The determination of whether to provide care at home or in the hospital environment rests almost solely on the patient's need for an acute level of care. In some instances families, either for emotional or physical reasons, are no longer capable of providing care. Typical reasons for admission to the hospital include intractable pain, intestinal obstruction, respiratory failure, persistent nausea and vomiting, peripheral vascular insufficiency, hemorrhage, seizures, and mental confusion. Once the patient's condition has been stabilized, an effort is made to return the patient home.

By employing principles and practices of sound hospice care and enlisting the help of family in providing certain elements of care, it is possible for the home health staff to render terminal care of the highest quality to patients in their homes.

In addition to home health department staff, other members of the hospice team, such as social workers, physical therapists, chaplains, and volunteers are available to make home visits as needed.

Table 15-1 shows the staffing assignment breakdown with respect to inpatient-outpatient responsibilities. In point of fact, however, responsibility and involvement are not sharply defined. The home health department nurses frequently visit patients while they are on the inpatient unit, and the inpatient personnel follow the

Table 15-1   Church Hospital Hospice Team Members' Responsibilities

Both Inpatient and Outpatient	Inpatient Only	Outpatient Only
Hospice physician	Clinical unit nurses	Home health nurses
Social worker	Clinical nurse-practitioner	Home health aides
Physical therapist	Clinical unit aides	
Chaplain	Clinical unit clerks	
Volunteers		

progress of hospice patients while they are out of the hospital. The key to successful coordination of inpatient-outpatient care is this kind of flexibility and good communication.

In this connection it is worth noting that with the possible exception of some of the volunteers, no one in the hospice care program is involved on a full-time basis. Everyone, including the hospice physician, inpatient nursing unit personnel, home health nurses, social workers, and chaplains, has other responsibilities. We feel that any disadvantages due to this lack of specialization are more than offset by the advantages of the spill-over of hospice concepts to other types of patient care. Minimization of staff stress is also a significant benefit.

Naturally, we have experienced a number of personnel changes over the years since the program began. Some of these have been in critically important positions. Reverend Dawson, who was truly the founder of our program, has left and is serving as chaplain at a large retirement community elsewhere in Maryland. Shortly after the inception of hospice at Church Hospital our home health director died. In the course of the history of hospice here we have had two hospice physicians and several head nurses on the inpatient unit. Of course, there has been appreciable turnover among other inpatient and outpatient personnel. Our CNP, who was involved in the initial development of the program, has left. Although some volunteers have been with us from the beginning, there have been some changes in this critical group also. In the last few years, we have been privileged to have the services of a clinical pharmacologist, which we have found most helpful; two different individuals have occupied this position. All of this is mentioned to emphasize that eternal stability of personnel is not an essential ingredient of successful hospice care.

Because we regard education about hospice as one of the important objectives of our program, provision is made for students who may be interested in an externship experience or a research paper. Such individuals are required to submit background information and objectives. The student is interviewed and discussions are held with his or her educational institution. Acceptance decisions are made by the hospice care committee. The student is assigned to a preceptor for supervision and support. A written evaluation of the hospice experience by the student is encouraged at the end of participation in the program.

Each week a *case conference* is held. At this time current cases, both inpatient and outpatient, are reviewed and discussed. Although this is fundamentally a patient care conference at which information is exchanged and decisions are made regarding individual cases, it naturally serves an educational function in a variety of ways. The principal conference designed primarily for *educational* purposes is our monthly *in-service program*, in which specific topics are covered and for which outside speakers occasionally are brought in.

As with all other aspects of patient care in the hospital, including other special programs such as hyperalimentation, the hospice care program is subject to the hospital mechanisms for quality assurance. This includes audits and other techniques of assuring optimal quality care. Evaluation of individual team members is discussed in Chapter 6. One of the advantages of a hospital-based program is that the mechanics of quality assurance are already in place; they ensure an element of independent review, since the departmental audit committees are made up largely of physicians having no direct involvement in the hospice program.

We have recently experienced an architectural change that affected our inpatient care. As a result of construction and remodeling, the nursing unit serving hospice inpatients has moved from a 50- to a 28-bed facility, a size modification all of us have endorsed. This was a strictly geographic change. Basically the hospice staff moved intact, although individual staff members were given the opportunity not to make the move.

Chapter 5 describes the way in which bereavement care is provided in our program, including matters such as the annual memorial service. In Chapter 6 and 7 additional details regarding the way in which our hospice team functions in this program are described. Chapter 10 describes administrative considerations.

Church Hospital is a provider member of the National Hospice Organization. As the hospital is accredited by the Joint Committee on Accreditation of Hospitals (JCAH), the hospice program is carefully evaluated as part of that agency's accreditation survey. We have felt that separate JCAH review of the hospice program would be redundant. After examining the alternatives, we have determined that participation in the hospice Medicare benefit option would be of no advantage to the hospital or its patients.

Over the years clinical and other data have been kept on all patients entered in the program and have been analyzed from time to time. Our techniques of data collection and presentation are still evolving. The hospice care committee reviews basic statistical information on the program regularly.

Clinical Experience

The following material has been derived from our data collection and is presented in an effort to provide a picture of the clinical experience of the Church Hospital hospice program.

In 1978 we took a close look at a sample of 100 consecutive patients admitted during that year (Zimmerman 1979). Shortly thereafter Breindel and Gravely (1980) carried out a detailed statistical and financial evaluation of our program. These studies provided useful facts about our experience. Current data give us an opportunity for comparison with information from those sources.

From the beginning the five most common sites of primary tumor have been lung, pancreas, colon and rectum, breast, and esophagus. A wide variety of other primary sites are represented. There have been a number of patients in whom the location of the primary tumor has never been established.

Presently an average of about nine patients per month (110 per year) are accepted into the program, with considerable day-to-day and week-to-week variation. There are approximately equal numbers of males and females. Patients have ranged in age from 14 to 93; roughly two-thirds have been in the seventh and eighth decades of life.

Knowledge about guidelines for admission to the program has become increasingly widespread. This, combined with liberal use of the informal informational system available to those who might be interested in the program, has tended to limit formal application to those with a reasonably good chance of acceptance. Thus figures relating to the percentage of applicants who are accepted are of little value. Insofar as possible, patients who do not meet the criteria for acceptance in this program are referred to other programs having criteria they do meet. About 4% to 5% of formal applications are rejected because, upon evaluation of all of the available information, it is evident that there is not a suitable caregiver in the home.

The total number of hospice patients on a given day varies, but it presently averages about 19. Of these, approximately 70% to 80% are at home and the remainder are in the hospital. Between July 1983 and June 1984, the average monthly inpatient census ranged from 1.9 to 7.2 patients, with an average of 4.56 for the year. Over the last five years, although the distribution between inpatients and outpatients has remained stable, the number of patients admitted to the program and the census have dropped slightly, by about 10 per year. This is probably related in part to the development of other hospice programs in the area. Also, as physicians have become increasingly familiar with the principles of symptom control under hospice care, some have opted to utilize these principles and the facilities of the home care department without formal entry of the patient into the program.

As noted earlier it is our preference to have all patients hospitalized for a brief period when they enter the program. Consequently, we have had relatively few patients who have never been hospitalized during their time on the hospice program. Because we are a hospital-based program, a sizable percentage of patients are already hospitalized at the time application is made. About 80% of our patients have a single hospitalization during their stay in the program, 15% have two admissions, and the remaining 5% have three or more hospitalizations.

In 1984 82% of all patients entering the program spent some time at home. This represents somewhat of an increase over the last five years. Naturally, because of case selection, a hospital-based program will have a higher percentage of patients who have never been at home than will a free-standing or home care based program. As noted, at any given time roughly three-fourths of all patients in our program are at home. During the time that our inpatient census averaged 4.56, our outpatient census averaged 13.98. Patients who are able to spend some time at home generally have a longer duration of life than those who do not. Currently, about 60% of our patients die at home. Of course, this figure tends to be lower for a hospital-based program than for others, again because of case mix.

Total length of stay in the hospice program during the last couple of years has averaged approximately 80 days, up substantially from 38 days in 1978. For patients who died during the last six months of 1984, the range in total length of stay was from 1 to 728 days, compared with a maximum stay of 320 days six years earlier. The increased total length of stay is doubtless related to the fact that as the experience of our medical staff with hospice care has increased, they have tended to refer patients at an earlier stage of disease.

Length of hospital stay for hospice patients has recently been 8.6 days, with a range of 1 to 53 days hospital stay for the 49 hospice patients who died during the last six months of 1984. This compares to an average in-hospital stay of 12.1 days among 45 patients entering the program in one three-month period in 1978. We believe that to some extent the reduction in hospital stay is the product of increased efficiency in the program, making earlier discharge to home care possible. Over the last several years, there has been a decrease in the average length of stay for all medical-surgical patients in the hospital.

It would be helpful to compare longevity and length of hospital stay between our hospice patients and a similar group of terminally ill patients outside the hospice program, but data for this comparison do not presently exist.

Our home care department, of course, handles both hospice and nonhospice patients. During the period from July 1983 through June 1984, the average daily patient load at any given time was approximately 76 patients, of whom 14 were hospice patients. Home care visits to hospice patients tend to be more frequent and longer than visits to nonhospice patients. Thus at a time when the hospice census represented approximately 19% of the entire case load, hospice visits constituted 35% of the total.

As noted, our arrangement with an independent nursing home facility has made it possible to place there some patients for whom the original plans for home care have for some reason not worked out. However, high census at the nursing home has limited the use of this program and has prevented its extension to allow admission to our hospice program of patients without an identifiable home caregiver at the time of entry into the program. Naturally, when few patients are admitted to the nursing home over a period of time the staff there tends to lose its skills in hospice care, particularly since there are personnel changes.

For approximately 60% of the patients entering the program, the referring physician has elected to continue as the attending physician. For patients of members of our medical staff this figure is 75%. For the remainder the hospice physician has served as attending physician during the patient's stay in the hospice program. There appears to be a gradual but definite increase in the percentage of patients for whom the referring physician has continued as the attending physician. Presumably, this is due to increasing familiarity with hospice principles and practice on the part of our medical staff; this is a trend that the hospice care committee has encouraged.

Approximately 80% of the patients entering the program have been referred by members of the medical staff at Church Hospital. Of the 20% who have entered the program on referral from other sources, roughly half, or 10% of the total, have been referred by the Oncology Center at the Johns Hopkins Hospital.

The average cost for hospitalized hospice patients in late 1979 was $174 per day or $1920 per admission. At the same time, the cost for general medical-surgical patients was $345 per day and $3431 per admission. In other words, hospice patients had a lower daily cost and lower average length of stay, which resulted in a substantially lower total expense per admission. The cost was somewhat lower for patients under the care of the hospice physician than for those under the care of other staff members. In the latter group it appeared that the more familiar a patient's physician was with the hospice program and the more frequently he or she served as the attending physician in it, the lower the patient's costs.

In 1983 we compared length of stay and costs for hospice patients under Medicare and those having other insurance. For the whole group the average total length of stay in the program was 80 days, approximately 80% of that time spent on home care with an average per case expense of $6822. However, Medicare patients had an average length of stay in the program of 135 days with an average expense of $8201, whereas non-Medicare patients had an average stay of 49 days and an average expense of $4754. The average percentage of time on home care was the same for both groups. During the last half of 1984, as in 1983, approximately 60% of our hospice patients were insured under Medicare.

Breindel and Gravely (1980) conducted a rigorous analysis of nursing time per patient day in the Church Hospital hospice program, comparing nursing hours per patient for hospice and nonhospice patients. For hospice patients, total personnel hours per day were 7.3, of which 3.9 were nursing personnel hours and 3.4 were volunteer and family hours. During the same interval, general medical-surgical patients received 4.4 hours of total personnel time, all of it by nursing personnel.

In the last several years, there have been some significant changes in health care delivery generally. We have entered a period of considerable concern with the cost of health care and the consequent development of various mechanisms to control those costs. Government, employers, unions, insurers, and others have made control of health care costs a priority. The resultant programs have reduced hospital admissions and length of stay, with consequent, sometimes dramatic, reduction in the hospital occupancy. These developments are beginning to have some effect on hospice. For example, with occupancy rates much lower than they were a few years ago, hospital medical staff members feel less threatened by unavailability of beds.

In the last few years, we have seen in this area, as elsewhere, the creation of a number of new hospice programs. These have been of various types and meet a variety of needs. This has inevitably had an effect upon the number and types of patients referred into our program.

A caveat should accompany all data on length of stay, locus in which care is provided (home versus hospital), nursing time per patient, and costs. A number of factors influence these figures. For example, the source of referral will affect the length of stay in the program. A hospital-based unit is more likely than a free-standing unit to accept patients who are acutely ill and have a short life expectancy. Therefore, hospital-based programs are prone to have a higher percentage of patients in the hospital and a lower percentage of patients dying at home. Physician understanding of and confidence in a program affect the nature of referrals and thus the length of stay. In addition, there tend to be changes in a number of measurements over a period of time in the early history of a program. For example, there is a shifting balance between inpatient and outpatient loads during the first year or two of a program's existence as effective discharge planning is developed and as the public and medical communities adjust to the home care option. Finally, there are subtle but important options in the methods of collection and analysis of data that may profoundly influence the results obtained.

For all of these reasons, one must be extremely cautious in the interpretation of data with respect to hospice programs; this is particularly true in making comparisons between different programs.

We have not analyzed information about the frequency with which various symptoms or problems have occurred. One interesting and surprising point, however, is that only 58% of patients in the program have required a potent analgesic such as morphine.

Assessing the success of symptom relief in a hospice program is difficult. Since symptoms are by definition subjective, there are difficulties in measuring them and documenting changes in them. The development of techniques that will permit objective assessment of results is one of the challenges for the future, for it is in this way that we will be able to evaluate alternative approaches. It is even more difficult, of course, to assess the results of hospice team efforts in dealing with psychological and social problems and in providing spiritual support.

As a consequence, we cannot speak of success rates either overall or with respect to individual problems. However, it is the uniform consensus of our hospice personnel, referring physicians, and families that the net effect achieved with patients in the program has been very strongly positive. No quantifying data are needed to demonstrate the comfort and relief brought to patients and their families by the sympathetic understanding and professional expertise of hospice workers as they deal with the psychological and practical problems of terminal illness. With respect to symptom relief, it is the author's impression that for certain symptoms, such as pain, depression, thirst, and constipation, results have been extremely good; however, in the treatment of other symptoms, such as weakness, anorexia, dyspnea, and dysgeusia, we have been far less successful.

Naturally, the least overall benefit was achieved by those patients who died soon after entry into the program. In retrospect, some of these patients could have been identified prior to acceptance. It is our conviction that patients with very limited life expectancy at the time of referral usually should be excluded from the program. Exceptions occasionally can be made where the benefit to the family will be substantial. As familiarity with the program increases further, we hope that physicians will continue earlier referral of patients.

There have been a few patients, particularly early in our experience, who have not remained in the program until death. Some of these were patients who were accepted into the program with the understanding that their home situation would permit home care but who, because of a change of status in their home situation such as illness of the caregiver, were required to enter a nursing home where it simply was not possible to continue hospice care. Others have been patients who have decided, or for whom the family or the attending physician has decided, that further effort at curative treatment should be undertaken. As our sophistication in the provision of hospice care has increased, the frequency of dropouts has declined.

A number of observations have been made about the impact of our hospice program upon nonhospice patients in the hospital and the interaction between hospice and nonhospice patients. Although there have been all types of interpersonal relationships between hospice and nonhospice patients — some positive, some negative, and some neutral — it is our impression that the positive have predominated in both directions. Very seldom have we had nonhospice patients complain about the special privileges permitted hospice patients or about being in a room with a dying patient. Efforts by our staff to explain the hospice program probably account in substantial measure for this. We have had a number of instances in which nonhospice patients have served an important role in the emotional support of hospice patients.

The overall effect of the hospice program on the care rendered to nonhospice patients is, of course, difficult to assess, and no formal study has been made at this point. Again, it is the impression of observers that the positive effects have predominated. There seems to be a spillover of hospice principles and practices into the care of nonhospice patients.

Church Hospital uses a patient classification system in making nursing assignments on a daily basis. This system relates staffing to severity of illness and the nursing needs of the patients. Since initiation of the hospice program, there has been no need for a major change in the number and type of nursing personnel assigned to the nursing unit in which the hospice patients are located. As noted, there has been some turnover among the staff, and the location of the inpatient unit has been moved.

It is safe to say that the problems of staff stress and morale that have been experienced are, as one might anticipate with this patient mix, related primarily to the general frustrations of patient care rather than specifically to factors arising from dealing with the dying patient. In the first two years of the program a few staff members on the inpatient nursing unit were transferred off the unit, some temporarily and some permanently, because of factors related to staff stress. Two years after assignment of all hospice patients to one nursing unit was begun, the director of nursing systematically interviewed each member of the nursing staff on that unit. These interviews proved very illuminating and helpful in identifying problems.

Lack and Buckingham (1978) and Walter (1979) have published extensive and detailed reports on a free-standing hospice in New Haven, Connecticut, and a hospital-based hospice unit in Hayward, California. Because of organizational and methodological differences, it is difficult at present to make meaningful comparisons among hospice programs. However, the similarities between Church Hospital's hospital-based program and the one at Hayward are evident.

Conclusion

Our experience at Church Hospital illustrates that hospice can be both stable and dynamic. While maintaining a constancy of underlying purpose, to provide optimal comfort for dying patients and their families, hospice can adapt to a changing environment. Personnel and physical facility changes within are not only inevitable but healthy. We can count on seeing changes in society at large and in health care delivery, some of which will be welcomed and some of which will not. However, by keeping informed of current developments, with a willingness to be flexible and with a firm commitment to the fundamental philosphy of hospice care, individual hospice programs should be able to adapt to changes from within and without.

References

Breindel CL, Gravely GE: *Costs of Providing a Mixed-Unit Hospice Program*. Working paper, Department of Health Administration, Medical College of Virginia, Richmond, 1980.

Kübler-Ross E: *On Death and Dying*. Macmillan, New York, 1969.

Kübler-Ross E: *On Children and Death*. Macmillan, New York, 1984.

Lack SA, Buckingham RW: *First American Hospice*. Hospice Inc, New Haven CT, 1978.

Walter NT: *Hospice Pilot Project Report* Kaiser-Permanent, Hayward CA, 1979.

Zimmerman JM: Experience with a hospice care program for the terminally ill. *Ann Surg* 189:683, 1979.

Chapter 16

Hospice Care for Terminal Illness Other Than Cancer

Jack M. Zimmerman

The selection of subject matter in this book reflects, for the most part, the principal objectives, practices, and experience of hospice programs. Because the majority of patients in most such programs are terminally ill from neoplastic disease, we have focused largely on that group of patients.

Historically, hospices also have dealt with individuals suffering from other conditions. Our Lady's Hospice in Dublin in the 1870s and St. Joseph's Hospice in London in the early twentieth century both accepted patients with long-term illness. This also has been true of the modern hospice from its inception at St. Christopher's. In the United States the Medicare hospice benefit is not restricted to any specific diseases. Although in current hospices people with nonmalignant disease constitute a relatively small percentage of patients, it seems prudent here to devote some special consideration to their care.

Such patients raise some interesting issues. For example, the definition of *dying* and of *terminal illness*, as suggested in Chapter 1, can be somewhat more complex than it is for the patient with cancer. In addition, as hospices deal with patients having nonneoplastic diseases, the relationship of hospice to the remainder of medicine can become somewhat closer. In providing hospice care to patients with nonmalignant disease, one often begins to move into the area of long-term or chronic care. Thus it can be a short additional step to the use of hospice principles in nonterminal illness. The implications of this for the relationship of hospice care to the remainder of medical care, as discussed in Chapter 14, are interesting and provocative.

Although there has been a moderate amount of experience, of which some has been recorded (Johnson 1982; Platts 1982; Saunders et al. 1981), not a great deal has been written about terminal care for patients with nonmalignant disease. In actuality, most published material describing hospice care for noncancer patients has dealt with a single disease entity or has considered the topic only briefly and peripherally. There has been a natural tendency in much of the literature on hospice to slide back and forth in discussions of terminal illness and cancer as though the two were the same.

Also, it is often recommended that in needs assessment for a hospice program, *cancer* death statistics should be used as a guide, and many workers have employed this approach even though it was their intent and practice to accept noncancer patients (Schraff 1984).

For the reasons outlined in Chapter 15, the Church Hospital hospice program has been restricted to patients terminally ill from cancer. It is thus with some misgivings that the author has tackled the topic addressed in this chapter. Unquestionably there are those who will feel that there is a "do as I say, not as I do" implication in what follows. On the other hand, others probably will be of the opinion that the approach is overly cautious. In truth, the theme of this chapter is that each hospice must determine, on the basis of its own needs and capacities, whether or not it should extend care to patients ill from diseases other than neoplasm, and if so, what diseases should be included. As with so much of hospice care, the decision must be an individual one based upon particular circumstances.

The Church Hospital hospice committee regularly reviews its policies and has from time to time considered expanding the admission criteria to include noncancer patients. Therefore, we have followed with interest the experience of other programs with such patients and have tried to keep abreast of developments in this area. Of course, the author and other members of our team have had moderate personal experience in the nonhospice setting with most of the diseases discussed here, and some team members have worked in other hospice programs that do accept patients with diseases other than cancer. It seems reasonable, then, to undertake a somewhat systematic analysis of the subject of hospice care for the patient with nonneoplastic disorders, trying to draw together the rather fragmentary information available from a variety of sources. The chapter is placed at this point because we have not had extensive clinical experience with these diseases in the context of hospice care.

The approach here will be to review some general considerations with respect to hospice care for patients with diseases other than cancer and then to discuss some of the individual disorders for which such care may be appropriate.

General Considerations

There are a number of reasons why cancer patients constitute the vast majority of individuals receiving hospice care. Malignant disease is, of course, among the leading causes of death. It is a disease occasioning not only a great deal of interest but also considerable fear. Although, as noted, there can be some difficult problems at the curative-palliative interface, the fact is that in most patients with cancer the distinction between curability and incurability is relatively sharp. Of great importance also is the time factor. Once a patient with cancer has developed metastases or incurable local recurrence, the duration of survival is reasonably predictable and is often relatively short — less than six months. DuBois (1980) has suggested that the availability of funding also may have played a role in preferential selection of cancer patients for hospice care.

Obviously there are may disorders aside from cancer that are progressive and for which at some point treatment directed at the disease offers no reasonable prospect of reversing or materially slowing it. The point at which this occurs varies from one disease to another. Some, such as certain neurological disorders (e.g., amyotrophic lateral sclerosis), are incurable from the time the diagnosis is first made. Diseases also vary in the speed of their progression once they are incurable. For example, most of neurological disorders have a protracted course, whereas AIDS progresses relatively rapidly.

Torrens (1985) has pointed out the importance of dealing with the question of *which* dying patients hospice should serve. Rational development of individual programs, and public policy with respect to hospice care generally, will depend upon the answer to this question. For example, different program models, policies, and practices will emerge depending upon whether hospices deal only with cancer patients or with certain other types of patients as well. Torrens also observed that in addition to a decision with respect to *diseases*, hospice programs must make other decisions with respect to the types of patients accepted. He notes that some consideration must be given to the issue of whether a hospice program will be designed for all dying patients or for those who are experiencing a "difficult death." Similar choices must be made regarding "heavy care" versus "light care" patients and regarding patients with and without primary caregivers.

It would appear that in actual practice most hospices have phrased their *admission criteria* quite broadly to include both patients with cancer and with other conditions. However, some, such as Church Hospital, have restricted themselves to handling patients with malignant disease. Others, such as St. Christopher's, have specified certain disorders, such as motor neuron disease, that they will accept. When one examines the *clinical experience* of hospice programs (Buckingham and Lupu 1982; Torrens 1985), it is evident that approximately 95% of the patients entering them are suffering from malignant disease. Among programs designed for children, the percentage of noncancer patients is materially higher (Burne et al. 1984). Naturally, there is considerable variation from one individual program to another.

As hospice care is applied to patients with nonneoplastic diseases, the objectives and the principles of the program remain fundamentally the same as they are for cancer patients. It is still the purpose of such care to provide an optimal balance of quantity and quality of life for each patient. The patient and family are the unit of care and an effort is made to provide all care in the most appropriate setting. The particular methods employed to implement hospice care are largely the same for patients having other diseases as they are for patients with cancer. The same rules apply with respect to truth telling and patient understanding. Copperman (1983) has pointed out that many of the symptoms seen in patients with advanced cancer are also present in those having other terminal illnesses. Nonetheless, each disease presents some of its own characteristic physical and psychological problems; appropriate methods must be designed and employed to deal with these.

When the decision is made to include patients with diseases other than cancer in a hospice program, some attention must be paid to the matter of definition of dying and terminal illness. As has been noted, for nonneoplastic diseases it is often somewhat difficult to determine at precisely what point the patient is to be considered terminal. Although many such conditions are incurable when first diagnosed, the course of the disease may be exceedingly prolonged and the onset of functional impairment may occur relatively late and quite gradually. One approach to this issue has been simply to evaluate each case on its individual merits. To an extent there always must be some element of this approach. However, an operational definition of terminal illness and some criteria will be necessary for a program that regards its primary purpose as providing care to patients who are *terminally* ill. Definition and criteria will also be necessary to ensure consistency and fairness in the use of limited resources. Finally, practical considerations such as reimbursement may necessitate the use of relatively stable guidelines.

As described in Chapter 1, Bayer et al. (1983) has proposed that the common element in terminal illness is a high probability that the patient will die within a relatively short time. This seems to be a practical definition but may require, in particular circumstances, some modification such as precise delineation of the length of time in which death is expected to occur. The Medicare hospice benefit specifies six months. Some have employed the term *preterminal*, but unless there is a clear definition of how it is distinct from *terminal*, its use only compounds as an already difficult situation.

With nonneoplastic diseases, then, problems at the curative-palliative interface may be even more difficult than they are in patients with malignant tumors. Also, for such disorders the distinction between hospice care and chronic or long-term care may become blurred. All of these are matters with which a hospice program accepting noncancer patients must deal, but obviously none are insurmountable problems.

When noncancer patients are included in a hospice program that deals mostly with cancer patients, certain issues must be considered. The medical problems related to the disease itself and to its treatment will be somewhat different from those seen in the patient with cancer. In addition, the set of psychosocial problems may well be different, in part because of the disease and its treatment, but also because the disease may affect a different age or social group. Many nonneoplastic diseases have an age distribution far different from cancer. For example, some incurable disorders involve largely, or even exclusively, children or young adults. This means that the hospice staff will be dealing not only with the psychosocial problems of young adults and children as patients but also as family members.

Young adults, for example, present some special concerns as patients, as caregivers, and as bereaved spouses and parents. Indeed, the basic problems of loneliness, isolation, fear, uncertainty, disappointment, frustration, anger, and depression know no age boundaries. However, they may have special meaning and expression in an individual in his twenties. As a group young adults are emotionally, socially, and financially investing in the future. They often are thinking ahead to further education, home purchase, and raising a family. Although at no age are we prepared while healthy for our own death, the change is much sharper for young people. Also, the social and financial disruption of death at this age can be particularly devastating.

Children of various ages, as patients and as bereaved, obviously require special consideration (Corr and Corr 1985). An interesting aspect of the issue of inclusion of noncancer patients in a hospice program is its impact on the feasability of a program designed for children. As has been pointed out, terminal illness among children is not a common occurrence. Except in a large metropolitan area, a program for dying children restricted to those with malignant disease would be quite small. However, the inclusion of nonneoplastic diseases such as cystic fibrosis and bile duct atresia may increase the potential population sufficiently to make a pediatric program practical.

The important point is that as diseases other than cancer are incorporated into hospice programs, attention must be paid to the need for staff members who are knowledgeable and comfortable with the medical and psychosocial problems of the patients who will be cared for. The overriding consideration is quality of care. Excellence must not be sacrificed. A program that accepts *all* types of terminal illness will, of necessity, be dealing with relatively few patients with certain diseases, and this always raises some quality issues. This is less so when certain *specific* diseases are selected. It should be pointed out in this connection that the increased expertise necessary to encompass diseases other than cancer should include the capacity to implement quality assurance mechanisms in whatever areas are covered.

The adoption of a particular organizational model of hospice care (e.g., hospital based, free standing) should not preclude, per se, handling patients with nonneoplastic diseases. Because hospice care for such patients does tend to merge with long-term and chronic care, facilities having excellent home care and ready access to some type of intermediate care facility may be more flexible in dealing with this type of patient than would, for example, a hospital-based program without access to an intermediate care facility. This is interesting from an historical and health care planning standpoint. As Starr (1982) has pointed out, it was just about a century ago that the growing emphasis on surgery and relief of acute illness brought about a redefinition of the purpose of hospitals toward such treatment in place of chronic care. Now hospitals, faced with excess beds, may at least begin to find ways to amalgamate chronic care into their structure. As this occurs it is to be hoped that our regulatory and reimbursement systems will favor the development of cohesive and coordinated arrangements rather than unhealthy and costly fragmentation.

Each hospice program must make its own decision regarding the diseases or categories of diseases that it will encompass. Up to this point almost every program in the United States has accepted patients with malignant disease, and this group has constituted the overwhelming majority of patients. Nonetheless, it is certainly conceivable that hospice programs can be designed and developed primarily, or exclusively, for patients with diseases other than cancer.

As decisions are made about the types of patients to be included, the advantages and disadvantages of the various options must be studied. A program confined to cancer patients that is considering expansion of its services to include other diseases might list the following in a benefits-burden approach:

Benefits
1. Hospice care can be offered to more patients.
2. The hospice program is likely to have a wider impact on surrounding medical care.
3. The greater diversity of patients may offer advantages to patients, family, and staff.

Burdens
1. The need for additional staff expertise in a new set of medical and psychosocial problems.
2. Wide disparity in length of stay in the program.
3. Possible need for different facilities.
4. Problems in defining terminal illness.

Torrens (1985) summarizes briefly some of the issues needing consideration as this kind of decision is addressed. Whatever decision a hospice makes with respect to the types of patients it will accept, it is probably prudent that the program leaders and staff review that decision from time to time.

Specific Conditions

There are several possible ways to classify diseases for which hospice care might be appropriate. One method is by major etiological or pathological category, e.g., congenital, traumatic, infectious, neoplastic, metabolic. Another method is categorization by organ system: nervous system, cardiovascular system, respiratory system, and so on. Also, it is possible to categorize diseases by age group involved, such as child, adolescent and adult, or even by smaller age subgroups. Obviously, the various systems of classification can be used together.

As each program reaches a decision about the diseases it will encompass, several options may be used. A program may elect to provide care for terminally ill patients with only one disease, or with several diseases, or with one category of diseases, or with no restriction on the type of disease. It is obviously somewhat simpler to deal with a single disorder or a small category of conditions. It does seem best that whatever choice is made, it be articulated in the objectives and policies of the program so that all involved understand it. The implications of extending care to patients with diseases other than cancer must be recognized and dealt with. The program must be prepared to meet the medical and psychosocial needs of the patients with those diseases. This includes preparation for coping with the problems of particular age groups among patients and family members.

The Church Hospital program has been established for adults and adolescent patients with cancer. Many other successful programs accept all types of disease entities. Some programs such as Helen House (Burne 1984) have been conducted for all types of terminal illness in children. In that program the largest group of patients has had central nervous system disorders, and neoplastic disease has constituted only the third largest group.

The following discussion of considerations in hospice care for a number of individual nonneoplastic conditions is in no sense complete. However, it does provide some examples of the issues involved.

Diseases of the Nervous System

Historically, it was conditions in this category to which modern day hospice concepts were initially extended beyond neoplastic disease. From the first at least 10% of St. Christopher's beds were designated for patients with motor neuron disease (Saunders et al. 1981). Amyotrophic lateral sclerosis, Lou Gehrig's disease, is a condition characterized by progressive wasting of the muscles. The rate of progress of the disease is quite variable, ranging from a matter of months to several years. It is a disorder of late middle life. Impairment of mobility, difficulty with speech, and respiratory failure are among the principal problems. Constipation, dysphagia, insomnia, fatigue, and excessive salivation are often seen. Handling the patient's physical infirmities and meeting the psychological needs of the patient and family can be demanding.

There are a number of other peripheral and central nervous system disorders that may well benefit from hospice care, although experience with this application has been limited. Dementia of various types, particularly of the Alzheimer's variety, comes immediately to mind, particularly in view of the immense strain that this condition places on family members (Mace and Rabins, 1981). Persistent vegetative state possibly presents another interesting application for hospice principles. Here, of course, the benefits would be derived almost exclusively by the family.

Heart Disease

There are a wide variety of cardiac conditions that can produce severe progressive illness. Among children, uncorrectable congenital heart disease is a significant cause of mortality. Acquired heart disease is a major source of disability in adults.

Among the categories producing serious problems are ischemic heart disease secondary to coronary atherosclerosis, valvular heart disease, and cardiac rhythm disturbances. Johnson (1982) reviews the problem of death, dying, and the cardiac patient. Lear (1980) has provided a graphic picture of terminal illness from ischemic heart disease, reviewing some of the medical and psychosocial problems.

Like cancer, heart disease is surrounded by fear. This includes fear of being crippled and dependent and fear of sudden death. Physical symptoms, of course, depend upon the type and status of the heart disease but include anginal pain, dyspnea, edema, and palpitations. Although ancient and modern technology have provided with us a variety of drugs to relieve some of the symptoms, and modern technology has made operations upon the heart and the use of pacemakers standard procedures, many patients reach a point where none of these measures provides any reasonable chance of reversing the disease process or of giving significant symptomatic relief. At this point morphine often offers the best sedation and the possibility of a relatively serene end.

Managing advance heart disease in the hospice setting poses a number of challenges. Among these is the fact, mentioned above, that we do indeed possess a number of pharmacological and other weapons in our fight to control cardiac symptoms. However, each of these produces a number of side effects. This presents problems in selection of drugs and in the need for monitoring the patient.

The author does not know of any hospice program that has had extensive experience in handling either children or adults terminally ill with heart disease.

Kidney Disease

Incurable chronic renal failure can be attributable to a number of causes including chronic pyelonephritis, polycystic kidney, and glomerulonephritis. Such conditions usually pursue a protracted course. During much of the time the patient is likely to be asymptomatic.

Dialysis, either peritoneal or hemodialysis, and transplantation offer a reasonable life expectancy to patients with chronic renal disease but at considerable cost — not only financial, but psychological and social. There are some patients who, for one reason or another, are not suitable for dialysis or transplantation. In these patients treatment must be directed to relief of symptoms once they occur. Platts (1982) has discussed this topic. She notes that the common symptoms of uremia are lethargy, nausea, pruritus, and dyspnea. The use of a low-protein diet can ameliorate some of the lethargy and nausea, and appropriate use of diuretics can decrease dyspnea. Itching, as discussed in Chapter 3, can be a very troublesome symptom. The social and psychological problems, particularly in young patients, can be most difficult.

Selection of patients for dialysis and transplantation raises some very difficult ethical and social problems including allocation of limited resources. Although these matters are beyond the scope of this book, those charged with the responsibility for providing palliative care to patients not selected for such treatment see the ramifications of these decisions in touching, often heart-wrenching, personal terms.

Throughout the United States there are numerous centers for the care of advanced renal disease. However, there does not appear to have been any large-scale application of hospice care principles to patients terminally ill from chronic renal failure.

Liver Disease

Biliary atresia, although relatively uncommon, is responsible for about 2% of all deaths in children under the age of 15. Helen House has had a limited experience with children suffering from this condition (Burne 1984). Although liver transplantation offers some promise, the limited supply of donor livers clearly will restrict this approach.

Hepatic cirrhosis unfortunately remains a relatively common condition among adults. Although other causes are not rare, alcohol abuse dominates the etiology of this complex and devastating disease. Its manifestations are varied and may include abdominal discomfort from hepatomegaly, abdominal enlargement from ascites, massive gastrointestinal bleeding from portal hypertension and varices, disorders of coagulation, jaundice, and often finally, hepatic encephalopathy with coma and death. For the patient whose cirrhosis is due to alcoholism, the liver pathology is often, to some extent, reversible through abstention from alcohol for a protracted period. As we know, most cirrhotic patients do not take this course. For them the terminal illness is a composite of the multiplicity of problems due to cirrhosis plus other physical and psychosocial manifestations of alcoholism.

Therapeutic measures to deal with symptoms in the cirrhotic patient vary in complexity, cost, and side effects. Psychosocial problems, particularly among relatives of alcoholics, can be exceedingly challenging.

As with heart, kidney, and lung disease, there seems to have been limited experience among hospice teams in dealing with advanced cirrhosis.

Lung Disease

Emphysema or chronic obstructive pulmonary disease (COPD) is among the common afflictions of middle-aged and elderly individuals, particularly heavy smokers.

The overriding symptom is, of course, progressive dyspnea, which initially produces gradual limitation of activity and finally becomes distressing at rest. In addition, cough, sputum production, hemoptysis, and recurrent pulmonary infections are often troublesome. Acute exacerbations of the disease are not uncommon. At times these are clearly the result of environmental factors such as air pollution, but at other times there is no evident cause. Thus repeated hospitalizations are a common phenomenon in these patients.

Cigarette smoking is the dominant etiological agent, but other factors such as occupational exposures can play a role. Lung cancer and pleural mesothelioma are more common in patients with COPD than in the general population. Synergistic action between smoking and other factors, such as anthracotic dust and asbestos, appear to play a role in some of the diseases related to COPD.

There do not seem to have been many hospices that have accepted patients terminally ill from COPD alone. However, because of its association with lung cancer, hospice workers have accumulated a substantial experience with the disease.

For this and other reasons, it is this condition that we have felt our program at Church Hospital might best include if we were to extend it to patients terminally ill from diseases other than cancer. Most of our hospital staff—nurses, physicians, and others—are quite familiar with the disorder and the principles of its management. In addition to being a relatively common concomitant of lung cancer, many of the symptoms are the same as those occurring in the patient with an advanced pulmonary neoplasm. Thus both the physical and psychosocial problems are not strange to our hospice staff nor to others in the hospital. Although repeated hospitalizations are not uncommon in patients with emphysema, the vast majority of care can be provided in the home setting. For reasons that are not totally clear, a high percentage of these patients do indeed have an identifiable caregiver in the home. This, then, seems like a particularly promising group if we are to expand the scope diseases that we will encompass.

One of the principal barriers to inclusion of COPD patients in a hospice program is a logistic one. At least in our setting, it is an exceedingly prevalent disease—much more so than neoplasm. Thus the inclusion of such patients would require intensive efforts at prioritizing applicants for hospice care. This is not a reason for their exclusion but simply illustrates the sort of issues raised by inclusion of non-cancer patients in a hospice program.

Acquired Immune Deficiency Syndrome (AIDS)

Acquired immune deficiency syndrome (AIDS) is a disease of the immune system. It has been recognized only recently as a disease entity and occurs primarily in certain groups, particularly homosexuals. There is no known treatment and it is frequently, if not invariably, fatal. Therefore, it is not surprising that AIDS has been the subject of considerable public concern and debate. For hospice programs it has presented some unusual medical, psychosocial, and organizational problems.

There have been throughout the United States several hospice programs that have accepted AIDS patients and many others that have the matter under consideration.

Developments with respect to this disorder have been rapid and our understanding about it is changing almost daily. The ground shifts so rapidly that it perhaps would be prudent to put not only a date but a time on this section. Nonetheless, an effort to review the current knowledge and thinking about AIDS and its relationship to hospice care seems worthwhile.

We address this subject in some detail for several reasons. AIDS raises a number of issues of current public concern and of interest to hospice workers. There has been appreciable attention to and controversy about the disease, not only among hospice workers and the general public, but also in the media. In addition, AIDS in many ways exemplifies graphically some matters of general importance to hospice care and of particular pertinence to such care for noncancer patients.

Anyone even slightly familiar with the topic of AIDS recognizes that it carries a very strong emotional charge. Discussions of it tend to be quite spirited.

In part this is because it is perceived by many as a threat to their personal health. Indeed, it is a disease that has spread with alarming rapidity, is incurable and uniformly fatal, and about which there are huge gaps in our knowledge. Such circumstances generally bring a less than placid response.

However, most of the fervor in our reactions to AIDS is unquestionably a product of the fact that the disease is related to homosexuality. Views of homosexuality occur along a spectrum. Points on that spectrum include: it is intrinsically sinful; it is a violation of reasonable rules of conduct; it is a disease; it is an acceptable alternate life-style. For a number of reasons, opinions on homosexuality tend to be strongly held and to have an emotional component. There is no question but that an individual's view of homosexuality profoundly affects his or her view of AIDS. For example, those who see homosexuality as a violation of the rules of society and those who consider it a completely acceptable alternate life-style are likely to differ immensely in their attitudes toward AIDS. This includes their opinions on the proportion of resources that society should commit to fighting the disease, both in research and in the care of patients. Emotional reactions are common among all sides in the controversies that arise. Those who see homosexuality as intrinsically sinful have a tendency to feel that AIDS patients "get what they deserve." On the other hand, those who view homosexuality as an acceptable alternate life-style have a tendency to feel that every limitation on AIDS research or patient care is the result of ignorance, bigotry, and fear.

It would be valuable at this point to review the facts about AIDS as we currently perceive them.

The first cases were identified in 1981; it is not clear why AIDS did not occur or was not recognized previously. Its cause was initially obscure, but before long a virus was implicated. It was recognized quickly that the virus was related to the human T-cell leukemia-lymphoma virus (HTLV-I) and to the HTLV-II virus that may cause hairy-cell leukemia. Thus the AIDS virus has come to be known as HTLV-III. It acts by attacking T-lymphocytes, and sometimes apparently B-lymphocytes, both of which are important components of the body's immune system. The virus is rapidly reproduced in the affected lymphocytes and ultimately destroys the cells, resulting in severe impairment of the body's defense mechanism. AIDS is thus an infection that itself reduces the body's capacity to fight infection.

As a consequence of the action of the virus on T-lymphocytes, the patient develops a variety of diseases customarily found only in individuals with compromised immune systems. The two most common disorders in this group are *Pneumocystis carinii* pneumonia and Kaposi's sarcoma. Precisely why these disorders occur in immunocompromised patients is not clear.

It is apparent that not all individuals infected by the HLTV-III virus develop AIDS. Most develop no symptoms or minimal symptoms. Such individuals do harbor the virus and are probably a persistent source of infection for others. Some who are infected by the virus develop a mild version of immune system depression. They experience malaise, anorexia, fever, weight loss, and lymphadenopathy. This syndrome is known as AIDS-related complex (ARC). Some patients with ARC develop full blown AIDS, but others apparently do not.

In response to the presence of the HTLV-III virus, the body produces an antibody. There is now an enzyme-linked immunosorbent assay (ELISA) for detection of this antibody. This test will determine whether or not an individual has at any time been infected by the HTLV-III virus. There is no test at present, however, that will determine whether or not an individual currently has AIDS.

Perhaps the most important, but unfortunately uncertain, aspect of HTLV-III virus infection is its mode of transmission. This uncertainty has led to much fear and controversy.

The virus is present in semen, blood, saliva, and tears. The details of the mechanisms of its spread are not clear.

There is no question but that the virus is transmitted by sexual contact and that it tends to be particularly likely to spread through male homosexual contact, although the precise mechanisms of this differential are not clear. AIDS can indeed be spread by heterosexual contact, apparently more readily from male to female than from female to male. In heterosexual transmission, at least, frequency of contact seems to be important, and thus the disease is usually spread between steady sexual partners. In some areas of the world, this seems to be the predominant mode of transmission. In the United States it is the homosexual or bisexual male who is at greatest risk.

However, like the hepatitis B virus, the HTLV-III virus can be spread through blood serum. Consequently, frequent intravenous drug users and those who receive blood transfusions or, most particularly, certain components of blood are also at risk. The blood component most likely to carry the virus is that used in treating hemophiliacs; thus they are at high risk.

Whether or not saliva and tears play any role in the spread of AIDS is uncertain. It does appear that the disease can be transmitted from mother to child during pregnancy or delivery. Most children with AIDS are either hemophiliacs or have received transfusions or were delivered when their mothers had AIDS.

When AIDS was first discovered in the United States, it appeared to occur principally in four groups: male homosexuals, drug users, hemophiliacs, and Haitians. The reason for its prevalence among Haitians remains unclear; it is uncertain whether the afflicted Haitians fell within the other high-risk groups.

Of course, a principal concern regarding contagion is the question of how much risk an AIDS patient constitutes to those who come in contact with him. At this point it would seem that a male homosexual partner or a steady heterosexual partner of an AIDS patient is at significant risk of contracting the disease, as are intravenous drug users and individuals who receive certain blood components. It appears now that others are not at measurable risk. However, it is important to note that in the United States there are perhaps as many as 3% to 6% of the total cases for which the origin is *not* explained by any of the known methods of spread. This is an area in which more is being learned all the time. Reasonable precautions in contact with AIDS patients, particularly with respect to secretions and serum, seem prudent.

On the basis of current data derived from the antibody test, it is estimated that 500,000 to 1,000,000 Americans carry the virus; there have been about 12,000 cases of AIDS reported. More alarming is the fact that the disease seems to be escalating rapidly in frequency.

The clinical picture is somewhat variable. Malaise, feverishness, sweats, anorexia, lymphadenopathy and weight loss are almost universal. Other symptoms have included cough, diarrhea, and candida infections. It would appear that there is often a long incubation period between infection with the virus and the development of symptoms. Once symptoms do occur, the course is one of steady progression but at a somewhat unpredictable and perhaps variable rate. Life expectancy from onset of symptoms to death appears to average in the range of 8 to 14 months. The cause of death is, almost invariably, uncontrolled sepsis.

As noted, there is presently no successful treatment. A variety of agents are being tested throughout the world. In addition, there is, of course, need for a vaccine that will offer some protection against the disease. It is important to note, however, that even if this were developed now, it would not completely remove the problem of AIDS because there are already many individuals who harbor the virus but have not yet developed the disease.

We are thus faced with a condition that is uniformly fatal after a relatively prolonged course. Therefore, from the time the diagnosis is made, the patient is incurable and thus, in a sense, terminally ill. The proper means of handling such patients has been a serious problem to caregivers and has been the subject of considerable debate.

Although the disease itself cannot be reversed or even retarded, some of the specific infections that the patient develops can be treated. Acute care for these episodes can be rendered in a hospital. However, when such an acute episode ends, some provision must be made for long-term care. As that care must be intensive and the communicability of the disease is not totally clear, there are some serious impediments to the provision of long-term care by family members. In addition, the lifestyle of the homosexual male is such that when he is known to have AIDS, he often does not have a potential caregiver living with him.

Lillard et al. (1984) has reviewed some of the measures useful in symptom control for AIDS patients, particularly in the home care setting. The dual direction of infection prophylaxis in AIDS patients must be borne in mind. Most public attention has focused on preventing the spread of AIDS from the patient to others. However, the nature of the disease is such that the patient's host defense mechanisms are seriously impaired, and therefore *he* must be protected from potential infections. A task force at the University of California has developed and published infection control guidelines for patients with AIDS (Conte et al. 1983). Local health departments can be of considerable help in securing information about various aspects of caring for the AIDS patient, including contact with local groups interested in the problem.

In view of the difficulties surrounding the terminal care of AIDS patients, it is not surprising that hospice programs have been touched by the issue in various ways. Although little has yet been published or formally presented, the author found, in informal conversation, widespread interest in the topic among hospice workers at St. Christopher's Third International Conference in London in June 1985 and at the International Hospice Institute Conference at Airlie House in August 1985.

The semantic, theoretical, and practical relationships between neoplasm and AIDS is worth commenting upon. Although Kaposi's sarcoma is truly a neoplastic disease, it is seldom in and of itself fatal and is almost never a major factor in the death of AIDS patients. However, the AIDS virus has clear-cut similarities to the HTLV-I and -II viruses, which are related to leukemia and lymphoma. In addition, another major cause—actually among the most common causes—of acquired deficiency in the immune system is antitumor therapy. Through their work with neoplasm, hospice workers are often familiar with the immunosuppression occurring in association with chemotherapy and radiation or that produced deliberately in patients receiving bone marrow transplantation. This clearly has some implications for extending the application of hospice concepts to AIDS patients.

As noted, many hospice programs throughout the world have given consideration to the inclusion of AIDS patients. A number have begun to accept such patients, and their experience is growing. The decision of each program is obviously an individual matter based upon specific circumstances. Many factors must be assessed in arriving at this decision. One consideration, for example, may be whether or not the program is already accepting other noncancer patients. Another will be the availability of facilities and resources suitable for the management of AIDS patients. Since many such patients have no indentifiable caregiver in the home, they cannot be properly accommodated in a program offering only hospital and home care, for during a substantial portion of the terminal illness the patient will probably not be suitable for acute care hospitalization.

Hospice programs that do accept AIDS patients must establish criteria for admission and procedures to deal with the special problems that such patients present. These include not only the need for dual direction prophylaxis, as mentioned above, but *fear* of contagion on the part of other patients and staff. A matter perhaps also to be considered is the establishment of separate facilities for AIDS patients. Although this carries with it the threat of further physical and psychological isolation for a group of patients who already feel alienated, it might offer some advantages. Infection prophylaxis in both directions would be simpler and the group dynamics in such a unit might be of help in meeting the unique psychosocial needs of AIDS patients.

As decisions are made with respect to dealing with AIDS patients, a number of ethical issues are faced (Jonsen 1985). Our professional obligation to treat those in need irrespective of our moral judgment about them should weigh heavily upon each of us. On the other hand, it must be recognized that we each face practical limitations in what we are able to do; fear and prejudice are not necessarily the only reasons for electing not to extend care to AIDS patients.

A final point that should be borne in mind by hospice programs as they make decisions with respect to AIDS patients is the public relations aspects of such decisions. There is presently, and there is likely to continue to be, a high level of public and media interest in the handling of AIDS patients. Also, as we have described, there is a potent emotional component to the issue. Consequently, the choices made by hospice workers in this area may receive much more public attention than decisions they have made in other matters. This attention is likely to include considerable controversy. Hospice programs generally have been treated well by the media and thus are particularly vulnerable to the "hero is *really* a bum" phenomenon. This is an affliction to which those unaccustomed to publicity are prone to expose themselves. We who are involved in hospice care usually prefer to make our decisions rationally and quietly, in the best interests of our patients and their families. We hope to continue to do what is best, irrespective of the way in which it may be portrayed, but realism requires that hospice workers at least be aware of the possible public relations ramifications of their decisions with respect to AIDS. In dealing with journalists it is also important to recognize that they generally develop a thesis (which may be true, partly true, or false) and then fit their facts and quotations to conform to the thesis. Lest this seem an unduly harsh criticism of reporters and columnists, it should be remembered that all of us, even those us who regard ourselves as clinical scientists, are prone to take a somewhat similar approach.

Congenital Disorders

For hospice programs that serve children, particularly those restricted to children, it may be possible and prudent to accept patients with lethal congenital disorders. Such conditions obviously can affect a variety of organ systems, and the program may wish to be selective in this regard, accepting children only with certain types of congenital conditions. As has been pointed out, when the span of terminal diseases is increased, the need for staff knowledge and skills increases. This is particularly true for congenital diseases because they are lethal at different rates, and thus different age groups of children may be involved. The diversity in needs of children from birth to age 10 can be immense. Corr and Corr (1985) deal in considerable detail with hospice care for children with various types of diseases.

Nonterminal Disease

Up to this point we have looked at hospice as a system of care for individuals who are terminally ill or dying. We have pointed out that for neoplastic diseases the distinction between potentially curable and incurable provides some information about life expectancy, where as for other diseases that may be incurable, the distinction between long-term or chronic care and terminal care may not be at all clear. Owen (1985) has examined the application hospice principles in the long-term care setting. Extension of hospice services to such patients naturally raises questions about its further extension to individuals who are not, in any sense, terminally ill. There are various categories that might be considered, for example, the severely handicapped or even those who are acutely ill. Would the application of the hospice concept of care to such patients be helpful? If hospice care was offered to patients who are going to recover, would this "really be hospice"? Perhaps some but not all of hospice principles are applicable in these circumstances. Maybe the real mission of hospice is to expand well beyond terminal care to affect the care of *all* patients. That this potential exists has been a major thesis of this book. Certain aspects of this were dealt with in Chapter 14, which looked at hospice in the larger context of medicine as a whole.

This entire arena of hospice care for nonterminal illness raises some interesting philosophical and practical issues.

Conclusion

Each hospice must define its own scope, i.e., what patients are to be served? One important dimension of this question is the determination of the diseases to be encompassed. The majority of patients in most hospice programs are dying of cancer, but hospice principles clearly have applicability beyond this group.

We have tried here to review some of the more significant issues involved in the inclusion of noncancer patients in hospice programs. Based upon its particular circumstances, each hospice must reach its own individual decisions. These will include whether or not to incorporate noncancer patients. If it is decided that such patients are to be cared for, decisions must be made with respect to which diseases are to be included. Policies, procedures, and staffing must then be developed to meet the particular needs of the patients and families to be cared for. There is no substitute for a thoughtful, careful analysis of the factors involved in such decisions. Nonetheless, the boldness and courage that have been characteristic of hospice should not be excluded from the decision-making process.

References

Bayer R, et al.: The care of the terminally ill: Morality and economics. *N Engl J Med* 309:1490, 1983.

Buckingham RW, Lupu D: A comparative study of hospice services in the United States. *Am J Public Health* 72:455, 1982.

Burne SR, Dominica F, Baum JD: Helen House—A hospice for children. *Br Med J* 289:1665, 1984.

Conte JE, et al.: Infection control guideline for patients with acquired immunodeficiency syndrome (AIDS). *N Engl J Med* 309:740, 1983.

Copperman H: *Dying at Home*. John Wiley and Son, New York, 1983.

Corr CC, Corr DM: *Hospice Approaches to Pediatric Care*. Springer, New York, 1985.

DuBois PM: *The Hospice Way of Death*. Human Sciences Press, New York, 1980.

Johnson AM: Death, dying and the cardiac patient. *In* Wilkes E (ed): *The Dying Patient*, 57. George A Bogden and Sons, Ridgeway NJ, 1982.

Jonsen A: Ethics and AIDS. *Am Coll Surg Bull* 70:16, 1985.

Lear MW: *Heartsounds*. Simon and Schuster, New York, 1980.

Lillard J, et al.: Acquired immunodeficiency syndrome (AIDS) in home care: Maximizing helpfulness and minimizing hysteria. *Home Healthcare Nurse*, p 11, November/December 1984.

Mace NL, Rabins PV: *The Thirty-Six Hour Day*. Johns Hopkins University Press, Baltimore, 1981.

Owen G: The application of hospice principles in longterm care. *In* Paradis LF (ed): *Hospice Handbook—A Guide for Managers and Planners*, 109. Aspen, Rockville MD, 1985.

Platts MM: Common problems in advancing chronic renal failure. *In* Wilkes E (ed): *The Dying Patient*, 81. George A Bogden and Sons, Ridgeway NJ, 1982.

Saunders C, Summers DH, Teller N: *Hospice: The Living Idea*. Edward Arnold, London, 1981.

Schraff SH: *Hospice the Nursing Perspective*. National League for Nursing, New York, 1984.

Starr P: *The Social Transformation of American Medicine*. Basic Books, New York, 1982.

Torrens PR: *Hospice Programs and Public Policy*. American Hospital Publishing, Chicago, 1985.

Chapter 17

Questions Commonly Asked About Hospice

Jack M. Zimmerman

As we have spoken with individuals and groups about our work in the care of the terminally ill, certain questions recur frequently. Some of these questions help to crystallize issues and problems. Others permit a different focus on some of the complex matters covered elsewhere in this text. For these reasons it seems useful to deal directly with these questions here.

Questions Regarding Hospice Care in General

Is there a means by which hospices are certified or approved?
    The name "hospice" has been used by various institutions for centuries and is still in use today by institutions that have little or nothing to do with the care of the terminally ill. In most places there is, as yet, no restriction on the use of this term.
    From the beginning the need for the development of standards for hospice care of the terminally ill and some means by which hospice programs could be certified was recognized by all concerned. The National Hospice Organization (NHO), which was formed by the leaders of hospice care in America, devoted early attention to this matter. As a result of work with the Joint Commission on Accreditation of Hospitals (JCAH), standards were agreed upon and a mechanism for survey of individual programs was established. Presently, accreditation is optional for hospices although it may be required for eligibility for certain types of reimbursement. State laws and regulations vary with respect to licensure for programs or for components such as home care. Each hospice must familiarize itself with local requirements. Most of us involved in hospice care have the conviction that standards should be set and accreditation provided, insofar as possible, by caregivers rather than by government agencies.
    No one can question the desirability of establishing criteria for adequate hospice care and of developing an accreditation mechanism. This is needed to prevent abuse of the hospice approach and development of substandard programs. It is also necessary to enable programs to be reimbursed through health insurance plans. However, we must remember that hospice care is a dynamic field and that there is still a great deal to learn. Innovation must be encouraged. Standards, therefore, must be sufficiently flexible to permit progress and avoid stagnation.

Hospice care is really not new, is it? Isn't it just a return to old values and approaches?

In some measure it is correct that hospice includes a return to traditional values and methods. It reestablishes the kind of personal concern and attention that we associate with a bygone era; this personal concern has decreased in many aspects of modern medical care, particularly in dealing with the dying. Much of the value of hospice care derives from its reemphasis on the traditions of caring that have been such an integral part of the medical and nursing professions.

However, there are some features of hospice care that are relatively new; they present an opportunity to apply modern techniques and approaches to the old traditions. The multidisciplinary nature of hospice care is an example; it applies in coordinated fashion the technology of many trained and skilled professionals. Certain specifics of patient care also are relatively new. From the work of Twycross (1974) and others, we have learned a great deal about pain control in the terminally ill. The technique described for managing intestinal obstruction in advanced malignancy without the use of nasogastric tubes and intravenous solutions represents a departure from conventional care. It utilizes drugs such as stool softeners and antiemetics, which were not available before the era of nasogastric tubes and intravenous fluids.

In a sense hospice care permits us to return to useful old values and techniques but with a much improved prospect for effectiveness (Zimmerman 1983).

Won't hospice care lead to the development of one more specialty and thus to further fragmentation in medicine?

It is too early to tell at this point to what extent hospice care will establish itself as a specialty. It certainly is an area in which some workers will concentrate their interest. To the extent that the terminally ill profit from this specialization, the benefits in care outweigh the disadvantages of fragmentation. Unquestionably, the developmment of anesthesiology as a specialty further fragmented medicine, but few of us would want to be put to sleep with an unskilled person administering our anesthetic.

In a very real sense, hospice care is holistic; one of its aims is to bring to the patient and family, in a coordinated fashion, the benefits of many disciplines. It may thus teach us something about how to deal with fragmentation in other areas of medical care.

Doesn't hospice care separate the patient from his or her physician?

This question is often asked both by patients and physicians. There is nothing intrinsic in hospice care that automatically leads to separation of a patient from his previous attending physician or to loss of control of the medical aspects of care by that physician if he or she wishes to retain control. Different hospices are obviously organized in different ways. Similarly, physicians in individual circumstances will vary in their desire for continuing involvement in the patient's care. A family practitioner who has followed the patient for many years may well wish a different approach from an oncologist who has played a specialized role in the patient's recent management.

Our experience has been with a model that permits maximum adaptability to different circumstances, and we feel that hospice programs should be designed with this in mind. For the attending physician who wishes continued active participation in the patient's care, the hospice team can serve in a largely consultative capacity. Conversely, if the current attending physician simply wants to be certain that the patient receives excellent care but does not want continued control over management, the patient can be placed under the care of the hospice physician. In other words, each case can be handled on the basis of the individual situation and in accordance with the wishes of the patient, family, and attending physician. In our experience patients need not fear being separated from physicians with whom they are comfortable, and physicians need not fear loss of their patients.

Isn't there a risk that patients with potentially curable cancer will be regarded as hopelessly ill and entered in a hospice care program?

In a patient with malignant disease, the decision that the condition is incurable must always be made cautiously and carefully. The existence of hospice care does not change this imperative.

Sometimes it is easily evident that a malignant tumor is beyond the point of cure. On other occasions it may be very difficult to make a decision. In such circumstances the availability of hospice care may actually make it easier to crystallize this decision. It is usually much more satisfactory to make a clear choice rather than to evade the issue.

With hospice care as an option, it becomes somewhat simpler to face the decision more forthrightly. Presently, there is sometimes a tendency to continue invasive, uncomfortable therapeutic measures directed against an incurable tumor simply because there is nothing else to do.

In those instances in which there is doubt about whether or not there is a reasonable chance for cure, the use of ample consultation and tumor board consideration can be valuable. Both the physician making referral to a hospice care program and the physicians operating the program must be certain that the available evidence indicates that further efforts at cure of the disease do not have a reasonable prospect of success.

We feel it is extremely important that management of the terminally ill through hospice care be a part of the continuum of medical care, rather than something outside the remainder of the health care system. This is necessary, in part, because this issue exists at the curative-palliative interface.

The rapid developments in the treatment of certain forms of malignant disease make it essential that hospice physicians remain informed about advances in oncology. Rarely, new treatment methods may convert a previously incurable patient into one who can be cured; such a patient should promptly be placed upon appropriate therapy for his or her disease. In short, hospice care does not mean that any patient with a reasonable chance of cure will be deprived of that chance.

Isn't hospice care really a form of euthanasia?

Not in the sense in which the term euthanasia is so often used, i.e., the hastening of death or "death by request." On the contrary, the aim of hospice is to make this type of euthanasia irrelevant for those who are terminally ill. Its goal is to make death as painless as possible. To the extent that dying is gentler and more comfortable, the issue of hastening death becomes less relevant.

We would be less than candid, though, if we did not say that the issue of providing palliation to the terminally ill must be looked at in two dimensions, both in terms of quantity of life and quality of life. The overriding objective in dealing with the terminally ill is to stretch life in both dimensions. However, hospice care is committed to the principle that in those instances where a choice *must* be made between making living more comfortable and extending life, the only rational decision is to do everything possible to improve the quality of life. Experience with hospice care suggests that this is a choice that very seldom has to be made.

One might also inquire whether the administration of relatively high doses of potent narcotics shortens life. This is unlikely since these drugs are administered in doses carefully adjusted to keep the patient not only quite conscious, but actually alert.

There is no evidence to suggest that patients in a hospice care program have a shorter life expectancy than similar patients treated outside of a hospice care program. We have some reason to suspect, in fact, that through the relief of symptoms, life is actually prolonged for some patients. Perhaps this occurs through that nebulous but very real "will to live".

How do you get physician support for developing a hospice program?

This question, which is usually asked by nonphysicians who are familiar with hospice concepts and wish to start a program in their community, recognizes the critical importance of physician support for such a program. It is virtually impossible to undertake any type of meaningful hospice care without the endorsement and involvement of physicians. It is futile to consider generating a hospital-based program without the active participation of the hospital medical staff.

To a large extent the answer to this question depends upon local factors and perhaps upon some intangibles. There is no substitute for the "right chemistry." We think, however, that certain measures are of great help. The first is identifying and enlisting the enthusiastic involvement of certain key physicians. Within the organization of any medical community, there are identifiable physicians who have a great deal of influence with their colleagues. From among these it is usually possible to interest and enlist several who will serve as catalysts.

It is important to recognize that physician involvement must occur early in the planning stages. Nothing discourages physician participation faster than for them to be presented with a virtually fully developed protocol for a program that has been developed without physician input. As soon as the key physicians are sufficiently familiar with hospice care, they should begin to involve other physicians in planning.

From the first, physicians must see hospice care as a tool to use in the care of their patients, not as a threat that will limit their therapeutic options, steal their patients, or entangle them in paperwork. This requires very careful descriptions of exactly what problems hospice care solves and the ways in which it does so. Factual presentation, not evangelism, convinces physicians.

In securing physician support, the option for the attending physician either to continue in the care of the patient or to turn the patient over to the hospice physician has been most helpful. In this way hospice care has been seen by a large number of physicians as something they could use to solve problems.

Finally, patience and perseverance are important. Physicians are besieged with new techniques that are purported to offer advantages and benefits. They have learned, for their own defense and that of their patients, to be skeptical about such proposals and to be cautious in their acceptance. More than we realize, all of us are the beneficiaries of this attitude.

The most effective means of securing physician support is to demonstrate repeatedly what hospice care will do for their patients. A few physicians will remain unconvinced until the experience is first hand. Some of the most skeptical doubters on our medical staff became avid supporters of the program once it was in operation. Incidentally, we owe a special debt to these physicians, for we learned much from their doubts.

What about malpractice suits in hospice programs?
Hospice care apparently has rarely led to malpractice suits; even more rare is a suit in which the plaintiff has been successful. Although the author has not made an exhaustive study of this topic, at this writing he does not know a judgment rendered against a hospice caregiver arising directly out of hospice care.

In the United States today, there are growing numbers of civil suits for damages in most fields. The paucity of such suits in England, where hospice care has been in operation longer, is of little comfort because the ground rules in both legal matters (where there is no contingency fee) and in the health care delivery system are strikingly different.

Furthermore, hospice care is in a sense at high risk because it literally deals with life and death situations, emotion-charged issues, and a circumstance in which "failure" is the normal outcome. The decision to undertake no further curative therapy and the delegation of responsibilities to volunteers and families unquestionably increase the medicolegal vulnerability of hospice workers. The existence of extended family, not all of whom may be identified during the terminal illness, raises some special problems.

Nonetheless, it is not surprising that malpractice suits have been a very uncommon experience for hospices. There is a great deal of evidence suggesting that a common denominator among the vast majority of malpractice actions is the lack of the very things that hospice care emphasizes: strong interpersonal relationships, deep sympathetic concern, and meaningful communication.

Doesn't the team approach reduce the patient's privacy?

If by privacy is meant the possibility for patients to be alone when they wish, the answer is firmly negative. Hospice workers generally are quite sensitive to the needs of patients and families to be left alone. The availability of team members in no way means that they force themselves upon the patient and family. They do respond as required.

However, the term privacy may be used in the sense of *confidentiality*. Strictly speaking, to the extent that patients and their families share their concerns and problems with team members, confidentiality will be decreased. However, such information should pass no further than the hospice team. Theoretically, there is perhaps more possibility for leak of information with team involvement than when the patient communicates only with one individual such as the physician. However, our experience has been that team members quickly understand the importance of confidentiality and are very unlikely to violate it. In practice, this is one of those matters in which the gains from the team approach clearly outweigh the loss.

What has been the reaction to your program?

The reaction has been overwhelmingly favorable. It has been seen on the faces and heard in the words of innumerable patients. It has been described in touching fashion by bereaved loved ones. Almost without exception the medical staff of the hospital, as individuals and as a group, has given its enthusiastic endorsement. Interest in the community has been substantial and is reflected in the initiation of other programs. Third-party payors and government agencies have reacted favorably in a number of ways. We have made no formal effort to measure and document reaction in these various groups and feel that efforts to do so would only prove the obvious.

What are the major problems your hospice faces today?

This is a question that doubtless would be answered somewhat differently by different members of our hospice care team. The following is the author's response and thus represents the perspective of the chairman of the hospice care committee.

Reimbursement for services is incomplete, which makes it difficult for the program to pay for itself. Most inpatient reimbursement formulas have been about as satisfactory for hospice as for nonhospice patients, but the situation is not as good with respect to outpatient expenses. For years health insurance has emphasized hospital benefits, and although the situation is improving, there are still many patients who have little coverage for outpatient and home care services. Generally speaking, insurance programs have provided better reimbursement for *procedures* than for other aspects of health care. This put a program that emphasizes personal attention and de-emphasizes technology at a disadvantage. Also, certain features of importance in hospice, such as bereavement care, are not covered under most health insurance policies. As always, finances are of critical importance, but lack of balance in the payment system presents some special impediments to ideal care for the terminally ill.

Work load and staff assignments require study and modifications. Breindel and Gravely's work (1980) has begun to provide some data that can be used for this purpose. As more members of our medical staff become familiar with principles of hospice care, we hope that more of them will serve as attending physicians for patients in the program and thus lighten the demands upon the hospice physician. Training of additional volunteers for evening and night duty would be helpful. In some measure there is a question of properly distributing personnel to meet the demands; we have not had the information to permit doing this in a rational way. For reasons evident from Breindel and Gravely's study, much of the frustration that personnel in the program experience is not specifically related to hospice care, but simply to the work load on the nursing unit to which hospice patients are assigned.

There is need for additional education programs, both for hospice personnel and for others whose work has an impact on the hospice program. Medical staff members who refer patients need a clearer perception of what the program offers. Members of the medical staff who serve as attending physicians for their patients in the program need continuing education in principles of hospice care. Nursing personnel and volunteers need continuing education as well.

For us to learn as much as possible from our growing experience, improved methods of data collection and analysis are needed. Through this we will learn by doing, and others can profit from our experience.

Our limited ability to deal effectively with certain symptoms such as anorexia and weakness is a source of frustration and dissatisfaction. We hope that clinical experience, properly investigated, will lead to some breakthroughs.

Won't the development of a cure for cancer make hospices obsolete?
Unfortunately, we are unlikely to see for some time that happy day when there is a uniformly effective method of prevention or treatment for cancer. Meanwhile, hospice care can accomplish an immense amount of good and can have a favorable impact on medical care in general. Even when cancer is no longer a threat, there are other diseases for which the application of hospice principles and practice will be useful.

What have been the major changes in hospice care since your program began?

There have obviously been important changes in the health care system generally with increasing interest in the matter of cost control. Hospice grew up in the United States in an era when there really was very little attention to medical care costs. Questions about selection of management were almost always answered in terms of quality only. The pendulum has now begun to swing, and this cannot help but have an impact — perhaps in unforeseeable ways — on hospice care.

Since the first edition of this book was written, an accreditation program for hospices has been developed by the JCAH and a number of states have passed hospice legislation of various types. Of course, most attention has been focused on the federal law that made a hospice benefit available to Medicare patients. That legislation and its implementation have been a great source of controversy, and many of its ramifications at this point remain uncertain.

There continues to be a growth in the number of hospice programs throughout the country. Diversity in organizational structure continues.

In our program we have had, as expected, considerable change in personnel and have been pleased that despite this the program remains strong.

Questions Regarding a Hospital-Based Hospice Program

How does a hospice program fit into the organizational structure and environment of a hospital?

Some have assumed that the objectives and methods of hospice are incompatible with those of a hospital and have thus suggested that the only way in which hospice can flourish is by being separate from hospitals.

We are committed to the belief that the basic objectives of hospice care conform to those of the hospital: the care of the sick. Methods employed for the treatment of the terminally ill may vary from those employed for other patients, but hospitals are certainly accustomed to dealing differently with patients having different types of problems.

A hospice program within a hospital can be readily fit into that hospital's organizational structure. Our program is under the direction of a committee of the medical staff, with broad representation from other fields. It functions much like other interdisciplinary programs such as hyperalimentation. A manual has been prepared and is periodically revised.

The inclusion of hospice patients on a general medical and surgical nursing unit has not in any way proved disruptive to that floor nor has it compromised the benefits of hospice care. Naturally, some modification of routines on the nursing unit is required. The two-way interaction between hospice care and nonhospice care on an inpatient nursing unit is described in Chapter 9.

What are the advantages of a hospital-based program?

This question is difficult to answer briefly because it involves a number of complex issues. To list them is cumbersome. Nonetheless, there are several points worth making.

A hospital-based or affiliated program can be developed within the framework of the present health care system in most communities. This has a number of very important advantages.

The transition from curative to palliative care often is easier if it does not require the patient to make an adjustment to a totally new setting or personnel. Since many patients enter a hospice program as inpatients, this is a particularly important consideration.

Similarly, once a patient is in a hospice program, the ease of access to more sophisticated forms of treatment may be an important factor in determining whether or not such measures are used. It is often argued that hospice care, by its nature, does not require much technological support. This is true, but we have found that circumstances do occur in which the ready access to facilities located in the hospital has been extremely helpful in providing palliation. This applies not just to antitumor therapy such as surgery, radiation, and chemotherapy, but also to other support measures such as intramedullary nailing to prevent pathological fractures and tracheotomy for upper airway obstruction. We feel that the ready availability of the entire spectrum of care that a hospital offers has improved the caliber of palliative care that we can offer.

Communication between those providing day-by-day hospice care and others who might contribute to the comfort of the patient is simpler and more effective in the hospital setting. For a patient with vertebral metastases from breast carcinoma who shows signs of impending paraplegia, on-the-spot consultation with the neurosurgeon, oncologist, and radiotherapist can be of inestimable value.

The most common criticism of hospital-based hospice programs has to do with the impersonal, inflexible, and frightening environment of the hospital and its institutional policies. It is said that only outside of a hospital can an environment be created in which patients can be comfortable and relaxed. Our experience indicates that this is simply not so. We make no pretense of being able to provide all of the comforts of home in our hospital, but then neither does any type of institution, be it hospital based or free standing. This is why we all believe so strongly in home care. Nonetheless, we have found it possible to create within the hospital a very suitable atmosphere for the proper rendering of hospice care. It is feasible to relax hospital regulations for hospice care patients sufficiently to permit comfort in a degree comparable to that achievable in any institutional setting.

In looking at free-standing and hospital-based programs, we prefer not to take an either/or approach. At this point either may be the preferable — or the only possible — place to begin, depending upon local circumstances. Neither can be regarded as totally meeting the needs of the terminally ill patient. The hospital-based program with home care is handicapped in handling the patient who does not require hospital care but whose home circumstances do not permit management there. The free-standing unit with home care is limited in its ability to handle the patient who would profit from inhospital care. Both types of units must strive to develop methods that permit them to cover the entire spectrum of care needed by terminally ill patients.

Even in a hospital-based program, wouldn't it be better to have a separate unit for hospice patients?
  This question can probably be dealt with best by looking at two aspects of the design of in-hospital hospice facilities. The first is patient care. There are no controlled studies to tell us whether patients are better handled in a separate unit or in one integrated with other hospital patients. We can say that the interaction between hospice and nonhospice patients on the nursing unit that houses our hospice patients has usually been positive in both directions. More frequently than not, hospice and nonhospice patients have each had a beneficial effect upon the other. There have been very few problems related to this arrangement. Furthermore, by not having a separate unit for hospice patients, our staff has been involved with both hospice and general medical-surgical patients. This has avoided some of the psychological problems that occur in many hospice programs in which personnel handle only terminally ill patients. It also has permitted some of the desirable features of hospice care to cross-fertilize general medical care in a way that would otherwise not have been possible.
  The other consideration is the matter of economics. The establishment of a separate facility, whether it is some place outside the hospital, on a specially designated floor of the hospital, or at the end of a corridor, necessitates some construction costs. But this is not the most important consideration. What is of critical importance, particularly for the medium-sized or small hospital, is flexibility in bed usage. To the extent that beds are set aside for specific purposes, a hospital's ability to utilize the total number of its existing beds is diminished. Since in a short period we may experience a variation in daily inpatient hospice census of from 1 to 12 patients, it is easy to see the impact that designated beds or a separate unit would have. Using a "swing bed" system, such as that at Church Hospital, probably makes having a hospice program feasible for many hospitals for which it would otherwise not be practical.
  In summary, if those of us who have been involved in the hospice program at Church Hospital were offered the opportunity to have a separate unit for our patients, there probably would be split opinion. We would be unanimous, however, in our response to the question of whether we would rather have a hospice program with swing beds or no program at all.

Aside from a separate unit and swing beds on a general unit, what other organizational options are there for a hospital-based hospice program?

So-called "scatter beds" may be used throughout the hospital. This approach has been employed with fair success by a number of programs. Its disadvantages are related to the dispersion of patients to widely separated areas throughout the hospital. This usually requires that the hospice team be a consultative service — a symptom control support team. Such an arrangement, although apparently the best approach under certain circumstances, lacks the cohesive impact of a hospice team functioning in a specific nursing unit with the option for the hospice physician to serve as the attending physician for some of the patients in the program.

What has been the attitude of other patients toward the hospice program?

On all general medical-surgical nursing units with semiprivate rooms, patients have been exposed to the terminally ill, so that this has presented no particular problem. Naturally, one of our initial concerns was whether nonhospice patients would resent the relaxation of hospital regulations for hospice patients. This simply has not been a problem; on the few occasions when questions have been raised, brief explanations by the staff have been well accepted. The two-way interaction between hospice and nonhospice patients has often been mutually profitable.

What has been the effect of the hospice program on the care of other patients?

At this point we have no data on this topic, only impressions. There is some reason to believe that the reemphasis of some of the traditional values of medical care, including the meaningful communication and sympathetic concern that are such an important part of hospice care, have rubbed off onto the care provided nonhospice patients. There might be a question as to whether the increased demand for personal attention to hospice patients on the part of staff might not diminish the attention directed to nonhospice patients on the same unit. This does not seem to happen.

Breindel and Gravely's data (1980) indicate that although hospice patients take more total personnel time than nonhospice patients, this increased time is given largely by volunteers and family. This suggests an explanation for the observation that attention to nonhospice patients has not decreased.

Questions Regarding Organization and Financing of a Hospice Program

How expensive is hospice care?

Among those who have observed hospice programs, there is no doubt that it is "care effective." Determining whether or not it is "cost effective" is a complicated matter. It may be an impossible task, since no one can find a means of placing a dollar value on human comfort.

In addressing this question, one must also take a look at the basis of comparison. If hospice care is compared to conscientious conventional treatment for the terminally ill, including prolonged hospitalization, numerous diagnostic tests, and the liberal use of radiation and chemotherapy, hospice care is almost certainly more economical. On the other hand, if hospice care is compared to virtually no care at all, it is clearly more expensive.

At this point there are no data that permit reasonable comparison of the management of terminal illness in conventional fashion and in a hospice care program. The following observations may be of some help, however.

For inpatients, hospice care is clearly labor intensive. Although it is a relatively low level of care technologically, with far fewer diagnostic and therapeutic maneuvers, it does require a high level of personal attention. A substantial portion of this attention, however, can be provided by volunteers and by family, once they have gained a certain level of understanding. Breindel and Gravely's data (1980) compare hospice patients with intermediate care general medical-surgical patients, the vast majority of whom are not terminally ill. Those data indicate that the average cost per patient day for hospice patients is approximately half that of nonhospice patients.

In addition, it is reasonable to presume that hospice care permits a far larger percentage of the terminal illness to be spent as an outpatient than would be possible under conventional care. Thus hospital stays are shorter. On the other hand, outpatient care costs are doubtless higher for hospice than for nonhospice patients.

The bottom line would seem to be that when somewhat lower daily inpatient costs and shorter hospital stays are combined with somewhat higher outpatient costs, hospice care offers an economically attractive alternative to traditional terminal care.

How do you get reimbursed for hospice care?
The answer to this question has to be a bit complex and equivocal. This is an area in which changes have occurred and will continue to occur. In addition, these changes will be different in different areas and for different patients.

The reimbursement situation varies somewhat according to the setting in which the patient is located: in the hospital, in an intermediate care facility, or at home. It also varies from one type of insurance to another.

Within the last two years, for example, Medicare beneficiaries have had the choice of selecting a hospice option *in place of* other benefits if they are terminally ill. Hospitals have concomitantly had the option of reimbursement for such patients under the traditional Medicare formulas or under hospice benefits. For patients and institutions there are pros and cons in these options.

What follows is based upon our growing experience with common health insurance reimbursement formulas.

For inpatients, reimbursement is the same as for nonhospice inpatients. Hospice patients who require hospitalization would require it whether or not they were in a hospice program. As a consequence, third-party payors use the same rules as they would for any other hospitalized patient.

Reimbursement for outpatient care is a more complex matter. Some patients possess home care coverage as part of their health insurance; for these, many services are reimbursed. For patients who do not have a home care provision in their health insurance, there is little or no reimbursement from third-party carriers. In such instances the patient is billed; any balance beyond what the patient can pay has to be secured from other sources such as grants and donations. To the extent that it cannot be recovered, it must be accepted as a loss.

But even for patients who possess insurance that covers home care, certain features of such coverage are often not suitable for hospice care. There are often stipulations, for example, that there must have been a prior period of hospitalization or that the patient be homebound. These are requirements that many hospice patients do not meet; as a consequence, home care service for them is not reimbursed. Furthermore, home care visits for hospice patients are usually longer than those for patients on other types of home care. Since reimbursement formulas do not take this into account, the provider of care is not fully compensated.

It is in the area of coverage for outpatients, then, that there is the greatest need for improvement. This incidentally, is a problem not confined to hospice programs. By and large, insurance carriers are offering increasing options for various types of home care coverage. There is need for a larger number of such policies covering more services. However, it is the purchasers of policies who will determine whether or not such options sell. Individuals and groups such as companies and labor unions need to be educated in the value of having insurance that covers home care services.

Bereavement and other counseling services present a special problem. It is difficult to imagine that in the foreseeable future such services will be covered by any type of health insurance. Other options must be found for financing this aspect of hospice care.

What changes will more liberal reimbursement for hospice care bring about?
Although it is difficult to predict whether or not more liberal reimbursement for hospice services will come about, there are a number of factors in the present environment that suggest it will. Exactly how this will affect hospice care depends, of course, upon the nature of the liberalization. There is a natural tendency for "services to follow reimbursement·" Stated conversely, services that are not paid for are difficult to provide. To the extent that increased payment is available for personal attention, including bereavement, the provision of these is likely to increase.

Across-the-board increase in financial support for hospice services would doubtless result in the increased availability of hospice care. However, it would be likely to bring some problems. For example, the role of the volunteer might be substantially altered and diminished, with serious adverse consequences. Also, the increased availability of reimbursement might well attract into the hospice field those with a more entrepreneurial than humanitarian interest in the terminally ill.

What factors should a hospice consider in deciding whether or not to seek JCAH accreditation?

If a hospice desires or needs heightened credibility as a legitimate health care provider, JCAH accreditation could indeed contribute significantly to its stature. As a competitive asset, JCAH accreditation is not generally perceived as a necessity nor is it a qualifying prerequisite for payment of any sort. Expenses associated with achieving accreditation may be significant for the non-hospital-based program. If reorganization or changes in policy are required to comply with the standards, additional costs may be incurred.

What factors should a hospice consider in deciding whether or not to participate in the Medicare hospice benefit?

The ability of the hospice management to identify accurately the relationship between its costs and the Medicare payment levels is the first step in evaluating this option. The question of stability and/or control in projecting expenses is also pertinent. For a hospice program already recognized as a Medicare provider, comparison with the revenue generated from the current payment system is applicable. For some hospice programs the Medicare hospice option may represent a new opportunity for payment where none existed before. For all programs any expense related to organization or policy changes as well as paperwork required to qualify for payment must be determined.

What role should physicians play in program management?

This depends upon the needs and resources of the particular program. Physician involvement is essential for successful hospice care, but the precise form this takes depends upon a number of factors. We feel that a hospital-based program should be under the purview of a medical staff committee but that day-to-day physician participation in the administrative details of operation is not necessary.

Have you added staff to the nursing unit that houses the hospice inpatients?

Little if any change was made in the staffing pattern on the general medical-surgical nursing unit when we began housing all hospice inpatients there. Study of nursing time per patient (Breindel and Gravely 1980) suggests that the overall staffing requirements are not greatly altered by having hospice patients on a nursing unit. Although more total personnel time is required in the management of hospice than nonhospice patients, this difference is largely made up by volunteers and family.

Thus, except for the addition of volunteers, there was little need to change the total number of personnel assigned to the unit. What did take place was some change in the individuals making up the staff. Some of the staff assigned to that nursing unit did not wish to be involved in hospice care, and some employees on other units requested assignment to the hospice floor. As far as possible these requests for changes were honored. Since that time, except for the customary turnover, personnel have remained the same but have moved from a 50- to a 28-bed unit. In addition, a total patient care model of nursing practice has been adopted for all patients on that unit.

What problems have you had with staff stress and burnout and what do you do about it?

Probably because personnel on the nursing unit containing hospice patients deal with both hospice and nonhospice patients, we have had few of the problems that arise from day-to-day exposure exclusively to the dying. As noted earlier, some staff members have found themselves unsuited to the care of the terminally ill; since this nursing unit has a disproportionate percentage of patients in this category, they have requested transfer to other units. Usually it has been the staff member him- or herself who has first recognized the desirability of transfer.

What almost every member of our staff has experienced in some degree is the common syndrome of overwork. In his 35 years in medicine, the author has not found a totally satisfactory solution to this problem. This is partly due to the fact that some of the satisfactions in taking care of patients are deeply intertwined with factors that lead to overwork.

General problems related to the work load have unquestionably been aggravated occasionally by specific difficulties related to providing care to the terminally ill. Fears regarding one's own death, grief over a patient with whom one has felt particularly close, and insecurity about one's role in the multidisciplinary team do occur.

We have not developed a formal structured system for dealing with staff stress. Although each member of the hospice team has doubtless been at some time very important to other members in coping with stress-related problems, the intimate involvement of our chaplains in the program has made them a particularly valuable resource in dealing with stress. At the weekly patient conference, staff members are encouraged to express any specific personal concerns or difficulties they may have had with the patients under discussion. This has often led to helpful sharing in the group.

The section on staff stress in Chapter 6 addresses this issue more systematically and in greater detail.

Questions Regarding Patient Care in a Hospice Program

How are patients selected for the program?

Our program is designed for patients who are under the care of members of our medical staff and who are terminally ill from malignant disease. Other hospice programs are accepting patients who are terminally ill from non-malignant disease. Some patients who are not under the care of the Church Hospital medical staff are accepted.

Any attending physician who has a patient whom he or she feels is suitable for entry into the program makes a referral to the hospice program. If the guidelines described in Chapter 15 are met, the patient is accepted. On occasion, the work load in the program is such that no additional patients can be accommodated, in which case an accepted patient is placed on a priority list according to the severity of symptom control problems.

Do you reject many patients who apply for the program?

As members of our medical staff and the community as a whole have become increasingly familiar with our program, there has been increasing familiarity also with the criteria for admission. In addition, it is easy for those who don't know a great deal about the program to make inquiry. As a consequence, we have relatively few formal applications from patients who do not meet the criteria for admission. Occasionally, it is learned only after the application and supporting material are reviewed that there is no suitable caregiver in the home and that the patient is thus not eligible.

Inquiries regarding the program are directed to the home care office so that they are handled by an individual who is familiar with community resources. Patients who do not meet the entry requirements for our program, whether because of the nature of their disease, their geographic location, or other factors, are referred to other appropriate agencies.

What are patients in your program told about their disease?

This question is difficult to answer both well and briefly. It could be the subject of a book itself. There are many ramifications and much need for individualization. However, a few points are worth making.

The first thing one must understand is that in dealing with the patient dying of advanced malignancy, it is much more important to *listen* than to *tell*. It is only when one perceives what the patient presently knows, wishes to know, and needs to know that one can provide meaningful help. One must listen carefully to what the patient tells; one must be sensitive to nonverbal language and to the real meaning of questions, as well as to questions not asked. Nothing worthwhile can be conveyed to a patient in a speech or lecture about his or her condition; genuine dialogue is essential.

On the one hand, most patients with advanced malignancy strongly suspect or really "know" what their situation is. It is difficult to be even mildly ill these days without imagining that one has incurable malignancy. Patients with cancer bring to their illness a background of awareness about malignancy and are usually quite sensitive to the verbal and other signals being sent by those around them.

On the other hand, almost all patients experience denial in some degree when first perceiving that they have an incurable disease. This denial must be appraised with respect to its intensity and its value as a defense mechanism. It must then be taken into consideration as one approaches the matter of discussing with patients their understanding of their situation.

For those patients who know, or almost know, the true situation, there are many benefits to be derived from having it confirmed in the right way at the right time. Often unpleasant truth is easier to bear than uncertainty. The truth opens avenues that permit patients to talk about and be reassured on those points that may be of concern to them. For example, a patient can bring out his fears about pain and death; this, in turn, makes it possible to deal with these fears. He can speak with his loved ones about the things most important to them and can cope with practical problems such as finances in a much more prudent fashion.

To me it seems a hoax of the cruelest and most absurd dimensions to refuse to discuss with a patient who already understands his situation the facts that he wants and needs to know. By listening carefully one can determine what the patient suspects, what he would like confirmed, and what additional information he needs to have. In addition, it is important to provide the information with kindly candor, telling the truth within the patient's ability to understand.

It is important to recognize that you can not tell people something they refuse to know. Attempting to convey the truth to patients who are not ready to accept that they are dying is futile. For patients who are not ready — and some are never ready, even at the moment of death — it is pointless and probably harmful to enter into vigorous efforts to get through to them.

What I have said so far is fine as a generalization, but if any matter requires individualization, it is this. There is an immense individuality in patients' capacity to know and understand their disease and its implications. Sensitivity of the highest order is required to detect a particular patient's readiness to talk. In addition, this readiness is not a static thing; it will change in either direction from day to day.

Two final comments should be made on this matter of patients' understanding of their status. First, the almost moment-by-moment variation in acceptance should be emphasized. This can be quite striking in some patients and is distinct from the patient's variable readiness to talk. It is not uncommon to have a patient, almost in sequence, discuss his impending death and describe plans for something four or five years in the future. The other point is to remember to be nonjudgmental with respect to the patient's level of understanding of his or her status. Many of us have an instinctive inclination to feel that the most realistic appraisal is the best. In truth, for some patients denial to the bitter end may be the best of all options.

What are the common problems that necessitate hospitalization of hospice patients?

The basic rule, of course, is that it is generally better to manage the patient at home if this can be done. Hospitalization, however, can be necessitated by a number of problems.

Many of our patients are in the hospital when they enter the program. The fact that they have terminal malignancy and are candidates for hospice care has been discovered while the patients are hospitalized. As soon as such patients can be managed at home, they are discharged from the hospital.

The single most common reason for admission to inpatient status is probably inadequate pain control. Although patients can be managed on very high doses of narcotic at home, the titration process by which the optimal pattern of narcotic administration is achieved requires close observation and frequent dosage changes that are difficult to execute outside the hospital.

Mental confusion often necessitates hospitalization. No matter what the home situation, it can be very difficult to manage a confused, restless, agitated patient at home.

Severe insomnia poses difficult problems for the caregivers at home. An uncomfortable, sleepless patient saps the strength of the others in the household; this may be the factor that tips the balance against remaining at home.

Sometimes a brief period of hospitalization is provided largely to give rest to an exhausted or sick caregiver at home. Admission to the hospital for this purpose may raise questions about reimbursement for inpatient care from third-party payors. For the hospital-based program with home care, this situation points out the value of having available an intermediate care facility in which hospice care can be provided without loss of continuity. Most hospital-based programs do not have such an arrangement. However, the issue seldom presents a practical problem. In most cases in which the primary purpose of hospitalization is to provide respite for a caregiver at home, the need occurs because of specific physical problems that the patient has; these legitimately can be cited as the reasons for hospitalization. One must concede that this is a gray area, but the author has no personal difficulty in justifying hospitalization in these circumstances because, over the long haul, hospice care is cost effective; this is simply one of the built-in costs. In other words, without hospice care such patients would probably have spent a much larger share of their terminal illness in the hospital under more costly circumstances.

Each patient and family are dealt with on an individual basis to determine in what setting optimal care can be rendered. Ready access to and smooth transition between various levels of care are essential to optimal management of the terminally ill, as are excellent communication and coordination between personnel providing care at those levels.

Using all that morphine, aren't patients knocked out and don't they become addicted?

Addiction is not a problem in the terminally ill. To begin with, the course of most patients is of such a nature that addiction is irrelevant. Furthermore, our experience, and that of others, has been that patients with chronic pain from advanced malignancy are able to reduce the dosage of narcotic without serious problem if, for some reason, pain is relieved by other means such as radiation therapy.

With respect to the use of drugs for relief of chronic pain in terminal illness, it has been observed repeatedly that for most narcotics there is a range of dosage within which the patient can be maintained free of pain and quite alert. The only drowsiness that most patients experience is during the initial period of dosage adjustment when they are being brought into that range.

In patients for whom severe pain has been a chronic problem, we begin by assuring them at the outset that we can relieve their pain without rendering them somnolent. We start with a quite heavy dosage of narcotic, which may produce drowsiness. We then gradually back off into that range of dosage that leaves them quite bright but pain free. From time to time advancing disease will result in increased pain, in which instance narcotic dosage usually can be increased to satisfactory analgesic levels without producing drowsiness. One really has to see hospice patients alert and comfortable on what we would ordinarily consider prohibitive doses of morphine to truly comprehend how well this works.

Aside from those in the process of initial dosage adjustment, the only drowsy, indolent patients are those who are extremely debilitated. Most of these patients are at a stage in their terminal illness at which they would exhibit lassitude even without narcotic administration. However, debility does seem to narrow that range of narcotic dosage within which the patient can be maintained pain free and alert.

Do you permit connubial visits?

Yes. In our program, however, this has rarely been a consideration because most patients who are well enough to be sexually active are not on the inpatient unit. For those few exceptions our hospice staff has discreetly demonstrated its imagination, ingenuity, and compassion in arranging connubial visits.

Do you let patients take drugs such as Laetrile?

We discourage the use of measures such as Laetrile on two grounds. First such substances appear to be medically useless and sometimes harmful. Second, condoning the use of what the patient sees as curative therapy runs counter to the type of adjustment that we are usually hoping the patient will make.

As a practical matter there is no way in which we can prevent a patient from popping an occasional Laetrile. However, this is usually not the fashion in which the drug is administered by its advocates. It is given as part of a program that includes special diets, megavitamins, and high colonic irrigations. We have found these measures to be quite incompatible with hospice care.

Currently, Laetrile is only the most highly publicized unapproved form of cancer treatment. There are many other similar programs available at various places throughout the world. Our attitude toward all of these is the same as toward Laetrile.

Why are we seeing more invasive procedures carried out on hospice patients? Is this done to justify hospital stay?
This is a question sometimes asked by our volunteers.

At present we do not have firm data to support or refute the assumption in the question; namely, that more invasive procedures are being carried out. The author shares the suspicion that they are.

There are several explanations for this. As familiarity with and popularity of the program has grown, there has been a tendency for patients to apply at an earlier stage of their disease. As a result we presently have a higher proportion of patients than we did a few years ago for whom some form of aggressive treatment, either anti-tumor therapy or other measures, might be appropriate. For example, the presence of vertebral metastasis with the potential for spinal cord compression would be dealt with quite differently for a patient with a life expectancy of several months than it would for one likely to die within a few days.

In addition, technological advances *have* had an impact on palliative care. Current techniques permit earlier diagnosis at a stage when problems can be prevented by relatively aggressive therapy. Computed tomography (CT) scan, radiation, and steroids can be used to deal with a small brain metastasis before it produces devastating and irreversible changes. Also some treatment measures have become substantially easier on the patient as the result of technical developments. For example, utilizing sonography and CT scanning, it is possible to insert a small tube into an intra-abdominal fluid collection with minimal trauma to the patient and often with a substantial increase in comfort. An application of this is the performance of nephrostomy, which previously would have required a moderately sizeable operative procedure, a large tube, and so forth.

In deciding about whether or not to undertake aggressive treatment of any kind in the terminally ill patient, we have employed a benefit-burden approach, weighing what is to be gained against the "costs." As pointed out in Chapter 14 (where this matter of invasive tests is discussed in some detail), it is not always easy to predict in advance the merits of a particular form of treatment. However, patient and family participation in this type of decision is of utmost importance.

The objectives of hospice care for the terminally ill remain the same: to make the dying process as comfortable as possible.

One hopes that the answer to the second half of the question is *never*. A good quality-assurance program should be in place in the institution, and one of the major thrusts of quality assurance is a close examination of the justification for the performance of procedures of all types. This should serve as a double check on the use of invasive procedures on hospice patients.

How do you decide about the use of tube feedings and intravenous fluids in hospice patients?

As a general rule tube feedings and intravenous fluids are seldom employed in our patients. Special circumstances do arise where the benefits of such treatment outweigh the burdens, but these are unusual.

It goes without saying that for mentally competent patients, these measures are never undertaken without their concurrence. Chapter 13 deals with the complex and controversial issue of making this decision for the incompetent patient.

We have found that in actual practice quality of life and quantity of life seldom come into conflict; but when they do, we have generally given the former priority.

Do you experiment on hospice patients?

Hospice patients are not used as the subjects of clinical studies of antitumor therapy. Even for symptomatic treatment, previously untested treatment schemes are not employed. However, we do try to learn as much as we can from our experience with each patient.

Why do patients drop out of the program?

Once entered, very few patients drop out of the hospice program. Because of the particular course of their disease, some patients require little or no hospice service over a protracted period of time. Such patients are at home and regular home care visits would be superfluous. Because many home care services are not reimbursed by third-party payors, the patient and family may request cesssation of home care services because of concern about expense. Such patients are maintained on inactive status. Contact with them is not lost, and they are returned to active status as soon as hospice care services are deemed warranted.

There are several reasons why a very small number of patients (less than 2%) have left the program before death. In spite of admission screening, which attempts to assure that the patient's home situation makes home care possible, the home situation may be misjudged or may change for some reason such as the illness or death of a family member. In such cases it may be necessary to place the patient in a nursing home, where all aspects of hospice care cannot be provided. Our program presently is capable of providing in-hospital care and care at home, but we have very limited capacity for continuing hospice care in an intermediate facility such as a nursing home. We are working to increase this capacity.

There are a few other reasons for withdrawal from the program. Error in diagnosis at the time of admission can occur. The importance of avoiding this if possible and of recognizing it promptly if it does occur is obvious. Although we have seen a number of instances of partial spontaneous remission of tumor in our hospice patients, we have not yet had an instance of complete and permanent spontaneous regression. Such a patient would probably be put on inactive status rather than dropped from the program. The same applies to unanticipated therapeutic remissions.

A few patients have been withdrawn from the program by their attending physicians. In one case this was for the purpose of instituting vigorous antitumor therapy, presumably in the hope of cure. In another instance the attending physician wished, very late in the patient's course, to provide vigorous supportive treatment in the form of endotracheal intubation and respiration support, aggressive treatment that was simply incompatible with the principles of hospice care.

After patients have been entered into the program they, or sometimes their families, may have a change of heart about accepting inevitable incurability and may decide to abandon the program to undertake antitumor therapy. Sometimes they do this through conventional avenues such as radiation or chemotherapy, but usually it has been to participate in unapproved treatments such as the use of Laetrile. A few patients leave a hospice program simply because they feel that they can handle the situation on their own.

Although we are naturally disheartened whenever patients are withdrawn from the program, we have learned a great deal from these experiences. The matter of withdrawal by the attending physician deserves some special comment. It is, in a sense, part of the price we pay for allowing referring physicians on our staff the option of continuing as the patient's attending physician in the hospice care program. It has been a small price for a valuable feature of the program and is a problem that can probably be corrected with additional physician education.

However, as can be seen from the two instances cited, the problem goes beyond the hospice care program. These patients at least entered the program. The real problem is to identify how frequently such decisions are made before entry into a hospice program, so that patients who might profit are kept out of the program. This is a matter that requires the attention of all physicians concerned with improving the care of the terminally ill. We are attempting to study this subject through our departmental audit committees and our quality-assurance program.

What about the special problems of the dying child?
Church Hospital has medical, surgical, and gynecological services. It does not have a pediatric service and does not admit children below the adolescent level. Therefore, we have not taken children into our hospice care program.

Many of the problems and principles of caring for the dying adult apply also to the dying child. However, there are naturally some special considerations in children.

Some hospice programs have had experience with children (Burne 1984, Corr & Corr 1985), but for the most part this has been quite limited. In part this is because terminal illness is relatively uncommon in children and adolescents. This means that it is unlikely for any one hospice program to gain a wide experience with children.

The work of Martinson (1976) indicates that the establishment of carefully developed home care programs offers the most promising approach in dealing with terminally ill children and adolescents and their families. Increased knowledge about the handling of death and dying and increased development of programs that utilize available existing knowledge are among the major needs in the years ahead.

What do you do about patients with other special problems such as alcoholism or drug addiction?

As has been pointed out, patients and families bring to terminal illness all of their preexisting medical, psychological, and social problems. Whatever their source and type, they are dealt with on an individual basis. Whether the problem is physical infirmity, dementia, or substance abuse, the measures taken are designed to be appropriate to the particular circumstances. There is, for example, no one right way to deal with all alcoholics who comes under hospice care. Different approaches are necessary for the active alcoholic as opposed to the recovered alcoholic, and different approaches are necessary for family members and for patients. For the patient with a history of drug addiction, the nature and types of drugs, e.g., heroin versus cocaine, may be of importance.

In any event, the multidisciplinary hospice team is well equipped to work with other individuals and groups who may be in a position to be of support to the patient and family.

What assurances are there regarding the quality of care that hospice patients receive?

Whether hospital based or otherwise, each hospice program should make certain that some quality-assurance mechanism is in place. The fact that the program calls itself hospice and that those involved in it are well intentioned does not ensure that care is optimal. Some form of extrinsic evaluation should be utilized. Precisely how this is done will vary from program to program, but it is an obligation to our patients and their families.

In the hospital the institution's quality-assurance program should encompass hospice care. Some special criteria and measures may be necessary. In this connection, it should be pointed out that the quality-assurance program should also look at the care of terminally ill patients who are not in the hospice program to determine that their care meets a standard comparable to that available in the program. If it does not, nonhospice care must be upgraded or means must be found to get these patients into the hospice program.

References

Breindel CL. Gravely GE: *Costs of Providing a Mixed Unit Hospice Program*. Working paper, Department of Health Administration, Medical College of Virginia, Richmond, 1980.

Burne SR, et al.: Helen House — A hospice for children: Analysis of the first year. *Br Med J* 289:1665, 1984.

Corr CA, Corr DM: *Hospice Approaches to Pediatric Care*. Springer, New York, 1985.

Martinson IM: *Home Care for the Dying Child*. Appleton-Century-Crofts, New York, 1976.

Twycross RG: Clinical experience with diamorphine in advanced malignant disease. *Int J Clin Pharmacol Ther Toxicol* 9:184, 1974.

Zimmerman JM: Hospice critics: Sheep in wolves clothing? *Md State Med J* 32:106, 1983.

Chapter 18

The Future of Hospice Care

Jack M. Zimmerman

The first edition of this book concluded with a look at what lay ahead for hospice care. We are now about four to five years into that future. This gives an opportunity not only to look back on what has happened, but to compare it to what we thought and hoped would happen.

The fact is that there has clearly been some change, a part of which could be considered progress. Nonetheless, many of the same issues remain. We must ask the same two questions: What is the future likely to do to us? What can we do to the future? Although it is important to examine the forces that are likely to shape our options, the focus of what follows is not upon where we are being taken, but upon where we need to go.

It is difficult to foresee circumstances under which there will not be continuing growth of hospice care programs. An increasing interest and willingness to confront the handling of death and terminal illness, coupled with the results of hospice care programs in action, constitute a compelling argument for the wider use of such programs. Most indications seem to point toward expansion of hospice care. The experience of our program and that of others indicate that there is continuing need for the development of additional hospice programs.

One of the major changes that has occurred in health care delivery generally has been the awakening of concern about cost factors. Whereas a few years ago little attention was directed to control of health care costs, this now has become an important item on the national agenda. A related issue, of course, is the allocation of limited health care resources. Hospice will affect and will be affected by these issues. In precisely what way is open to question.

Diversity of form and style has been one of the strengths of hospice care thus far (Osterweis and Champagne 1979; Buckingham and Lupu 1982). Successful hospice programs have adapted to local needs. This should continue. Some free-standing hospices have obviously been enormously productive and have provided valuable knowledge regarding the care of the terminally ill. In some instances they will be the best means of meeting community needs. However, the Church Hospital hospice experience and that of other hospital-affiliated programs confirm that the hospital-based hospice is not only a possible but also desirable alternative approach.

There are philosophical, organizational, and financial reasons for promoting the growth of hospital-based units. We hope to see the development and expansion of various types of hospital-based programs. Some will possess a separate facility for hospice patients; some, like Church Hospital's, will have hospice patients integrated with nonhospice patients on a nursing unit; others will have hospice patients distributed throughout the hospital, under treatment by a palliative care team. As new programs are contemplated, those responsible for starting them should examine the options carefully and should design the program best suited to their particular circumstances. Standards for hospice care must be drawn to permit diversity.

As time passes it would perhaps be good if the distinctions between free-standing and hospital-based hospices are blurred. Possibly each hospice program will continue to have a locus at which its administrative function is centered. This may be in a hospital, in a free-standing unit, or in a home care program. However, hospitals, free-standing units, and home care programs serve patients at different levels of care. What is most needed for optimal care of the terminally ill are programs that are truly comprehensive in that they offer continuity of care as the patient shifts from one level to another. In other words, hospice programs should be organized to enable the application of hospice principles and practice across the entire spectrum.

It will be imperative for hospital-based programs to offer care not only in the hospital but in the home, as well as to patients who require institutionalization in an intermediate care facility. For many the term nursing home carries very unpleasant connotations. However, there is nothing that makes it categorically impossible for the finest type of hospice care to be available within a nursing home setting. Just as there is nothing that mandates that a hospital providing acute general care cannot offer excellent hospice care, so there is nothing that dictates that a nursing home facility providing care to other patients cannot also render hospice care of the highest caliber. Hospital-based hospice programs should seek to develop suitable arrangements so that they can provide care at the intermediate and home care levels. Often this will require arrangements with existing intermediate care facilities. Decline in hospital occupancy rates as a consequence of cost containment measures may free up some hospital beds for other use. It is not inconceivable, given appropriate financial incentives, that hospitals will opt to develop in-house intermediate care facilities of their own.

Similarly, free-standing hospice units will need to develop formalized arrangements that will permit the preservation of continuity of care when patients require acute hospital care. They will also have to cultivate the types of relationships that permit easy transition between levels of care. They must be certain that patients who would profit from some of the techniques that hospitalization allows are not denied the advantages this would permit.

Programs that begin with a home care base will need to find the means whereby patients can receive care in intermediate facilities and in hospitals without loss of continuity of care.

In other words, whatever the origin and whatever the center of operations, the ultimate aim of hospice programs will have to be the provision of comprehensive care. Otherwise, hospice will run the danger of perpetuating the kind of fragmentation that has plagued the conventional approach it seeks to supplement.

The economics of health care are undoubtedly going to shape the way in which we deal with the terminally ill. Conversely, hospice can have an impact on health care costs. There is an increasing general recognition of the fact that hospice care is an avenue worth exploring in our effort to reduce expenditures for health care without reduction in the quality of that care. There unquestionably will be continued study of this approach, and our experience thus far indicates that hospice care will fare well as a result. However, there is an increasing recognition by many that our financial and other resources for health care are limited and that there must be some thought given to the way in which those resources are allocated, if not rationed. We would be naive if we didn't believe that this poses some threat to the care of the terminally ill.

Cost restraints of various types have already led to declining occupancy rates in many hospitals and have fostered competition in the health care field. These developments cannot help but have an effect upon hospice programs. Unless hospital bed closures follow the declining occupancy rate, the increase in empty beds will remove at least one concern that the medical staffs of hospitals have expressed about hospice programs, namely, that they will attract increased numbers of terminally ill patients and thus threaten bed availability. Competition will stimulate hospitals and physicians alike to offer care as comprehensive as possible.

Clarification of cost and reimbursement issues must be concomitant with resolution of organizational problems in hospice care. Decisions in these areas are matters of public policy and will have to be addressed in this arena. Health consumers will have to determine for what they wish to pay. The role of hospice leaders is to inform the public of what is available so that consumers can make intelligent choices.

There are a number of questions to be dealt with. Is care of the terminally ill important, or should our financial resources be directed primarily at curative and rehabilitative medicine? If we are to reimburse for terminal care, what services should be reimbursed? Should bereavement counseling be reimbursable? At what level should services be reimbursed? What sort of organizational format should we require of those providing terminal care in order to be eligible for reimbursement? Should only hospital-based programs or only free-standing programs be eligible? What stipulations and restrictions should be placed upon the delivery of care at home? Should it be necessary that the patient be homebound?

It is the legislatures and insurance companies, presumably on the basis of public preference, that establish the services to be reimbursed and the formulas for that reimbursement. They need to be particularly well informed about issues relating to the care of the terminally ill.

The experiences of free-standing and hospital-based programs and of third-party payors such as Blue Cross have provided some data about costs and reimbursement problems in hospice care. Some lessons were learned through the Health Care Financing Administration demonstration projects. There is need, however, for continued careful study that will provide information upon which decisions can be based.

The resolution of cost and reimbursement issues may result in other problems. In its formative years, hospice care has been characterized by a high level of altruism among its personnel. As hospice services become reimbursable, the potential for exploitation is inevitable. This is going to require the vigilance of conscientious hospice leaders.

As hospice systems evolve and matters of reimbursement are settled, the role of volunteers in hospice care will require close scrutiny and careful thought. The contribution of volunteers to the success of hospice has been enormous. This contribution has in part been through the provision of services that have made the volunteers effective extensions of the professionals on the health care team. This has had a tremendous financial impact. In some instances it has made hospice care possible, for it is only in this way that the high level of personal attention that hospice care requires could be provided. But, in addition, volunteers have contributed in another important respect; they have brought values and viewpoints that have refreshed and strengthened hospice programs.

As hospice care becomes more integrated into the health care system, as accreditation of hospice programs develops, and as reimbursement for hospice care becomes more widely available, there clearly will be a threat to volunteer involvement in hospice. The necessary steps must be taken to preserve volunteer participation.

Among those of us who have looked carefully at hospice care, one of the principal concerns has been the relationship between hospice care in particular and medical care in general. There are innumerable forms that this relationship could take. At one extreme is the frightening prospect of a totally separate system for the care of the terminally ill, entirely outside of and completely unrelated to the rest of health care. Serious hospice workers would be less than realistic if they considered unthinkable the development of a cultlike phenomenon for the care of the terminally ill. At the opposite extreme is the thought that within the hospice concept are the seeds of a healthy self-destruction, in the course of which hospice care would become completely amalgamated into general medical care, perfusing many of its precepts into the management of acutely ill patients. In truth, it is improbable that the future will take us to either of these extremes. As is often the case, the central part of the spectrum seems not only more sensible, but also more likely.

Some features of the care of the terminally ill suggest that management of such patients will be, in some respects, a specialty, but one comfortably within the framework of the traditional medical care system. The unique problems faced by the dying are such that they merit the special attention of certain physicians. There will always be a sizeable number of physicians who, when confronted with patients at the terminal stage of disease, do not wish to be responsible for the continuing care of the patient. Surgeons, radiotherapists, and oncologists are particularly likely to fall in this group. Their reasons for not wishing to continue in the care of the patient are usually sound, and we would be prudent to honor them.

Thus the need to provide and improve terminal care will direct us toward the development of a specialty in the care of the terminally ill. This specialty will be particularly fortunate to have had founders of unusual depth, compassion, and character. These leaders have provided a legacy that should be the foundation of an honorable history.

Specialties come in all degrees. Whether care of the terminally ill will become so discrete and well developed as to have its own certifying board depends upon a number of imponderables. Whatever direction it takes, it is clear that hospice care will have a major impact upon this specialty. Hospice care is not likely to evaporate, leaving no trace of itself. In this connection we must remember that care of the terminally ill and hospice care as we know it today are not synonymous.

Entirely outside of and completely unrelated to hospice care, there seem to be some healthy changes taking place in dealing with malignant disease and terminally ill patients. For example, in the surgical literature there has been a subtle but definite shift in emphasis regarding the treatment of patients with lesions such as esophageal carcinoma. A few years ago results of treatment were reported in terms of cure rates, usually concluding with an overall figure in the range of a 5% to 10% five-year survival rate. Nothing was said about the 90% to 95% of patients who were not cured. Recently, there has been an increasing recognition that our present modes of treatment for esophageal carcinoma are best looked at in terms of the palliation they provide, with cure being achieved in a minority of patients. This in no way denies the importance of a continuing search for techniques that will result in cure.

It is the author's impression that we really do not *frequently* see a senseless prolongation of life without reason or meaning, even outside of hospice care. Such cases do occur, but when viewed in context, they are relatively uncommon. This does not alter the fact that when they occur they pose some of the most difficult questions we are called upon to answer. It has been the author's experience that the situation usually has arisen because there was a point in the patient's course when resuscitation and rehabilitation seemed advisable. Once having begun the use of life support systems, it is very difficult to discontinue them.

Several years ago the American Medical Association adopted a resolution pledging to actively encourage and implement continued education of the practicing physician in the most effective methods "for meeting the symptomatic, rehabilitative, supportive and other needs of the cancer patient." In conformity with this resolution, the *Journal of the American Medical Association* has carried a series of articles on the care of the patient with advanced cancer (Moertel 1980).

The point is that in the management of the terminally ill, there are healthy changes taking place entirely apart from hospice care. To some extent these are a product of the same forces that have given birth to and shaped hospice programs.

If care of the terminally ill is to develop as some form of specialty, hospice care is likely to be a part of it. Hospice care possesses some features that make it different from any other medical specialty. One of these is the liberal use of many disciplines and of volunteers. Nonmedical people have played an immense role in the development and conduct of hospice care. They bring to those of us in medicine some perspectives and insights we would not otherwise have. It is to be hoped that they will continue to give of themselves so generously and that the response of physicians and other medical people will be positive. We must watch for and avoid two dangers. Nonmedical people interested in seeing hospice care develop may become so strident that they discourage the participation of medical people and then so frustrated that they decide to move outside the existing health care system. Conversely, medical people may become defensive about what they see as criticism of the way in which they are doing things; they may cease to listen.

Perhaps preservation of the name *hospice* is not the overriding consideration; however, the philosophy and principles that it embodies are. Thus, for those of us interested in the humane care of the terminally ill, our purpose would be achieved if the objectives of hospice were achieved: a clear-cut decision that the patient is incurable, followed by the institution of effective palliation designed to relieve symptoms in the broadest sense for patient and family in the optimal setting, utilizing all of the resources of the multidisciplinary team.

The matters of standards and certification deserve and unquestionably will receive considerable attention in the years ahead. Care of the terminally ill and hospice care are not alone in this. However, because they are relatively recent as identifiable areas for attention, and because they possess certain features that are particularly prone to abuse, those involved will have to deal with some special issues. Problems related to the lack of restriction on the use of the term hospice also raise some unusual questions.

The National Hospice Organization (NHO) has taken the initiative in developing standards for hospices. This is a most important matter and should be pursued vigorously. Several considerations must be borne in mind as standards for hospice care are formulated. As in all areas of medical care, standards must not become an impediment to progress, stamping everyone into a mold of mediocrity. It is particularly important in hospice care that there be enough flexibility to permit diversity and innovation. It is equally important that the initiative for setting and enforcing standards remain with those in the field of hospice care, rather than in the hands of government agencies.

Even within this framework an issue that will have to be faced by hospital-based hospices is the relationship between the NHO and the Joint Commission on Accreditation of Hospitals (JCAH). It is hoped that suitable arrangements can be made to prevent overlapping and conflicting requirements or the need for two separate certifications. Actually, cooperation betwen the two agencies can strengthen the accreditation process as it relates to the care of the terminally ill.

In addition to certification or accreditation of hospices, there is the issue of assessing the quality of care within hospices. The JCAH requires that all hospitals have a mechanism for assuring quality of care. It is important that each hospital that treats terminally ill patients apply these mechanisms to the evaluation of care of those patients whether or not it has a hospice care program. Quality assurance through audit can be a demanding and time-consuming process, but hospital-affiliated hospice programs should be certain that they are included in the medical care evaluation process in the hospital. This requires the setting of criteria and review of data.

The first encounter between hospices and regulations with teeth has not been a totally happy one. The hospice benefit available to Medicare beneficiaries effective in October 1983 resulted in the development of requirements for the participation of patients and hospice programs that many programs found unacceptably cumbersome and restrictive. As a consequence there has thus far been limited participation of hospices in this arrangement. It is to be hoped that some lessons have been learned.

Hospice care is clearly maturing. Whether it is in its infancy, childhood, or adolescence is not entirely clear. What is clear is that it still has some growing up to do. It must begin to learn to face the responsibilities of adulthood.

Like all of medical care, hospice care contains a large measure of art. Artistic skill requires development through discipline and learning. There is still much progress to be made in the art of hospice care; what follows is in no way intended to de-emphasize this aspect of the care of the terminally ill.

What must receive careful attention from hospice workers in the future, however, is the care of the terminally ill as a developing science. The groundwork in most scientific fields has been descriptive. However, to grow, flourish, and make contributions to humanity, a science must go beyond this. Hospice care is ready to do this and needs to do it. Up to this point, much of hospice care has been defined in anecdotal terms. It is now time to begin gathering and analyzing data by the scientific method and to test hypotheses.

This raises in many minds, most particularly in those of nonmedical people interested in hospice care, the issue of experimentation. All of us in hospice care must learn not to be ashamed of the word "research." Only through research can we reach full fruition. There is no reason why the terms research and experimentation should connote for the hospice worker images of cruel and grueling treatment, for research can be conducted with the utmost human compassion. Research in the care of the terminally ill will be demanding, but it will be demanding of the researchers, not of the patients.

An early step that will be particularly challenging will involve the development of measurement tools. This will at times seem to defy efforts. The objective of hospice care is the control of symptoms in the broadest sense. Symptoms, whether physical or psychological, are by their nature subjective. Measurement of subjective phenomena is difficult, but not impossible. Hospice workers, who have the advantage of already being geared to a multidisciplinary approach, must be ready to draw upon a variety of fields in which subjective factors are measured. Techniques applicable to hospice patients have already been developed (Eisman 1981; Spitzer et al. 1981). The time has come for their application. The capacity to assess the degree of relief of pain, weakness, nausea, anxiety, and depression will open important vistas for hospice care.

As in all scientific endeavor, the adequacy of measurement tools is the subject of endless debate. This is particularly true of measurement tools used to assess subjective phenomena. We must indeed preserve our skepticism and continue to question the methods we employ; that is part of science. However, we must not allow that debate to stop all progress. We can not allow ourselves to say that because we cannot measure something precisely, we should not measure it at all.

Measurement tools that relate to the organization and cost of hospice care also need to be developed. Some new techniques for quantification of personnel time and program component costs should be developed. Many of these techniques already exist and only need to be applied, perhaps with some modification.

As measurement tools are developed, they can and should be applied by hospice workers to study a number of problems. There clearly needs to be comparison of hospice care with other forms of care for the terminally ill. Up to this point, our efforts to promote the development of hospice care have been hinged largely on our descriptions and anecdotes. Those we are trying to convince will soon rightfully be demanding more from us. They will want some data; we should be ready to provide them. It is only in this way that growth of hospice care can be unfettered.

There is even greater need, however, for the application of research techniques within hospice care; there is a need for the comparison of various techniques of hospice care. Although we have done better with some symptoms than others, we have not yet reached perfection in handling any. We must apply acceptable measurement tools to the study of alternative methods for treating symptoms. When this is done, then we can begin to reap the full fruits of what hospice care has to offer.

We also need to apply our measurement tools to the relative merits of different organizational structures within hospice care. It is through such study that we can begin to make more rational decisions regarding the selection of a model of hospice care for a given community.

An area to which some investigative effort should be directed is the question of the effect of hospice care on the quantity of life. Since the overall goal of a program for the care of the terminally ill is the expansion of both the quantity and quality of life, the impact of various treatment measures on duration of survival can be useful information in making clinical decisions. The effect of various forms of therapy on survival duration has, of course, a financial as well as clinical dimension; knowledge about this can be helpful.

Some other areas of investigation relating to the care of the terminally ill suggest themselves. For example, we know little today about the mechanisms by which malignant disease produces symptoms or even about the mechanism of death from advanced malignancy. Some of us believe that there is reason to question the widely accepted view that pneumonia is the final common pathway to death in most patients with advanced cancer.

Some beginnings have been made in the application of the scientific method to the care of the terminally ill in general and to hospice care in particular. Recognizing that in no field will science solve all of our problems by giving us definitive answers to our most important questions, we must move ahead in our effort to answer as many questions as possible.

Just as hospice care must be, fundamentally, a medical program in order to reach its full potential, it must also have its roots firmly in science. We are in an era when there indeed has been "flight from science" (Editorial 1980). Historically, methods of alternative medicine have made some of their heaviest inroads in the area of care of the terminally ill. Hospice care owes much of its success to basic and clinical science and will do well to keep its attachments to them.

Conversely, this is also an era in which increasingly prevalent regulatory mechanisms have emphasized an extremely technological and disease-oriented approach to the treatment of patients. Our reimbursement systems are increasingly ignoring the contribution of personal attention to medical care (Burnun 1979). This development bears watching by hospice workers in the years ahead.

One interesting and anomalous feature of hospice care is that, as mentioned in Chapter 14, it has developed largely outside our academic institutions, both in England and the United States. This is surprising because seldom in the last several decades has medicine seen something as valuable and with as much potential impact as hospice care develop with so little input from major medical centers and universities. There is some evidence that interest in and use of death education for students in American medical schools is increasing (Dickinson 1981). In addition, Mathew and co-workers (1983) have shown that a hospice program can be effectively integrated into an acute care teaching hospital. However, notwithstanding the closer relationship of the Canadian hospices or palliative care programs to medical schools, and recognizing the role of a few institutions in the United States, the lack of involvement on the part of American teaching centers is striking.

It is interesting to speculate upon possible reasons for this; understanding them may contribute to correcting what can only be seen as an unfortunate situation. Nonetheless, the only point to be made here is the desirability of university involvement in hospice care in the future. Some might say that if we have gotten this far without them, we do not need them now; they may just complicate things. For several reasons, we do need their interest, support, and involvement. University medical centers are the repositories of resources that hospices need. They possess educational capabilities. It is through the introduction of medical students and house officers to hospice care as a part of the fabric of medical practice that we hope to see the widespread application of hospice principles to the terminally ill. University medical centers have the research capacity, expertise, and experience that can be so valuable to the future care of the terminally ill. This is not to suggest that every university hospital needs to open a hospice unit. There are various means by which academic centers can become involved in hospice care; such involvement would be to the advantage of both the universities and hospices. Put another way, academic institutions and major medical centers possess talents and a stature in our society that can only be ignored at some peril.

The influx of topflight talent into a given field is largely dependent upon the morale of those already in the field (Gardner 1961). Although problems of stress have been very real among those caring for the terminally ill, hospice programs have developed, and must continue to develop, ways of dealing with this stress. With the multidisciplinary approach they are in an excellent position to take steps to minimize the wear and tear on team members. The satisfactions experienced by hospice personnel combined with the infinite challenges in making the dying comfortable should serve as impetus for other qualified individuals in all disciplines to enter this field.

It will be exciting to see in the years ahead the type of role that hospice will play in the care of the dying. In addition to providing care to the terminally ill and their families and serving as teaching and research centers, hospice also should function as a catalyst in the community to promote excellence in all of health care (Rees 1982).

There is evidence that those serving in hospice programs are developing an increasing consciousness of the years ahead. The first annual American Conference on Hospice Care, scheduled to take place in Boston later this year, is entitled "Forging the Future of Hospice."

Experience thus far indicates that the approach embodied in the philosophy and practice of hospice programs offers the potential for better care of the terminally ill at a reasonable cost. Hospice programs are likely to increase in numbers and in quality. Both the art and science of hospice care will grow as experience is gained. Such care can reach its full potential as it becomes an integral part of our medical care system. Dying patients and those who love them deserve no less.

References

Buckingham RW, and Lupu D: A comparative study of hospice services in the United States. *Am J Public Health* 72:455, 1982.

Burnun JR: Scientific value of personal care. *Ann Intern Med* 91:643, 1979.

Dickinson GE: Death education in U.S. medical schools 1975 through 1980. *J Med Educ* 56:111, 1981.

Editorial: The flight from science. *Br Med J* 280:1, 1980.

Eisman P: The second dimension. *Arch Surg* 116:11, 1981.

Gardner JW: *Excellence: Can We Be Equal and Excellent Too?* Harper & Row, New York, 1961.

Mathew LM, et al.: Attitudes of house officers toward a hospice on a medical service. *J Med Educ* 58:772, 1983.

Moertel CG: Care of the patient with advanced cancer. *JAMA* 224:175, 1980.

Osterweis M, Champagne DS: The U.S. hospice movement; Issues in development. *Am J Public Health* 69:492, 1979.

Rees WD: The role of hospice in the care of the dying. *Br Med J* 285:1766, 1982.

Spitzer WO, et al.: Measuring the quality of life of cancer patients. *J Chronic Dis* 34:585, 1981.

Suggested Further Reading on Terminal Illness and Hospice

Jack H. Zimmerman

The preceding chapters have been intended to be not only clear, candid, and concise, but also comprehensive. Nonetheless, if we have done our job well, readers should reach this point feeling unfulfilled and with the desire for further information. Each of the following publications has been selected because this author found that it provided more scope or depth than we had been able to encompass here. Some of the suggested readings provide greater detail, another perspective, or even a differing view. Some have been chosen partly because they contain excellent reference lists and thus can themselves be used as leads to additional sources of information. Most have been selected because their range is relatively broad. The references listed in the individual chapters of this book and those within the suggested readings often cover more specific topics.

It is hoped that this admittedly subjective listing will be helpful to the reader.

Terminal Illness and Death

Blumberg B, Flaherty M, Lewis J: *Coping with Cancer,* publication 80-2080. National Institutes of Health, Bethesda MD, 1980.

Brim OG: *The Dying Patient* Russell Sage Foundation, New York, 1970.

Burne SR: Hospice care for children. *Br Med J* 284:1400, 1982.

Cassileth BR, Cassileth PA: *Clinical Care of the Terminal Cancer Patient.* Lea & Febiger, Philadelphia, 1982.

Cohen KP: *Hospice — Prescription for Terminal Care.* Aspen Systems, Germantown MD, 1979.

DeSpelder LA, Strickland AL: *The Last Dance — Encountering Death and Dying.* Mayfield Publishing, Palo Alto, CA, 1983.

Erle HR: Terminal care — The national scene and the individual patient. *Med Clin North Am* 66: 1161, 1982.

Grollman EA: *Concerning Death: A Practical Guide for the Living.* Beacon Press, Boston, 1974.

Gyulay J: *The Dying Child.* McGraw-Hill, New York, 1978.

Hamilton MP, Reid HF: *A Hospice Handbook.* William B Eerdmans Publishing, Grand Rapids MI, 1980.

Hickey RC: *Palliative Care of the Cancer Patient.* Little, Brown and Company, Boston, 1967.

Hofman AD, Becker RD, Gabriel HP: *The Hospitalized Adolescent.* The Free Press, New York, 1976.

Horan DJ, Mall D: *Death, Dying and Euthanasia.* University Publications of America, Washington DC, 1977.

Kastenbaum RJ: *Death, Society and Human Experience.* CV Mosby, St. Louis, 1977.

Kopperman H: *Dying at Home*. John Wiley & Sons, New York, 1983.

Kübler-Ross E: *On Death and Dying*. Macmillan, New York, 1969.

Martinson IM: *Home Care for the Dying Child — Professional and Family Perspectives*. Appleton-Century-Crofts, New York, 1976.

Nelson TC: *It's Your Choice — The Practical Guide to Planning a Funeral*. Scott, Foresman & Company, Glenview IL, 1983.

Rando TA: *Grief, Dying and Death — Clinical Interventions for Caregivers*. Research Press, Champaign IL, 1984.

Robbins J: *Caring for the Dying Patient and the Family*. Harper & Row, New York, 1983.

Saunders C, Summers DH, Teller N: *Hospice: The Living Idea*. Edward Arnold, London, 1981.

Walker AE: *Cerebral Death, ed 3*. Urban & Schwarzenberg, Baltimore, 1985.

Wanzer SH, Adelstein AJ, Cranford RE, et al.: The physician's responsibility toward hopelessly ill patients. *N Engl J Med* 301:955, April 1984.

Wilkes E: *The Dying Patient — The Medical Management of Incurable and Terminal Illness*. George A Bogden and Sons, Ridgewood NJ, 1982.

Hospice

Blues AG, Zerwekh JV: *Hospice and Palliative Nursing Care*. Grune & Stratton, Orlando FL, 1984.

Burne: *Br Med J* 284:1400, 1982.

CA, Vol 34, July-August 1984.

Cohen KP: *Hospice — Prescription for Terminal Care*. 1979.

Corr CC, Corr DM: *Hospice Care: Principles and Practice*. Springer, New York, 1983.

Corr CC, Corr DM: *Hospice Approaches to Pediatric Care*. Springer, New York, 1985.

DuBois PM: *The Hospice Way of Death*. Human Sciences Press, New York, 1980.

Hamilton MP, Reid HF: *A Hospice Handbook*. 1980.

Koff TH: *Hospice — A Caring Community*. Winthrop Publishers, Cambridge MA, 1980.

Miller SC: *A Medical Record Handbook for Hospice Programs*. Foundation of Record Education of the American Medical Record Association, Chicago, 1984.

National Hospice Organization: *NHO Bibliography of General Articles on Hospice*. NHO, Arlington VA.

NHO Bibliography of General Reading on Hospice. NHO, Arlington VA.

How to Start A Hospice Program in Your Community. NHO, Arlington VA, 1982.

Standards of A Hospice Program of Care. NHO, Arlington VA, 1979.

Saunders CM: *The Management of Terminal Malignant Disease, ed 2*. Edward Arnold Ltd, London, 1984.

Schraff SH: *Hospice: The Nursing Perspective*. National League for Nursing, 1984.

Stoddard S: *The Hospice Movement — A Better Way of Caring for the Dying*. Stein and Day, Briarcliff Manor NY, 1978.

Torrens PR: *Hospice Programs and Public Policy*. American Hospital Publishing, Chicago, 1985.

Wilkes: *The Dying Patient*. 1982.

Cancer and Physical Symptoms

Abeloff MD: *Complications of Cancer — Diagnosis and Management*. Johns Hopkins University Press, Baltimore, 1979.

Blues and Zerrwekh: *Hospice and Palliative Nursing Care*. 1984.

Calabresi P, Schein PS, Rosenberg SA: *Medical Oncology: Basic Principles and Clinical Management of Cancer*. Macmillan, New York, 1985.

Cassileth BR: *The Cancer Patient — Social and Medical Aspects of Care*. Lea & Febiger, Philadelphia, 1979.

Copeland EM: *Surgical Oncology*. John Wiley & Sons, New York, 1983.

DeVita VT, Hellman S, Rosenberg SA: *Cancer – Principles and Practice of Oncology*. JB Lippincott, Philadelphia, 1982.

Dietz JH: *Rehabilitation Oncology*. John Wiley & Sons, New York, 1981.

Hickey RC: *Palliative Care of the Cancer Patient*. Little, Brown & Company, New York, 1967.

Koszarowski T, Kulakowski A, Luewinski T: *Cancer surgery*. Urban & Schwarzenberg, Baltimore, 1982.

National Institutes of Health: *Coping with Cancer — an Annotated Bibliography of Public, Patient and Professional Information and Educational Materials*, Publication 80-2129, National Institutes of Health, Bethesda MD, 1980.

Nealon TF: *Management of the Patient with Cancer*, ed 2. WB Saunders, Philadelphia, 1976.

Saunders: *The Management of Terminal Malignant Disease*. 1984.

Spitzer WO, et al: Measuring the quality of life of cancer patients. *J Chronic Dis* 34:585, 1981.

Twycross RG, Lack SA: *Symptom Control in Far Advanced Cancer: Pain Relief*. Pitman, London, 1983.

Twycross RG, Lack SA: *Therapeutics in Terminal Cancer*. Pitman, London, 1984.

Wilkes E: *The Dying Patient*. 1982.

Public Policy, Economics, and Administration

Buckingham RW, and Lupu D: A comparative study of hospice services in the United States. *Am J Public Health* 72:455, 1982.

Davidson GW: *The Hospice: Development and Administration*. Hemisphere Publishing, Washington DC, 1978.

Hamilton and Reid: *A Hospice Handbook*. 1980.

Koff: *Hospice — A Caring Community*. 1980.

McDonnell AM: *Quality Hospice Care: Administration, Organization and Models*. National Health Publishers, Owings Mills, Maryland, 1985.

Miller: *A Medical Record Handbook for Hospice Programs*. 1984.

Paradis LF: *Hospice Handbook—A Guide for Managers and Planners*. Aspen, Rockville, MD, 1985.

Proceedings from the First National Conference on Hospice Finance and Administration, London, 1981.

National Hospice Organization: *The National Hospice Reimbursement Act: How a Hospice and a Home Health Agency Can Structure Their Relationship to Meet the Core Service Requirements for Nursing*. NHO, Arlington VA.

————: *The National Hospice Reimbursement Act: How a Hospice and a Hospital Can Structure an Agreement to Provide In-Patient Hospital Services*. NHO, Arlington VA, 1984.

Torrens: *Hospice Programs and Public Policy*. 1985.

Psychosocial Issues, Including Bereavement

Blues and Zerwekh: *Hospice and Palliative Nursing Care*. 1984.

Brooks AM: *The Grieving Time*. Delapeake, Wilmington DE 1982.

Cassileth BR, Cassileth PA: *Clinical Care of the Terminal Cancer Patient*. 1982.

Cassileth BR et al: *Psychosocial Correlates of Survival in Advanced Malignant Disease?* N. Engl. J. Med. 312:1551, June 1985.

DeSpelder and Strickland: *The Last Dance*. 1983.

Garfield CA: *Psychosocial Care of the Dying Patient*. McGraw-Hill, New York, 1978.

Grollman EA: *Explaining Death to Children*. Beacon Press, Boston, 1967.

Martinson: *Home Care for the Dying Child*. 1976.

Nelson: *It's Your Choice*. 1983.

Osterweis M, Solomon F, Green M: *Bereavement — Reactions, Consequences and Care*. National Academy Press, Washington DC, 1984.

Rando: *Grief, Dying and Death*. 1984.

Saunders: *The Management of Terminal Malignant Disease*. 1984.

Schneider J: *Stress Loss and Grief — Understanding Their Origins and Growth Potential*. University Park Press, Baltimore, 1984.

Schoenberg B, Carr AC, Peretz D, Kutscher AH (eds): *Psychosocial Aspects of Terminal Care*. Columbia University Press, New York, 1972.

Wilkes: *The Dying Patient*. 1982.

Worden JW: *Grief Counseling and Grief Therapy*. Springer, New York, 1982.

Ethical and Legal Considerations

Bayer R, et al.: The care of the terminally ill: Morality and economics. *N Engl J Med* 309:1490, 1983.

Beauchamp TL, Childress JF: *Principles of Biomedical Ethics,* ed 2. Oxford University Press, New York, 1983.

Blum JD: Withdrawing life support: A legal assessment and a possible response. *Hosp Med Staff, p 17, April 1984.*

Cassileth and Cassileth: *Clinical Care of the Terminal Cancer Patient*. 1982.

Cohen: *Hospice — Prescription for Terminal Care*. 1979.

Culver CM, Gert B: Seminars in neurology — Basic ethical concepts in neurologic practice. *Semin Neurol* 4:1, 1984.

DeSpelder and Strickland: *The Last Dance*. 1983.

Graber GC, Beasley AD, Eaddy JA: *Ethical Analysis of Clinical Medicine: A guide for Self-Evaluation*. Urban & Schwarzenberg, Baltimore, 1985.

Lo B, et al: 'Do Not Resuscitate' Decisions. *Ann Int Med* 145:1115, June 1985.

National Hospice Organization Ethics Committee: *Decisions in Hospice*. NHO, Arlington VA, 1985.

Pence GE: *Ethical Options in Medicine*. Medical Economics Company, Oradell NJ, 1980.

President's Commission for the Study of Ethical Problems in Medicine and Biomedical and Behavioral Research: *Deciding to Forgo Life-Sustaining Treatment*. US Government Printing Office, Washington DC, 1983.

Ramsey P: *The Patient as a Person*. Yale University Press, New Haven CT, 1970.

Robertson JA: *Rights of the Critically Ill*. Ballinger Publishing, Cambridge MA, 1983.

Siegler M: Decision-making strategy for clinical-ethical problems in medicine. *Arch Intern Med 142:2178, 1982.*

Steinbrook R: Decision making for incompetent patients by designated proxy. *N Engl J Med* 142:2178, 1982.

Suber DG, Tabor WJ: Withholding of life-sustaining treatment from the terminally ill, incompetent patient: Who decides? *JAMA* 248:2250, 1982.

Torrens: *Hospice Programs and Public Policy*. 1985.

Torrey EF: *Ethical Issues in Medicine*. Little, Brown & Company, Boston, 1968.

Wanzer, et al: *The Physician's Responsibility Toward Hopelessly Ill Patients*. *N Engl J Med* 301:955, 1984.

Index

Italic numbers refer to tables or illustrations.